The ABCs of Antihypertensive Therapy

Second Edition

The ABCs of Antihypertensive Therapy

Second Edition

Edited by

Franz H. Messerli

Ochsner Clinic and Alton Ochsner
    Medical Foundation
New Orleans, Louisiana

Authors' Publishing House
New York

 LIPPINCOTT WILLIAMS & WILKINS

A **Wolters Kluwer** Company

Philadelphia • Baltimore • New York • London
Buenos Aires • Hong Kong • Sydney • Tokyo

Although every effort has been made to ensure that the indications and doses for the various drugs are correct, the ultimate responsibility for the correct use of drugs lies with the prescribing physician. Likewise the institutions with which the authors are associated have no direct nor indirect responsibility for the contents of this book nor for the mode in which any drugs in this book are used.

This book has been offered for mass purchase to a number of pharmaceutical companies. Any such purchase, by a specific pharmaceutical company, in no way implies endorsement of any particular product, nor are the contents of the book in any way modified for any particular mass purchase.

ISBN: 1-881063-07-0

CONTENTS

CONTRIBUTING AUTHORS

George L. Bakris, MD
Rush-Presbyterian-St. Luke's Medical Center
Rush University Hypertension Center
Chicago, Illinois 60612

D. Gareth Beevers, MD
University Department of Medicine
Dudley Road Hospital
Birmingham B18 7QH
United Kingdom

Hans R. Brunner, MD
Division of Hypertension
Department of Medicine
Centre des Hopitaux Universitaires Vaudois
Lausanne, Switzerland

Murray Epstein, MD
Department of Medicine
Division of Nephrology
University of Miami School of Medicine
Miami, Florida 33125

Danilo Fliser, MD
Department of Internal Medicine
D-6900 Heidelberg
Germany

William H. Frishman, MD
Department of Medicine
New York Medical College
Valhalla, New York 10595

Thomas D. Giles, MD
Department of Medicine
Louisiana State University School of Medicine
New Orleans, Louisiana 70112

Ehud Grossman, MD
Department of Internal Medicine
The Chaim Sheba Medical Center
Tel-Hashomer 52621
Israel

Lennart Hansson, MD
Department of Geriatrics
University of Uppsala
S-75002 Uppsala
Sweden

Hope D. Intengan, PhD
Clinical Research Institute of Montreal
Montreal H2W 1R7
Canada

A. Ironi, MD
Department of Internal Medicine
The Chaim Sheba Medical Center
Tel-Hashomer 52621
Israel

Stevo Julius, MD
Department of Internal Medicine
University of Michigan Medical School
Ann Arbor, Michigan 48109

Norman M. Kaplan, MD
Department of Internal Medicine
University of Texas Southwestern Medical Center
Dallas, Texas 75235

S. Khoury, MD
Department of Endocrinology, Metabolism,
    Hypertension and Vascular Biology
Wayne State University
Detroit, Michigan 48201

John B. Kostis, MD
Robert Wood Johnson Medical School
New Brunswick, New Jersey 08903

John H. Laragh, MD
Cardiovascular Center
The New York Hospital-Cornell Medical Center
New York, New York 10021

M. Lester, MD
Department of Endocrinology, Metabolism,
    Hypertension and Vascular Biology
Wayne State University
Detroit, Michigan 48201

Gregory Y.H. Lip, MD
Department of Medicine
City Hospital
Birmingham B18 7QH
United Kingdom

Per Lund-Johansen, MD
Department of Heart Diseases
University of Bergen School of Medicine
Bergen 5016
Norway

Franz H. Messerli, MD
Ochsner Clinic
New Orleans, Louisiana 70121

Marvin Moser, MD
Department of Medicine
New York Medical College
Valhalla, New York, 10595

Kevin O'Malley, MD
Department of Clinical Pharmacology
Royal College of Surgeons in Ireland
Dublin
Republic of Ireland

Shawna Nesbitt, MD
Department of Internal Medicine
The University of Michigan Medical Center
Ann Arbor, Michigan 48109

Eoin O'Brien
Department of Clinical Pharmacology
Royal College of Surgeons in Ireland
Dublin
Republic of Ireland

Olaf B. Paulson, MD
Department of Neurology
The National University Hospital
DK-2100 Copenhagen
Denmark

Eberhard Ritz, MD
Department of Internal Medicine
University of Heidelberg
D-6900 Heidelberg
Germany

Ernesto L. Schiffrin, MD
Clinical Research Institute of Montreal
Montreal H2W 1R7
Canada

Roland E. Schmieder, MD
Department of Medicine
University of Erlangen Nurnberg
90471 Nurnberg
Germany

Bashar A. Shala, MD
Health Science Center
University of Tennessee
Memphis, TN 38163

Yehonatan Sharabi, MD
Department of Internal Medicine
The Chaim Sheba Medical Center
Tel-Hashomer 52621
Israel

Virmeet Singh, MD
Las Vegas, Nevada 89115

Peter Sleight, MD
Department of Cardiovascular Medicine
John Radcliffe Hospital
Oxford OX3 9DU
United Kingdom

James R. Sowers, MD
Division of Endocrinology, Metabolism
   and Hypertension
Wayne State University
Detroit, Michigan 48201

J. David Spence, MD
Stroke Prevention and Atherosclerosis
   Research Centre
Siebens-Drake/Robarts Research Institute
London N6G 2V2
Canada

Svend Strandgaard, MD
Department of Medicine and Nephrology
Herlev Hospital
DK-2730 Herlev
Denmark

Jay M. Sullivan, MD
Division of Cardiovascular Disease
University of Tennessee
Health Science Center
Memphis, Tennessee 38163

Anders Svensson, MD
Department of Geriatrics
University of Uppsala
Uppsala S-75002
Sweden

Michael A. Weber
Veterans Administration Medical Center
Long Beach, California

Alberto Zanchetti, MD
Centro do Fisiologia Clinica e Ipertensione
Universita di Milano
Ospedale Maggiore Milano 20122
Italy

FOREWORD

This new edition of the *ABCs of Antihypertensive Therapy* bears witness not only to the success of the first edition, but also to the continuous progress and evolution of antihypertensive therapy.

Since the first edition of this volume was published, several expert reports and guidelines on antihypertensive treatment have been issued by official organizations and scientific societies, namely the *Fifth and Sixth Reports of the U.S. Joint National Committee on Detection, Evaluation and Treatment of High Blood Pressure* in 1993 and 1997, the *World Health Organization/International Society of Hypertension Guidelines on Management of Mild Hypertension* in 1993, the *World Health Organization Report on Hypertension Control* in 1996, and the *Recommendations of Prevention of Coronary Heart Disease of the European Societies of Cardiology, Atherosclerosis, and Hypertension* in 1994.

Although some discrepancies among these various guidelines and recommendations are noted, it is important to stress that many more similarities than dissimilarities exist. All guidelines insist on the importance of both systolic and diastolic blood pressures when evaluating risk for cardio-vascular disease, a significant change from only a few years ago when attention was almost exclusively focused on diastolic blood pressure. All guidelines recommend evaluating the overall or global cardiovascular risk factors, such as age, diabetes, hypercholesterolemia, renal dysfunction, and previous cardiovascular events, etc., all of which may considerably increase the risk of a mild blood pressure elevation. Consequently, all guidelines also suggest calculating not only the relative risk of being hypertensive (the percent increase in the likelihood of having a cardiovascular event) and the relative benefit of antihypertensive therapy (the percent reduction of cardiovascular events to be expected from antihypertensive therapy), but also absolute risk and absolute benefit (the number of cardiovascular events to be expected in a given number of years in patients with a given profile of risk and the number of patients to be treated for a given number of years in order to prevent a cardiovascular event, respectively). All guidelines unanimously insist on the benefits of lowering blood pressure and on the concept that benefits are proportional to the absolute risk of the patient; but all guidelines wisely avoid establishing any arbitrary threshold of absolute risk below which treatment should be avoided.

In the time between the first and the present editions of this volume, greater knowledge has been gathered on the benefits of lowering blood pressure in the elderly, and treatment of elderly hypertensive patients has now become particularly pressing. The recent *European Study on Isolated Systolic Hypertension in the Elderly* has confirmed the benefit of treating this form of hypertension and extended the drugs to be used in its treatment from diuretics (essentially supplemented by beta-blockers) to include calcium antagonists (essentially supplemented by ACE inhibitors).

In recent years, more information has been accumulated on some classes of antihypertensive agents that were still relatively new at the time of the first edition, and a new class, the angiotensin II receptor antagonists, has been added.

While we still have relatively little prospective information about this new class of drug, several interesting potentialities are suggested from basic research, and a lot of clinically relevant data has developed from investigations on ACE inhibitors and calcium antagonists. The ACE inhibitors have been shown to be effective not only for hypertension, but for other hypertension-related conditions such as congestive heart failure, acute myocardial infarction, as well as in left ventricular hypertrophy. As for calcium antagonists, a very hot debate has developed regarding their safety. This debate has just been put into its proper frame by the report of an Ad-Hoc Committee established by the World Health Organization and the International Society of Hypertension, stating that not one of the studies raising the issue of calcium antagonist safety had sufficient power or characteristics to achieve meaningful conclusions. Furthermore, the debate should have reached a term with the recent demonstration by the Syst-Eur trial of significant reduction of cardiovascular events by treating isolated systolic hypertension in the elderly with a dihydropyridine calcium antagonist. At any rate, the debate has been productive and has suggested a better distinction between short-acting, abrupt onset calcium antagonists and the more recent calcium antagonists with longer duration and slower onset of action. It has also given new impetus to initiate large trials comparing different classes of antihypertensive agents.

Indeed, the end of the 1990s and the first years of the new century will see a new era of comparative trials investigating the possible benefits of ACE inhibitors, calcium antagonists, and angiotensin II receptor antagonists versus diuretics and between blockers and the more recent classes of drugs. The new era of megatrials will also see the beginning of prospective rather than retrospective meta-analyses of randomized trials, thus avoiding the biases of not taking into account unreported trials and of post-hoc selection of criteria for including trials into meta-analyses. By the year 2003 or shortly thereafter, we shall have data on more than 200,000 hypertensive patients and the almost 1,000,000 patient-years of follow-up.

For the time being, until the results of all these trials and their meta-analyses provide firmer evidence on the relative benefits of the various classes of antihypertensive agents in patients with a number of different risk profiles, we must learn how to best use all available drugs without preconceptions and theoretical or financial exclusions. This is what the *ABCs of Antihypertensive Therapy* does with great success and effectiveness. If we consider that despite the unanimous recommendations of many expert bodies and the large array of efficacious antihypertensive drugs, blood pressure is still poorly controlled in general practice in all parts of the world. This means that volumes like this one are greatly needed and may help practitioners to cope with the experts' guidelines, thus providing the hypertensive patient with the full benefits promised by the continuous progress in antihypertensive therapy.

Alberto Zanchetti

SUGGESTED READING

1. Joint National Committee on Detection, Evaluation and Treatment of High Blood Pressure. The fifth report of the Joint National Committee on detection, evaluation and treatment of high blood pressure (JNC V). Arch Intern Med 1993; 153:154–183.

2. Joint National Committee on Prevention, Detection, Evaluation and Treatment of High Blood Pressure. The sixth report of the Joint National Committee on prevention, detection, evaluation and treatment of high blood pressure (JNC VI). Arch Intern Med 1997;157:2413–2446.

3. Guidelines Sub-Committee. 1993 guidelines for the management of mild hypertension: memorandum from a World Health Organization/International Society of Hypertension meeting. J Hypertens 1993;11:905–918.

4. WHO Expert Committee. Hypertension control. WHO technical report series 862, World Health Organization, Geneva, 1996.

5. Pyorala K, De Backer G, Graham I, Poole-Wilson P, Wood D. Prevention of coronary heart disease in clinical practice. Recommendations of the Task Force of the European Society of Cardiology, European Atherosclerosis Society and European Society of Hypertension. Eur Heart J 1994;15: 1300–1331.

6. Zanchetti A, Mancia G. Strategies for antihypertensive treatment decisions: how to assess benefits. J Hypertens 1997;15:215–216.

7. Staessen JA, Fagard R, Thijs L, Celis H, et al. Randomized double blind comparison of placebo and active treatment for older patients with isolated systolic hypertension. The Systolic Hypertension in Europe (Syst-Eur) Trial Investigators. Lancet 1997;350:757–764.

8. Ad-Hoc Subcommittee of the Liaison Committee of the World Health Organization and the International Society of Hypertension. Effects of calcium antagonists on the risks of coronary heart disease, cancer and bleeding. J Hypertens 1997;15:105–115.

9. World Health Organization/International Society of Hypertension Blood Pressure Lowering Treatment Trialists' Collaboration. Protocol for prospective collaborative over-views of major randomized trials of blood pressure lowering treatments. J Hypertens 1998;16: in press.

10. Horton R on behalf of the Medical Editors' Trial Amnesty. Medical editors' trial amnesty. Lancet 1997;350:756.

11. Zanchetti A, Mancia G. Editors' corner: Searching for information from unreported trials—amnesty for the past and prospective meta-analyses for the future. J Hypertens 1998;16: in press.

12. Mancia G, Sega R, Milesi C, Cesana G, Zanchetti A. Blood-pressure control in the hypertensive population. Lancet 1997;349: 454–457.

PREFACE

Over the past few years we have witnessed an exceedingly rapid evolution in the treatment of many cardiovascular disorders. This is particularly true for the treatment of arterial hypertension and its cardiovascular complications. Although many new drugs offer real progress in treatment options, the only requirement of the Food and Drug Administration for approval of a new pharmaceutical entity is documents attesting to its efficacy and safety, but not to superiority over similar drugs. This results in the marketing of numerous "me too" drugs, thereby creating an embarrassment of riches. The *ABCs of Antihypertensive Therapy* was put together to give the practicing physician some guidelines on how to select the most appropriate antihypertensive drug therapy for a given patient based on clinical, pathophysiologic, and epidemiologic findings.

The basic objectives of this second edition of the *ABCs of Antihypertensive Therapy* are the same as those of the first edition, namely, to provide a practical and authoritative guide to the drug treatment of hypertension. The second edition has been completely revised. A total of four new chapters were added that discuss modern antiadrenergic therapy, combination therapy, hypertensive emergencies and urgencies, as well as angiotensin receptor blockers. Several chapters were shortened and others omitted.

We know that this text will continue to be a useful, comprehensive, day-to-day source of innovation and education for practicing physicians, general internists, and other health professionals.

The ABCs of Antihypertensive Therapy

Second Edition

CHAPTER 1

Antihypertensive Therapy: Past, Present, and Future*

Franz H. Messerli
John H. Laragh

THE PAST

For nearly half a century, hypertension, although easily identified in clinical practice because of the ingenious invention of Riva Rocci, remained an incurable disease invariably leading to stroke, heart attack, congestive heart failure, and renal insufficiency.

In retrospect, it is perhaps a matter of opinion whether the dawn broke with the discovery of chlorothiazide by Karl Beyer and his colleagues at Merck, Sharp & Dohme or earlier with the development of ganglion blockers by Plonker and Zaimis, reserpine by Wilkins, hydralazine by Jonkman and guanethidine by Plummer (both at Ciba), or bretylium tosylate by Burroughs Wellcome. The thiazide diuretics were used first alone and later in combination with reserpine or methyldopa. These discoveries led to the honeymoon phase of antihypertensive therapy during which clinical evidence of benefits was convincing and clearly outweighed the cost of leaving patients untreated. Hypertensive encephalopathy disappeared, pulmonary edema melted away, and retinopathy with papilledema, hemorrhages, and cotton wool spots resolved in parallel with the fall in arterial pressure. Even in patients with less severe hypertension, evidence of left ventricular hypertrophy on chest x-ray and electrocardiogram decreased, proteinuria became less pronounced, and patients subjectively experienced improvement.

Although this early period of drug treatment of hypertension was (like most honeymoons) heroic and exciting, it must be remembered that most antihypertensive drugs were not developed from the outset with the goal of lowering arterial pressure. The antihypertensive properties of most of these agents were discovered accidentally by clinicians. Sulfanilamide, when used as an antimicrobial drug, was demonstrated to have beneficial effects in congestive heart

* Modified with permission from Messerli FH, Laragh JH. *Cardiovascular Drug Therapy.* Philadelphia: Saunders, 1990.

failure; clinicians subsequently showed that it lowered blood pressure. The antihypertensive effects of methyldopa were first observed in control subjects in a study designed to evaluate its effect as a decarboxylase inhibitor in carcinoid syndrome. The antihypertensive properties of clonidine were discovered when a patient to whom it was given for the treatment of allergic rhinitis fell asleep because of sedation and hypotension. The beta-blockers and calcium antagonists entered the antihypertensive arsenal after they had been used for the treatment of angina pectoris and arrhythmias for many years when alert clinicians discovered their antihypertensive potential. Thus, pharmacologists have had a poor record in identifying antihypertensive drugs in the laboratory. Actually, only captopril, an orally active angiotensin-converting enzyme inhibitor, was discovered through an extensive search by Squibb after the blood pressure lowering properties of the venom of the Brazilian snake Bothrops Jararaca had been documented in humans. Therefore, captopril can possibly be considered the first "designer drug" that opened the gates to modern pharmacotherapy of essential hypertension.

THE PRESENT

When the Veterans Administration study led by Freis clearly documented the benefits of antihypertensive treatment not only in severe but also in mild essential hypertension, the modern era of antihypertensive drug treatment began. Proponents of the so-called stepped-care approach marched triumphantly throughout North America and other continents. The stepped-care approach was touted as safe, efficacious, and so simple that it could be used even by nurse practitioners and physicians who did not regularly treat hypertensive patients, such as gynecologists, psychiatrists, or dentists. Numerous studies attest to the fact that antihypertensive treatment by the stepped-care approach reduces cardiovascular morbidity and mortality.

However, it soon became apparent that stepped care was not the ultimate solution to essential hypertension. First, the reduction in morbidity and mortality was related mostly to a decreased incidence of strokes and perhaps renal failure, but little or no reduction in endpoints of coronary artery disease was observed. Second, patients with mild essential hypertension who were asymptomatic before treatment suddenly complained about a variety of symptoms induced by antihypertensive therapy and often were unwilling to trade a statistical increase in life expectancy by a few years for a substantial loss of quality of life for the remainder of their days. Third, it became obvious that the pathogenesis of essential hypertension was multifactorial; therefore, a "cookbook" approach with a single recipe for all (i.e., stepped care) was in many instances likely to fail or to be intrusive.

This latter line of thought was initiated by Laragh and colleagues in the early 1970s, when they were able to demonstrate clear-cut differences in blood pressure responsiveness that depended on the activity of the renin-angiotensin-aldosterone system. Patient profiling according to renin status was a simple, straightforward way to identify a predominant mechanism of pressure elevation, vasoconstriction in patients belonging to the high-renin category, or volume expansion in patients belonging to the low-renin category. These pioneering observations were subsequently extended to the adrenergic nervous system, systemic and regional hemodynamics, and cellular sodium and calcium transport.

Elucidation of these mechanisms has already defined the heterogeneity of essential hypertension and provided the basis for individualized drug regimens. While the cause(s) have not yet been revealed, continuing research within these new guideposts holds promise of bringing us closer to definitive solutions to this elusive problem. Meanwhile, it has been demonstrated that essential hypertension is a heterogeneous disorder and that mechanisms of pressure elevation vary from patient to patient. Clearly, therefore, antihypertensive therapy must be tailored to the individual patient. A "cookbook" approach, proposed by the Joint National Committee in the 1980s, left no room for individualization and led to dissatisfaction of patients and physicians alike. In subsequent reports up to JNC VI, the committee has changed its approach very little.

THE FUTURE

Given that essential hypertension is a heterogeneous disorder and that mechanisms of pressure elevations vary from one patient to another, it follows that no single drug recipe will be effective and safe in all patients with essential hypertension. Long-standing hypertension leads to target organ disease (i.e., left ventricular hypertrophy, coronary artery disease, congestive heart failure, renal failure, and cerebrovascular damage). Each of these target organ diseases often follows a course of its own that is no longer related to the level of arterial pressure. For example, left ventricular hypertrophy, which increases by sixfold to sevenfold the risk of dying suddenly of acute myocardial infarction, may be diminished, unchanged, or increased by antihypertensive therapy, depending on the mechanism by which the drug lowers pressure. The same holds true for patients in whom hypertension has led to nephrosclerosis, renal failure, coronary artery disease, congestive heart failure, or cerebrovascular disease.

Hypertension can no longer be considered a simple hemodynamic disorder. A host of metabolic abnormalities can be documented in the uncomplicated hypertensive patient, some of which further increase the cardiovascular risk profile. Antihypertensive therapy, therefore, should not only lower arterial pressure but diminish or at least not worsen associated risk factors. Mild essential hypertension is an asymptomatic disorder and should remain so when treated. Fortunately, the newer antihypertensive agents, such as angiotensin-converting enzyme inhibitors and calcium channel blockers, are remarkably free of side effects and may even give patients a feeling of increased well being, perhaps because they maintain or improve blood flow to target organs. Indeed, the latest drug class, the angiotensin II receptor blockers, exhibit practically no side effects and are a welcome addition to the other two anti-renin system classes of drugs: beta blockers and converting enzyme inhibitors.

Ample evidence suggests that lowering arterial pressure diminishes cardiovascular morbidity and mortality and thus prolongs life. However, we are just now learning that diminishing millimeters of mercury is not the ultimate goal in the treatment of hypertension. The antihypertensive approach of the future should demonstrate efficacy of drug therapy in preventing or reducing target organ damage and should preserve or improve organ function. At the same time, therapy should diminish concomitant risk factors for cardiovascular disease and should improve the quality of life. So far only the anti-renin system agents have proven value in clinical trials for protecting from or arresting subsequent myocardial infarction, heart failure, and kidney failure. Although the reduction in strokes and cardiovascular events in the Syst Eur study is very impressive, more data are required to define the cardioprotective benefits, if any, of the various types of calcium antagonists.

Notwithstanding, as available pharmacologic agents are now more potent and specific and have fewer side effects than ever before, we have reached a new level of therapeutic expertise. This expertise can enable us to achieve for greater numbers of patients than before the primary goal of antihypertensive therapy, using the fewest number of drugs in the lowest possible dose for the lifetime commitment that antihypertensive therapy may require. For increasing numbers of patients, monotherapy achieved by a rational process is a realizable goal. This modality will surely mean fewer side effects and a better quality of life for many patients, with reduced toxicity and optimal protection from heart attack and stroke.

CHAPTER 2

Evolution of Hypertension and Hemodynamics

Per Lund-Johansen

Our knowledge about the etiology and pathophysiology of the most common form of hypertension—primary or essential hypertension—is still far from complete. However, an increased systemic arterial blood pressure reflects a disproportion between the cardiac output and total peripheral resistance, the major factors determining the blood pressure.[1,2] Other factors, such as blood viscosity, also seem to play a role.[3] Blood pressure and cardiac output are measured most accurately by invasive methods such as intra-arterial pressure recordings and dye or thermodilution methods. During rest, blood pressure may be recorded reasonably accurately by methods based on the cuff method, and cardiac output may be measured by the echo or Doppler technique. During exercise, however, invasive methods are necessary for accurate recordings.

Total peripheral resistance (TPR) is calculated as the ratio between mean arterial pressure (MAP) and cardiac output (CO).

$$TPR = MAP/CO$$

The hemodynamic alterations responsible for increased blood pressure vary and depend on the age of the subject and the stage of the hypertensive disease.

Central Hemodynamics in Borderline and Mild Hypertension

It is always a dilemma to identify patients who are in the starting phase of essential hypertension. If one includes subjects who are too young or who have blood pressure elevations that are too mild, many of them will not turn out to be hypertensive over the years. If one waits too long, the starting phase may be missed. Most studies in the 1960s and 1970s concentrated on young subjects in their twenties to forties with borderline-to-mild hypertension and compared them with normotensive age-matched controls.[4]

During rest, the characteristic findings in such subjects with mild hypertension (diastolic arterial pressure 90 mm Hg to 105 mm Hg) were a high cardiac index, a high heart rate, and a numerically "normal" calculated peripheral resistance.[4,5] In most of these studies, the mean blood pressure has been about 15% higher than in normotensive controls. The variations in cardiac index may be great, however. More recent studies have demonstrated a pattern of high cardiac index in a substantial proportion of subjects with mild hypertension. By noninvasive methods, however, some investigators have found normal cardiac outputs and slightly increased TPR values in patients with mild hypertension.

Are Children with High Blood Pressure Particularly Hyperkinetic?

Studies in children and young adolescents have usually shown no marked increase in cardiac index and thus a slightly increased or normal TPR index. Studies in offspring from hypertensive parents have usually not disclosed particularly high cardiac indices in such subjects, who usually have slightly increased cardiac outputs.

From a pathophysiologic standpoint, the initial interest in possible disturbances in cardiac output was related to the theory that essential hypertension might be triggered by a high cardiac output due to increased sympathetic tone. According to the whole body autoregulation theory, this should lead to an overperfusion (luxury perfusion) in most vascular beds. This should again trigger vasoconstriction, which later would maintain the increased blood pressure when cardiac output fell. Because most studies have shown that oxygen consumption is also increased in early essential hypertension, the whole body autoregulation theory cannot explain the chain of events seen in human hypertension, as there is no luxury perfusion in the beginning.

Exercise Studies

In order to obtain accurate measurements of hemodynamics during exercise, invasive methods are necessary. Using such methods, we found that in young subjects (ages 20 to 40 years) with mild hypertension, cardiac index during rest tended to be slightly higher than in controls, but during 100-watt and 150-watt exercise, the cardiac outputs were subnormal, as was the blood flow related to oxygen consumption.[5] The cause of the subnormal cardiac index during exercise was an insufficient increase in stroke volume in transition from rest to exercise. This could be due to increased stiffness in the left ventricle (decreased compliance) and decreased ventricular diastolic filling. More recent studies by echocardiography have shown that this is an early phenomenon in essential hypertension, which might actually be seen before there is any increase in septal or posterior wall thickness.[6] It is also possible that insufficient myocardial perfusion during exercise could be responsible for the subnormal exercise stroke volume, but large studies of the coronary circulation during exercise in young subjects with uncomplicated hypertension are lacking.

Exercise studies also reveal that TPR is not falling to the same low levels as in normotensive controls, indicating that the resistance vessels are also affected in the early stage of essential hypertension.

ESTABLISHED AND SEVERE HYPERTENSION

Studies at rest and during exercise usually show that in this stage (diastolic blood pressure permanently > 105 mm Hg) cardiac output is subnormal, particularly during exercise, and TPR is markedly increased. Stroke volumes are subnormal, particularly during exercise. Patients with severe hypertension (diastolic blood pressure > 115 mm Hg) who are in the end stage of hypertensive disease are characterized by very high resistance values and low cardiac outputs. When heart failure is present, high filling pressures and high pulmonary wedge pressures are typical. In patients with severe hypertension, Omvik and Lund-Johansen reported enormously increased resistance values up to 6,000 dyn • sec • cm^{-5} • m^2, or almost three times normal values.[5]

SPONTANEOUS CHANGES IN CENTRAL HEMODYNAMICS OVER 20 YEARS

The previously described patterns of hemodynamic changes in essential hypertension are based on cross-sectional studies. Ideally, longitudinal studies in the same population should be investigated.

We studied 77 male patients (initially aged 17 to 66 years) with mild-to-moderate essential hypertension recruited from the Bergen population survey.[5] All subjects had blood pressure above 140/90 mm Hg at the screening in 1965 and at two follow-up examinations over a period of six months. All patients younger than age 60 were in World Health Organization stage I or II. All hemodynamic recordings were obtained with invasive procedures performed in the same laboratory.

During follow-up at 10 and at 20 years, there was a fall in cardiac output in all age groups, at rest as well as during exercise, mainly due to a fall in stroke volume.[5] TPR increased decade by decade. Figure 1 shows the changes in cardiac index, blood pressure, stroke index, and TPR index at rest and during exercise over 20 years in the group initially 17 to 29 years old.

Comparison of the Hemodynamic Pattern in the Young and in the Old

If we compare the mean values of the hemodynamic parameters at the first study in the youngest age group, 17 to 29 years of age, with those seen after 20 years of hypertension (although treated, but off drugs for two weeks) in the oldest group, 60 to 69 years of age at the re-study, marked contrasts are seen. Incidentally, the two groups had almost the same MAP at rest in the sitting position, about 114 mm Hg.

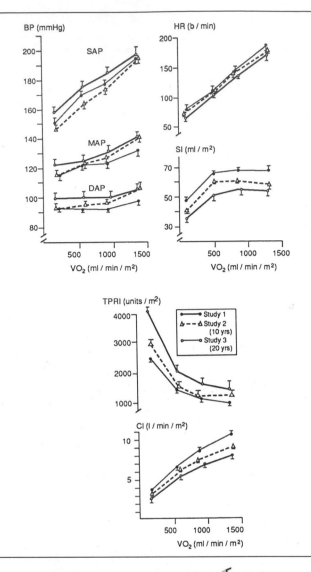

Figure 1. *Central hemodynamics at rest and during exercise in age group 1 (17 to 29 years) at initial study and at 10 and 20 years' follow-up. Mean values (n=14) and standard error of mean (SEM). HR, heart rate; CI, cardiac index; SI, stroke index; SAP, systolic arterial pressure; DAP, diastolic arterial pressure; MAP, mean arterial pressure; TPRI, total peripheral resistance index; VO_2, oxygen consumption. Note the marked increase in TPRI and fall in SI during the follow-up period.*

However, in the oldest group, systolic arterial pressure was higher and diastolic arterial pressure was lower than in the youngest group. The increase in MAP during exercise was much steeper in the older than in the younger group, and the TPR index during rest was about twice as high. In contrast, at 150-watt exercise, cardiac index was 11.1 $l/min/m^2$ in the youngest group at the first study and was approximately only half of this value, 5.94 $l/min/m^2$, in the oldest group. Thus, although the two groups had the same MAP at rest, central hemodynamics at rest as well as during exercise were very different in these groups, representing the early phase and the late phase of essential hypertension. Figures 2 and 3

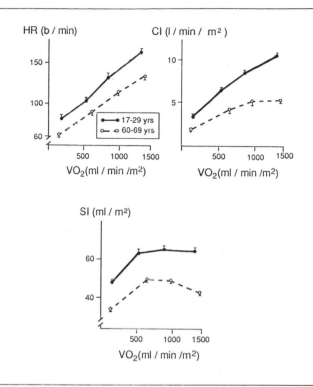

Figure 2. *Central hemodynamics at rest and during exercise in young hypertensives (n=14) versus older hypertensives (n=19). Mean values and SEM. HR, heart rate; CI, cardiac index; SI, stroke index; VO₂, oxygen consumption.*

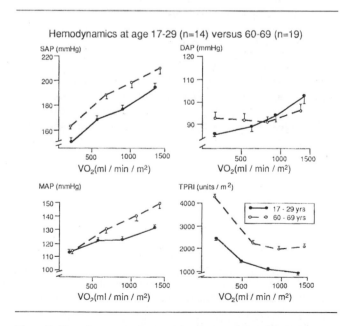

Figure 3. *Hemodynamics at rest and during exercise in young hypertensives (n=14) versus older hypertensives (n=19). Mean values of SEM. SAP, systolic arterial pressure; DAP, diastolic arterial pressure; MAP, mean arterial pressure; TPRI, total peripheral resistance index; VO₂, oxygen consumption.*

show the hemodynamic patterns in these two groups. The arteriovenous oxygen difference is much higher in the oldest group and the reserve of oxygen in venous blood is reduced.

REGIONAL CIRCULATION

The regional circulation is more difficult to study than central hemodynamics. Messerli and coworkers have performed simultaneous studies of cardiac output and renal and splanchnic blood flow in different age groups of hypertensive patients.[4] They found a correlation between cardiac output and renal blood flow and thus found that renal blood flow was normal in the early phase and was reduced in the late phase of hypertension. Renal vascular resistance increased as hypertension progressed. Several other investigators have stated that, with increasing blood pressure and deterioration of the hypertensive disorder, renal blood flow falls and resistance increases. In the early phase of hypertension, blood flow in the skeletal muscles tends to be higher than in normal subjects, but when hypertension becomes established, the resistance increases and the blood flow falls.

Most interesting is the coronary circulation, which, unfortunately, can only be assessed with rather invasive procedures. For this reason, the information about coronary hemodynamics in hypertensive heart disease in different ages and stages is incomplete. Strauer has shown that even in the early stage of hypertension, there appears to be a reduction in coronary reserve (measured after injection of dipyramidole).[7] In recent years, it has been shown that even in the absence of stenotic lesions in the visible coronary arteries in hypertensive patients, exercise blood flow may be reduced. Some of these patients develop angina pectoris.

Pulmonary Circulation

Somewhat surprisingly, it was shown about 15 years ago that patients with established hypertension tended to have slightly higher blood pressure in the pulmonary circulation than did normal subjects, even in the uncomplicated stage. This is due to an increased resistance in the pulmonary arterioles, as pulmonary blood flow is not increased.

MECHANISMS BEHIND THE HEMODYNAMIC ALTERATION IN ESSENTIAL HYPERTENSION

Most investigators believe that the high heart rate, high cardiac output, and subsequent increase in TPR could initially be caused by an overactivity in the sympathetic nervous system. In particular, studies have demonstrated that the noradrenaline spillover rate is increased in many organ systems in hypertensive subjects. Why the sympathetic nervous system is overactive in subjects with essential hypertension is still unknown. It is often claimed that the stress of everyday life in industrialized societies is responsible for the increase in blood pressure seen over the years, but the problem with this theory is that only a small fraction of the many subjects exposed to stress develop hypertension. Nevertheless, in this context it is interesting that among nuns from a secluded order, who had a very quiet life and no contact with the rest of the world, there was practically no change in the blood pressure over a 30-year period, in contrast to a similar group of women living in society under normal conditions. In recent years, it has been shown that the effect of stress hormones, such as the catecholamines, seems to be dependent on the sodium ion. Sodium-sensitive hypertensives have been found most sensitive to neurogenic stimuli.

Sooner or later during the hypertensive process, the left ventricle and the resistance vessels will undergo structural changes. In the heart, remodeling of the wall with an increase in the amount of collagen is typical, as has been demonstrated in many animal models.[6,8] The increased collagen content will result in a stiffer left ventricle and reduced compliance. This can be demonstrated in humans by echocardiography at a very early stage of essential hypertension and may also lead to a disturbance of ventricular filling. Thus, the atrial component becomes more important than the early filling; the so-called E/A-ratio decreases. Folkow and Mulvany[2,9] have demonstrated structural changes in the arterioles consisting of increased wall thickness and reduced lumen. These changes also occur relatively early in the hypertensive process. An increase in the aortic rigidity index (the ratio between pulse pressure and stroke index) was seen in our patients in the 20-year follow-up study.

SUMMARY AND CONCLUSION

The hemodynamic disturbances associated with the increased blood pressure of hypertension vary tremendously. In a 70-year-old patient, cardiac output may be just half of the cardiac output seen in a man in his twenties, although both persons may have the same MAP during rest. The peripheral resistance is much higher in the older patient. When hypertension is left untreated, there is an increase in TPR and blood pressure and a fall in CO and stroke volume over the years.

Ideally, prevention of these alterations should necessitate drugs causing permanent reduction in TPR and normalization of the left ventricular wall.[10] It would seem logical to start treatment at an early stage, before the structural changes are too pronounced and difficult to reverse. However, although great advances have been made in the development of antihypertensive drugs during the last 40 years, all drugs have side effects, and there are still no data showing that drug treatment of very mild hypertension in adolescents will arrest the hypertensive process and maintain normal organ function and structure over the following years.

REFERENCES

1. Conway J. Hemodynamic aspects of essential hypertension in humans. Physiol Rev 1984;64:617–660.

2. Folkow B. Physiological aspects of primary hypertension. Physiol Rev 1982;62:347–504.

3. Hofman A, Grobbee DE, Schalekamp MADH. The early pathogenesis of primary hypertension. In: Hofman A, Grobbee DE, Schalekamp MADH, eds. Excerpta medica. Amsterdam: International Congress Series 737, 1987: 1–219.

4. Messerli FH, DeCarvalho JGR, Christie B, et al. Systemic and regional hemodynamics in low, normal and high cardiac output borderline hypertension. Circulation 1978;58:441–448.

5. Lund-Johansen P, Omvik P. Hemodynamic patterns of untreated hypertensive disease. In: Laragh, JH, Brenner BM, eds. Hypertension: Pathophysiology, diagnosis, and management, New York: Raven, 1995:323–342.

6. Messerli FH. Messerli FH, ed. The heart and hypertension. New York:Yorke Medical Books, Cahners, 1987.

7. Strauer BE. Coronary vascular changes in the progression and regression of hypertensive heart disease. J Cardiovasc Pharmacol 1991:18(Suppl. 3): S20–S27.

8. Weber KT, Brilla CG, Cleland JG, Cohn J, Hansson L, Heagerty AM, Laragh JH. Cardioreparation and the concept of modulating cardiovascular structure and function. Blood Pressure 1993, 2:6–21.

9. Mulvany MJ. Are vascular abnormalities a primary cause or secondary consequence of hypertension? Hypertension 1991;18 (Suppl. 1):S52–S57.

10. Lund-Johansen P. Newer thinking on the hemodyamics of hypertension. Curr Opin Cardiol 1994;9:505–511.

CHAPTER 3

Evolution of Hemodynamic and Neuroendocrine Changes in the Course of Hypertension

Stevo Julius
Shawna Nesbitt

In Chapter 2, Lund-Johansen illustrated the important principle that hypertension is a dynamic process and that, depending on the stage of the disease, the underlying pathophysiology changes. In a large proportion of patients, the blood pressure elevation is initially associated with a high cardiac output, but later in the course of the disease a high vascular resistance predominates. These hemodynamic changes are also associated with alterations in responsiveness of various cardiovascular organs and with changes in many metabolic variables. I will argue that changes in the hemodynamics and in the organ responsiveness become a major factor in the later development of metabolic changes. Altered responsiveness of the cardiovascular system is also responsible for a gradual change of the autonomic nervous tone in the course of hypertension; in its early phases, there is a clear association between hypertension and signs of increased sympathetic tone, but, as hypertension advances, the autonomic nervous hyperactivity becomes less evident. Finally, I intend to show that an understanding of these dynamic interrelationships in the course of hypertension may be helpful in clinical practice.

THE HYPERKINETIC-HYPERADRENERGIC STATE

The high cardiac output observed in early phases of hypertension is due to increased sympathetic stimulation and decreased parasympathetic inhibition of the heart. This has been proven by acute pharmacologic blockade; after intravenous atropine and propranolol, the cardiac output in patients with borderline hypertension ceases to be higher than in control subjects.[1] The classic data on hemodynamics in borderline hypertension[2,3] have been collected with brachial artery puncture and cardiac catheterization. It was, therefore, possible that the high cardiac output may have reflected these patients' emotional reaction to the procedure and not their baseline physiologic state. Furthermore, patients studied in specialized laboratories tend to be self-selected, concerned individuals not representative of a typical patient with hypertension. However, in Tecumseh, Michigan, the hemodynamic procedures were noninvasive and studies were performed on unselected subjects from the general population.[4] In this population, whose average age at the time of the examination was 32 years, a hyperkinetic state was found in 37% of all subjects with borderline hypertension; they had elevated plasma norepinephrine levels, the blood pressure of their parents was elevated, and their blood pressure as children and young adults, decades before the current examination, was consistently elevated. Hyperkinetic, neurogenic borderline hypertension is frequent, appears in subjects with a background of hypertension, and is a reproducible, lifelong characteristic of these persons.

Further evidence that blood pressure elevation is neurogenic in a large proportion of young patients with borderline hypertension comes from studies of pharmacologic blockade of the alpha-adrenergic vascular tone,[5] measurements of norepinephrine turnover,[6] and with direct microneurographic recording of traffic in sympathetic fibers of the peroneal nerve.[7]

The cumulative evidence for a strong neurogenic component in blood pressure elevation in younger subjects with borderline and mild hypertension is overwhelming and undeniable. However, there is some confusion about the significance of the nervous system in hypertension because it is widely believed that neurogenic hypertension is present only in subjects with labile or "white coat" hypertension. There is no factual support for such a belief; actually, the blood pressure elevation in neurogenic-hyperkinetic borderline hypertensives is permanent and their blood pressure reactivity is not excessive.[8] A further source of confusion about the importance of the nervous system in hypertension comes from studies in more advanced hypertension. At that stage, the hypersympathetic state is less evident, but, as will be explained later, an abnormality in autonomic control of the circulation remains an important component of the pathophysiology of the disease.

Adding to the confusion is the notion that tachycardia, the hallmark of hyperkinetic hypertension, is an innocuous condition. This belief stems from the need to stabilize blood pressure measurements in clinical practice. Whereas it is true that a large proportion of patients with tachycardia may be "nervous" and that their blood pressure might come down after a period of rest, this does not mean that tachycardia denotes a particularly good prognosis. We have recently reviewed the topic,[9] and there is no doubt that tachycardia is, in fact, a predictor of poor cardiovascular outcomes. In normotensive subjects, a fast heart rate predicts future hypertension. Fast heart rate is also a predictor of poor coronary outcomes, sudden death, and of an increase in all causes of mortality. Importantly, tachycardia is not a marker of other co-morbidity (congestive heart failure, anemia) as it predicts fatal events that occur 10 to 30 years after the initial heart rate measurement.

The effect of tachycardia on cardiovascular morbidity and mortality reflects, in part, the mechanical deleterious effect of the frequent pulsatile flow on the vasculature and/or repeat myocardial contractions on the heart. The mechanical effect of the heart rate on the development of coronary atherosclerosis has been documented in experimental animals,[10] the fast heart rate decreases vascular compliance and increases the mean arterial pressure. The increased heart rate reflects the underlying increase of the sympathetic tone and a decrease of the parasympathetic tone.[1] This aberration of the autonomic tone has a major effect on cardiovascular morbidity and mortality. Sympathetic overactivity is associated with numerous coronary risk factors: insulin resistance, dyslipidemia, increased hematocrit, enhanced platelet activity, tendency for arrythmias, and sudden death, as well as vascular and cardiac hypertrophy.[11] Decreased parasympathetic tone is conducive to fatal arrythmias.[12] A detailed overview of the literature in support of these statements is given in a recent editorial review.[13]

ALTERATION IN THE RESPONSIVENESS OF CARDIOVASCULAR ORGANS

Long-term blood pressure elevation leads to hypertrophy and to alteration of organ functions in the circulation. Additionally, over a prolonged period, the excessive sympathetic tone in its own right contributes to changes of function and structure of cardiovascular organs. The sum total of these influences has an opposite effect on the two major components of the circulation; the heart is rendered hyporesponsive, whereas the resistant vessels tend to become overresponsive.

Patients who no longer have an elevated cardiac output but still show borderline hypertension uniformly have a decreased stroke volume.[14-16] The low stroke volume in these patients reflects a decreased cardiac compliance leading to a lesser end-diastolic distention and decreased Starling forces of ejection. A decreased diastolic cardiac function is an early consequence of blood pressure elevation and can be detected before signs of left ventricular hypertrophy are evident. In addition to a decreased stroke volume, patients with normal cardiac output-type of borderline hypertension also show decreased beta-adrenergic chronotropic responsiveness.[16] Apparently in a fashion similar to that of other organs exposed to repeated sympathetic activation, the heart downregulates its responsiveness to the stimulus.

We believe that in the course of hypertension the combined decreased stroke volume and the lesser heart rate response to beta-adrenergic stimulation eventually return the previously elevated cardiac output into the normal range. It ought to be noted that while numerically in a normal range, the regulation of the cardiac output in these patients is not physiologically normal. If one removes the autonomic influences on the heart in these patients with blocking agents, their cardiac output is clearly decreased.[16] The blockade uncovers an underlying pathophysiologic abnormality; in these patients, excessive autonomic drive is needed just to keep the cardiac output in the normal range.

While blood pressure related changes of the heart tend to decrease cardiac output, an excessive pressure load on the resistance vessels has the opposite effect. As Folkow has shown,[17] vascular hypertrophy in resistance vessels increases their responsiveness. If a resistance vessel is hypertrophic, the vessel's thicker wall encroaches upon the lumen. In a vasodilated state, the thicker wall does not have a major effect on vascular resistance. However, when the vessel constricts, the encroachment of the wall on the lumen becomes disproportionally greater and there is a steep increase in vascular resistance. The thicker wall of a hypertensive resistance vessel becomes an amplifier of all vasoconstrictive responses.

The mechanism of the hemodynamic transition from a high cardiac output to a high-resistance state in the course of hypertension can be explained by the pressure-related increase in vascular and decrease in cardiac responsiveness. However, this hemodynamic transition also provides a reasonable explanation of two other phenomena: the gradual decrease in sympathetic tone in the course of hypertension and the association of hypertension with insulin resistance and hyperlipidemia.

HEMODYNAMIC TRANSITION AND SYMPATHETIC TONE IN HYPERTENSION

In achieving a blood pressure response, the autonomic nervous system has access to all cardiovascular organs; a pressor response can be mediated either through an elevation of cardiac output or through an increase in vascular resistance. These responses tend to be stereotypical; for example, the increase in blood pressure that occurs with mental effort is effected through a rise in cardiac output, whereas the pressor response to noise is an increase of vascular resistance. However, abnormal circumstances can affect the direction of the hemodynamic components although they do not alter the magnitude of the blood pressure response. If the responsiveness of an organ is decreased, the autonomic nervous tone will be directed toward the other, more responsive organ system in order to secure the desired blood pressure elevation. It appears as if the nervous system "seeks" a certain blood pressure and will do "what it takes" to achieve the desired blood pressure level. Figures 1 and 2 are examples of such a behavior of the central nervous system.

In Figure 1, the subject's alerting response was elicited through quiet speaking.[18] This stimulus is similar to mental arithmetic; under normal circumstances, the blood pressure increases through elevation of cardiac output. As the open bars in Figure 1 show, there was a 20 mm Hg increase in blood pressure associated with a 1.5 l/min increase in cardiac output, while the vascular resistance decreased about 8 arbitrary units. When Ulrych gave patients beta-adrenergic blockade (shaded bars), the blood pressure increase was identical; however, because the unresponsive heart could not increase its output, the pressor response was mediated through an elevation of vascular resistance. The central nervous system shifted the autonomic tone from the heart to the blood vessels in order to achieve the desired blood pressure elevation. A similar change of the underlying hemodynamics can be observed after myocardial infarction (Figure 2).

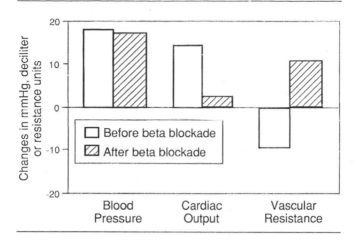

Figure 1. *Hemodynamic components of the blood pressure response to speaking. Before beta-adrenergic blockade, the response was mediated by an increase in cardiac output (open bars). After blockade, the magnitude of blood pressure increase was not changed, but, instead of an increased cardiac output, the response was mediated by increased vascular resistance (shaded bars). Adapted from Ulrych M. Changes of general haemodynamics during stressful mental arithmetic and non-stressing quiet conversation and modification of the latter by beta-adrenergic blockade. Clin Sci 1969;36:453–461.*

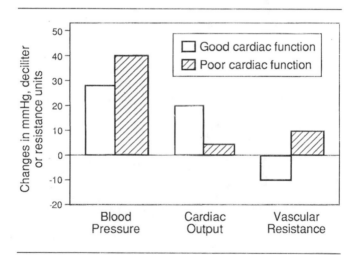

Figure 2. *Hemodynamic components of the blood pressure to isometric exercise in patients with good cardiac function (open bars) and poor cardiac function (shaded bars). Patients with good cardiac function responded by a cardiac output-mediated increase in blood pressure, whereas those with a poor cardiac function maintained blood pressure elevation through an increase in vascular resistance. Adapted from Baccelli G, Valentini R, Gregorini L, et al. Haemodynamic effects of isometric handgrip exercise in patients convalescent from myocardial infarction. Clin Exp Pharmacol Physiol 1978;5:607–615.*

Baccelli et al.[19] utilized the response to isometric exercise to evaluate cardiac function. Isometric exercise is always associated with a substantial elevation in blood pressure, which normally is due to an increase in cardiac output. It was expected that patients with poor cardiac function, unable to increase cardiac output, might fail to increase blood pressure. However, the blood pressure increase to isometric exercise as a test to assess cardiac function has failed; patients with a poor cardiac function (shaded bars) actually had a larger blood pressure increase. Again, the central nervous system shifted the sympathetic tone from the heart to the blood vessels to maintain the expected blood pressure increase through a rise in vascular resistance.

The fact that the cerebral cardiovascular centers can direct the autonomic tone to various organs provides an insight into the functional organization of autonomic control of the circulation. When a circulatory response is required, the central nervous system permits large variations of cardiac output and vascular resistance but very tightly regulates the pressure response. In order to achieve such a tight regulation of blood pressure, the brain must receive precise *feedback* information about the *achieved* blood pressure level. The ease by which a given blood pressure will be reached greatly depends on the responsiveness of the heart and the blood vessels. As described earlier, as they develop hypertrophy, hypertensive vessels become overresponsive to sympathetic vasoconstriction. Under these circumstances, less sympathetic drive is needed to elevate blood pressure. If, in a certain proportion of patients with hypertension, the central nervous system maintains elevated blood pressure levels, and if the brain is capable of "sensing" whether these higher levels have been achieved, a decrease in sympathetic tone in the course of advanced hypertension is fully expected. As the vasculature of these patients becomes hyperresponsive, blood pressure feedback to the central nervous system tends to decrease sympathetic outflow. The sympathetic tone of these patients resets itself toward similar numerical values as in normotensive subjects, but in its relationship to vascular reactivity this tone is excessive; although it may not be readily evident, hypertension in such patients remains neurogenic.

HEMODYNAMIC TRANSITION AND INSULIN RESISTANCE IN HYPERTENSION

Another frequently present abnormality in hypertension, insulin resistance, may also be largely dependent on the evolution of increased vascular resistance in hypertension. Epidemiologic studies show a strong relationship between higher blood pressure levels and/or hypertension and insulin resistance.[20,21] This is of great interest because insulin resistance is frequently associated with elevated plasma insulin levels and increased plasma insulin is a predictor of future development of atherosclerotic complications.[22,23] Furthermore, patients with insulin resistance are usually overweight and frequently have dyslipidemias. This close association of hypertension with other coronary risk factors may be one reason why antihypertensive treatment is not very efficacious in preventing coronary heart disease in hypertension. It is now well recognized that the effect of antihypertensive treatment on the reduction of coronary heart disease is much less dramatic than its effect on stroke reduction.[24]

Insulin affects glucose metabolism through its effects on liver, fatty tissue, and skeletal muscle. It has been well documented that skeletal muscle is the major site of insulin resistance in hypertension.[25] Whereas some of this resistance may be due to a receptor/transport protein abnormality and also an abnormality in the type of skeletal muscle fibers,[26] we recently suggested that hemodynamic factors also may affect insulin-induced glucose utilization in skeletal muscles.[27,28] Glucose utilization depends on nutritional blood flow; if an inadequate amount of glucose is delivered to metabolically active skeletal muscle cells, glucose metabolism will be negatively affected. Glucose delivery, in turn, depends on the capillary network around the muscle cells. If the capillaries in a skeletal muscle are less dense and there is a less favorable capillary-to-fiber ratio, nutrients will traverse a longer distance from the blood to metabolically active cells. The capillary-to-fiber distance will particularly affect utilization of substances, which, like glucose, are not freely diffusible.

Functional studies strongly suggest that vasodilatory reserve in skeletal muscles of patients with hypertension is diminished,[28,29] and there are also anatomic studies to demonstrate a decreased capillary-to-fiber ratio in the skeletal muscles of hypertensive patients.[30] One of the processes that may contribute to this vascular rarefaction in hypertension is the previously described medial layer hypertrophy in the resistance vessels.[17] As the vascular wall becomes thicker and encroaches upon the lumen, at some critical point the lumen can close and smaller blood vessels downstream may be excluded from the circulation.[31]

The strongest argument for a hemodynamic component in the association of hypertension and insulin resistance is in the effect of antihypertensive drugs on insulin resistance. It is well known that some antihypertensive drugs further aggravate insulin resistance, the patient's lipid profile, or both. Instead of accepting this as a fact of life, when treating hypertension one should ponder a couple of interesting questions: Why should drugs that lower blood pressure have a negative effect on lipids and plasma insulin levels? And, why should such pharmacologically different drugs as diuretics and beta-blockers[32,33] lead to the same result? The common denominator of both classes of antihypertensive agents, which aggravate insulin resistance and dyslipidemia in hypertension, is that they decrease cardiac output and increase vascular resistance. If one accepts that there may be a hemodynamic cause for insulin resistance in hypertension, then a decrease of the blood flow and a vasoconstriction in the skeletal muscle is fully expected to aggravate metabolic parameters in patients with hypertension.

The converse is also true; antihypertensive medications that improve insulin sensitivity[33,34] and have a positive effect on lipids[35] tend to be vasodilators. Again, the mechanism of vasodilation is quite different, but the effect on insulin sensitivity is similar. Physical exercise also improves insulin sensitivity,[36,37] and it is known that physical training increases capillary numbers in the exercising muscle groups.[38]

CLINICAL IMPLICATIONS

Because the association of hypertension with metabolic abnormalities starts early, it is important to assess both blood pressure and metabolic risk factors in patients with even the mildest blood pressure elevation. We have shown that subjects with "white coat" hypertension in Tecumseh have dyslipidemia and an elevated plasma insulin level.[39] Such patients may not need pharmacologic treatment to lower blood pressure, but their metabolic abnormalities and mild blood pressure elevation require medical attention. Because such patients often also show signs of circulatory hyperactivity, are overweight, and have increased sympathetic tone, ideal management would aim at improving all components of this pathophysiologic mosaic.

The first step in management of these patients must be a program of regular dynamic physical exercise. The effects of exercise are ideally suited to offset almost all negative factors in patients with mild hypertension. Physical training lowers the blood pressure; improves insulin sensitivity; and decreases cardiac output, heart rate, and sympathetic tone.[40] Exercise is also useful in weight control. Surprisingly little exercise is needed to achieve the desired effect.[40] In terms of blood pressure response, a patient will benefit maximally if he or she regularly exercises half an hour every second day at a load that increases the heart rate to about 120 beats/min. More vigorous exercise programs seem to be no more beneficial in terms of blood pressure.

Before deciding whether a patient with hypertension in the clinic should be treated with drugs, we recommend utilizing home blood pressure measurements. In our Tecumseh blood pressure study, we have found that having a home blood pressure of greater than 128 and 83 mm Hg has a sensitivity of only 48% while it has a specificity of 93% for predicting hypertension after three years of follow-up.[41] In contrast, a home blood pressure of less than 120 and 80 mm Hg had a sensitivity of 45% and a specificity of 91% for predicting normotension after three years. Based on this we have suggested an algorithm of follow-up (Figure 3).

If the decision for pharmacologic treatment has been made and a patient shows metabolic and neurohumoral abnormalities in addition to blood pressure elevation, vasodilating antihypertensive agents that do not cause a strong sympathetic counter-regulatory response (no tachycardia) are the most reasonable drugs. For instance, angiotensin-converting enzyme (ACE) inhibitors may control both blood pressure and insulin resistance,[33] whereas alpha-adrenergic blocking agents additionally may also have a positive effect on plasma lipid values.[35]

It must be stressed, however, that the benefit of blood pressure reduction is proven. In all trials, even with agents that tend to increase plasma insulin and lipid levels, because of the reduction in strokes and congestive heart failure the effect of treatment on overall mortality is beneficial. Thus, the primary goal of antihypertensive treatment continues to be reduction of blood pressure. It must be kept in mind that all modern antihypertensive agents effectively lower blood pressure in about 65% of patients. Consequently, using a com-

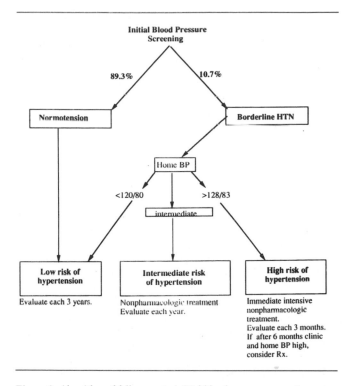

Figure 3. Algorithm of follow-up to initial blood pressure screening.

pound with ancillary beneficial properties in a given patient is justified as long as that drug is an effective antihypertensive agent in that individual. This truism is sometimes forgotten in clinical practice, and occasionally a physician uses a modern drug for its theoretical ancillary advantages and minimizes the importance of optimal blood pressure control.

REFERENCES

1. Julius S, Pascual AV, London R. Role of parasympathetic inhibition in the hyperkinetic type of borderline hypertension. Circulation 1971;44:413–418.

2. Julius S, Schork N, Schork A. Sympathetic hyperactivity in early stages of hypertension: The Ann Arbor data set. J Cardiovasc Pharmacol 1988;12(Suppl. 3):S121–S129.

3. Lund-Johansen P. Hemodynamics in early essential hypertension. Acta Med Scand 1967;482(Suppl.):1–105.

4. Julius S, Krause L, Schork N, Mejia A, Jones K, van de Ven C, Johnson E, Sekkarie MA, Kjeldsen SE, Petrin J, Schmouder R, Gupta R, Ferraro J, Nazzaro P, Weissfeld J. Hyperkinetic borderline hypertension in Tecumseh, Michigan. J Hypertens 1991;9:77–84.

5. Esler M, Julius S, Zweifler A, Randall O, Harburg E, Gardiner H, DeQuattro V. Mild high-renin essential hypertension: Neurogenic human hypertension? N Engl J Med 1977;296:405–411.

6. Esler M, Jackman G, Bobik A, Leonard P, Kelleher D, Skews H, Jennings G, Korner P. Norepinephrine kinetics in essential hypertension. Defective neuronal uptake of norepinephrine in some patients. Hypertension 1981;3:149–156.

7. Anderson EA, Sinkey CA, Lawton WJ, Mark AL. Elevated sympathetic nerve activity in borderline hypertensive humans: Evidence from direct intraneural recordings. Hypertension 1989;14:177–183.

8. Julius S, Schork N, Johnson E, Jones K, Krause L, Nazzaro P. Independence of pressure reactivity from blood pressure levels in Tecumseh, Michigan. Hypertension 1991;17(III):13–19.

9. Palatini P, Julius S. Heart rate and the cardiovascular risk. J Hypertens 1997;15:3–17.

10. Beere P, Glgov S, Zarins CK. Retarding effect of lowered heart rate on coronary atherosclerosis. Science 1984; 226:180–182.

11. Julius S. Sympathetic hyperactivity and coronary risk in hypertension (Corcoran Lecture). Hypertension 1993;21:886–893.

12. Lown B, Verrier RL. Neural activity and ventricular fibrillation. N Engl J Med 1976;294:1165–1170.

13. Julius S. Coronary disease in hypertension: a new mosaic. J Hypertens 1997;15:S3–S10.

14. Lund-Johansen P, Omvik P. Hemodynamic patterns of untreated hypertensive disease. In Laragh JH, Brenner BM, eds. Hypertension: Pathophysiology, diagnosis, and management. New York, Raven, 1990; 305.

15. Julius S, Jamerson K, Mejia A, Krause L, Schork N, Jones K. The association of borderline hypertension with target organ changes and higher coronary risk. Tecumseh Blood Pressure Study. JAMA 1990;264:354–358.

16. Julius S, Randall OS, Esler MD, Kashima T, Ellis CN, Bennett J. Altered cardiac responsiveness and regulation in the normal cardiac output type of borderline hypertension. Circ Res 1975;36–37(Suppl. I):I-199–I-207.

17. Folkow B. Physiological aspects of primary hypertension. Physiol Rev 1982;62:347–503.

18. Ulrych M. Changes of general haemodynamics during stressful mental arithmetic and non-stressing quiet conversation and modification of the latter by beta-adrenergic blockade. Clin Sci 1969;36:453–461.

19. Baccelli G, Valentini R, Gregorini L, Cellina G, Mancia G, Ludbrook J, Zanchetti A. Haemodynamic effects of isometric handgrip exercise in patients convalescent from myocardial infarction. Clin Exp Pharmacol Physiol 1978;5:607–615.

20. Modan M, Halkin H, Almog S, Lusky A, Eshkol A, Shefi M, Shitrit A, Fuchs Z. Hyperinsulinemia. A link between hypertension obesity and glucose intolerance. J Clin Invest 1985;75:809–817.

21. Florey CV, Uppal S, Lowy C. Relation between blood pressure, weight, and plasma sugar and serum insulin levels in schoolchildren aged 9–12 years in Westland, Holland. Br Med J 1976;1: 1368–1371.

22. Ducimetiere P, Eschwege E, Papoz L, Richard JL, Claude JR, Rosselin G. Relationship of plasma insulin levels to the incidence of myocardial infarction and coronary heart disease mortality in a middle-aged population. Diabetologia 1980;19:205–210.

23. Welborn TA, Wearne K. Coronary heart disease incidence and cardiovascular mortality in Busselton with reference to glucose and insulin concentrations. Diabetes Care 1979;2:154–160.

24. Collins R, Peto R, MacMahon S, Hebert P, Fiebach NH, Eberlein KA, Godwin J, Qizilbash N, Taylor JO, Hennekens CH. Blood pressure, stroke, and coronary heart disease. Part 2, short-term reduction in blood pressure: Overview of randomized drug trials in their epidemiological context. Lancet 1990;335:827–838.

25. Natali A, Santoro D, Palombo C, Cerri M, Ghione S, Ferrannini E. Impaired insulin action on skeletal muscle metabolism in essential hypertension. Hypertension 1991;17:170–178.

26. DeFronzo RA, Ferrannini E. Insulin resistance: A multifaceted syndrome responsible for NIDDM, obesity, hypertension, dyslipidemia, and atherosclerotic cardiovascular disease. Diabetes Care 1991;14:173–194.

27. Julius S, Gudbrandsson T, Jamerson K, Shahab ST, Andersson O. Hypothesis. The hemodynamic link between insulin resistance and hypertension. J Hypertens 1991;9:983–986.

28. Julius S, Gudbrandsson T, Jamerson K, Andersson O. The interconnection between sympathetics, microcirculation, and insulin resistance in hypertension. Blood Pressure 1992;1:9–19.

29. Conway J. A vascular abnormality in hypertension. A study of blood flow in the forearm. Circulation 1963;27:520–529.

30. Juhlin-Dannfelt A, Frisk-Holmberg F, Karlsson J, Tesch P. Central and peripheral circulation in relation to muscle-fibre composition in normo- and hyper-tensive man. Clin Sci 1979;56:335–340.

31. Greene AS, Tonellato PJ, Lui J, Lombard JH, Cowley AW Jr. Microvascular rarefaction and tissue vascular resistance in hypertension. Am J Physiol 1989;256:H126–H131.

32. Pollare T, Lithell H, Morlin C, Prantare H, Hvarfner A, Ljunghall S. Metabolic effects of diltiazem and atenolol: Results from a randomized, double-blind study with parallel groups. J Hypertens 1989;7:551–559.

33. Pollare T, Lithell H, Berne C. A comparison of the effects of hydrochlorothiazide and captopril on glucose and lipid metabolism in patients with hypertension. N Engl J Med 1989;321:868–873.

34. Pollare T, Lithell H, Selinus I, Berne C. Application of prazosin is associated with an increase of insulin sensitivity in obese patients with hypertension. Diabetologia 1988;31:415–420.

35. The Treatment of Mild Hypertension Research Group. The Treatment of Mild Hypertension Study. A randomized, placebo-controlled trial of a nutritional-hygienic regimen along with various drug monotherapies. Arch Intern Med 1991;151:1413–1423.

36. Tonino RP. Effect of physical training on the insulin resistance of aging. Am J Physiol 1989;256:E352–E356.

37. Krotkiewski M, Bylund-Fallenius A-C, Holm J, Bjorntorp P, Grimby G, Mandroukas K. Relationship between muscle morphology and metabolism in obese women: The effects of long-term physical training. Eur J Clin Invest 1983;13:5–12.

38. Saltin B, Henriksson J, Nygaard E, Andersen P. Fiber types and metabolic potentials of skeletal muscles in sedentary man and endurance runners. Ann N Y Acad Sci 1977;301:3–29.

39. Julius S, Mejia A, Jones K, Krause L, Schork N, van de Ven C, Johnson E, Petrin J, Sekkarie MA, Kjeldsen SE, Schmouder R, Gupta R, Ferraro J, Nazzaro P, Weissfeld J. "White coat" versus "sustained" borderline hypertension in Tecumseh, Michigan. Hypertension 1990;16:617–623.

40. Jennings G, Nelson L, Nestel B, Esler M, Korner P, Burton D, Bazelmans J. The effects of changes in physical activity on major cardiovascular risk factors, hemodynamics, sympathetic function, and glucose utilization in man: A controlled study of four levels of activity. Circulation 1986;73:30–40.

41. Nesbitt SD, Amarena JV, Grant E, Jamerson KA, Lu H, Weder A, Julius S. Home blood pressure as a predictor of future blood pressure stability in borderline hypertension. The Tecumseh study. Am J Hypertens 1997;10:1270–1280.

Target Organs in Hypertension: The Vascular Tree

Hope D. Intengan
Ernesto L. Schiffrin

Elevated peripheral resistance to blood flow is the hallmark of essential hypertension.[1] When the profile of blood pressure fall across the vascular tree is examined (Figure 1), a large part of this fall occurs in what are usually known as resistance arteries, indicating that these are a major site of generation of vascular resistance.[2] Resistance arteries comprise small arteries with lumen diameters between 100 and 300 μm, and arterioles, with lumen diameters smaller than 100 μm. It has been proposed that small arteries play a significant role in the pathogenesis of hypertension.[3] The fundamental cause of increased peripheral resistance to blood flow in hypertension is a decrease in lumen diameter of these small resistance vessels. According to Poiseuille's Law, resistance varies inversely with the fourth power of the blood vessel radius, so that a small decrease in the lumen markedly increases resistance to the flow of blood through resistance arteries.

In hypertension, the vascular changes that produce this decreased lumen size may be ascribed to structural and/or functional abnormalities. This chapter reviews first the structural and functional alterations of small arteries, their consequences, and the effects therein of antihypertensive therapy. The role of arterioles and conduit and medium-sized muscular vessels in hypertension is discussed in a second and third part of this chapter.

SMALL ARTERIES

Structural Abnormalities of Small Arteries in Hypertension

Structural remodeling in small arteries. In patients with mild essential hypertension, small arteries manifest structural alterations characteristic of "eutrophic remodeling."[4,5]

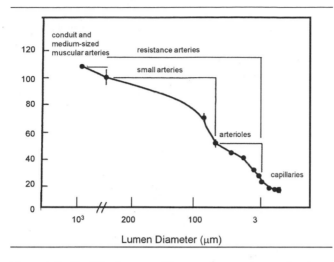

Figure 1. *Profile of blood pressure fall across the vascular tree, showing conduit and medium-sized muscular arteries, and resistance arteries, including small arteries and arterioles, where most of peripheral vascular resistance is generated.*

These arteries exhibit a reduced lumen and external diameter, usually without any difference in the cross-sectional area of the media relative to equivalent vessels of normotensive subjects.[6] It has been hypothesized that in these vessels, smooth muscle cells are rearranged around the lumen to decrease its size.[4,5] As hypertension becomes more severe, and in some special populations both in humans and in experimental animals with certain forms of hypertension, hypertrophy of the vessel wall predominates, and the change found, which typically includes an increased media cross-sectional area, is then called "hypertrophic remodeling."[4,5] The different forms of remodeling of small arteries are shown in Figure 2. All forms of remodeling resulting in changes that place them above the dashed line joining inward hypotrophic and outward hypertrophic remodeling result in increased media to lumen ratio, whereas those that are below this line have a reduced media to lumen ratio. The mechanisms involved in eutrophic remodeling are as of yet unclear. It is as well unknown whether these alterations of small vessel structure are a consequence rather than a primary cause of hypertension. These changes could serve to maintain elevated blood pressure and could also contribute to end-organ complications. There is evidence that small artery disease contributes to microvascular angina in hypertensive patients, and may as well participate in cerebrovascular disease, and through nephroangiosclerosis in the progression to renal failure. Alternatively, vascular remodeling, in concert with functional abnormalities, may contribute to the genesis of hypertension. Vasoconstrictor and growth-promoting hormones such as angiotensin II and endothelin-1, changes in cell adhesion, and altered interactions of cells with fibrillar or nonfibrillar extracellular matrix components may be key factors in the mechanisms of remodeling. Recent data suggests that alterations in the intercellular matrix, in the collagen and elastin content, may be more prominent than changes in smooth

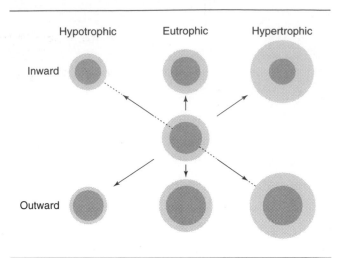

Figure 2. Classification of remodeling of resistance arteries. All forms of remodeling resulting in changes which place them above the dashed line joining inward hypotrophic and outward hypertrophic remodeling result in increased media to lumen ratio, whereas those that are below this line have a reduced media to lumen ratio. Modified from ref. 6.

muscle cells. The change in the composition of the intercellular matrix may contribute to the rearrangement of smooth muscle cells which is found in "eutrophic remodeling," and to the growth of the cross-sectional area of the media found in "hypertrophic remodeling."

Functional Consequences of Structural Remodeling of Small Arteries. The structural modifications of small arteries may be a protective adaptation in the face of elevated blood pressure. For example, wall stress is decreased by the augmented wall thickness at each level of circumferential tension (stress = tension/wall width). Thus, blood vessel wall thickening may buffer the damaging effects of high blood pressure on the vascular wall.

Reduced lumen diameter will also result in decreased wall stress according to the Law of Laplace as a consequence of the smaller circumferential wall tension occurring at each level of transmural pressure (tension = pressure x radius). Therefore, if the radius of the lumen of the vessel is smaller, the circumferential tension resulting from each level of pressure will be smaller, and the circumferential stress will accordingly be smaller too. However, the reduction in lumen diameter may have detrimental effects, inasmuch as reduced wall stress is achieved at the expense of increased resistance to blood flow, which may compromise tissue irrigation in critical vascular beds, such as in the heart, brain or kidney. According to the Law of Laplace, the transmural pressure against which a vessel must contract is inversely related to its radius (transmural pressure = tension/radius). Hence, despite reductions of active media stress developed in response to constrictor agents, vasoconstrictor responses will be amplified, and even if they are blunted by impaired signal transduction as responses to most of these agents are except for those to angiotensin II, they will be normalized, or enhanced. For example, whereas tension responses elicited by endothelin are decreased in subcutaneous arteries from mild hypertensive patients, maximum pressure responses are comparable to those observed in normotensive controls. The structural reduction in lumen diameter may thus contribute to maintain elevated blood pressure by amplifying responses to circulating vasoconstrictors, whether the intrinsic smooth muscle cell response to these is increased or not, solely on structurally-based amplification of vasoconstrictor responses. Figure 3 shows based on the mathematical model of Bjorn Folkow how the structural reduction in lumen diameter (with increased media to lumen ratio) in "hypertrophic remodeling" (H) will result in increased resistance to blood flow for the same level of smooth muscle contraction in comparison to vessels from normotensive subjects (N). In "eutrophic remodeling" (E), resistance to blood flow at each level of contraction of smooth muscle cells is predicted to be even greater than in "hypertrophic remodeling." In many studies it has been suggested that responses to vasoconstrictors are increased in hypertension. Responses of resistance arteries are in fact usually unchanged or reduced, except for reactivity to angiotensin II. Thus, enhanced response to most vasoconstrictors other than angiotensin II is structurally-based. The mechanism for enhanced responses of smooth muscle cells to angiotensin II is as yet unclear, but it appears to be secondary to postreceptor changes in signalling, which may be associated with modification in the phenotype of smooth muscle cells in blood vessels in hypertension.

Antihypertensive Therapy and Small Artery Structure. To improve clinical outcome in hypertensive patients, it has been hypothesized that therapy must induce regression of vascular remodeling. The failure to produce

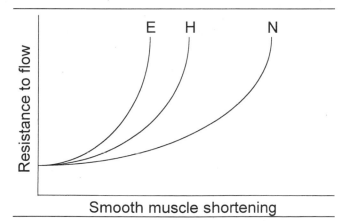

Figure 3. Effect of increased media to lumen ratio of resistance arteries in hypertension, on resistance to flow during contraction of smooth muscle in the vascular wall, in presence of either hypertrophic remodeling (H) or eutrophic remodeling (E), in comparison to the normotensive situation (N). Modified from ref. 15.

consistent regression of vessel wall changes may explain the limited success in preventing hypertension-related coronary events when blood pressure lowering is the sole therapeutic aim.

Several studies have examined the beneficial effects of antihypertensive agents on small artery structure. Angiotensin-converting enzyme inhibition with cilazapril[7] or perindopril[8] normalized structure of gluteal subcutaneous small arteries from essential hypertensive patients. Calcium channel blockade may also normalize small artery structure.[9] In contrast, antagonism of beta-adrenoceptors with atenolol appears ineffective in improving small artery structural abnormalities.[7,8]

Whether the reversal of structural abnormalities demonstrated in gluteal subcutaneous arteries will result in improved clinical outcome remains to be determined. However, regression of structural and functional abnormalities of gluteal subcutaneous arteries appears to be associated in hypertensive patients with improved structure and function of other more critical vascular beds such as the coronary microcirculation, as shown by indirect measurements.[10]

Functional Abnormalities of Small Arteries in Hypertension

Functional Changes in Small Arteries. Altered small artery function in hypertension also increases peripheral resistance by further decreasing lumen diameter. Functional abnormalities either enhance constriction or impair relaxation. As discussed previously, augmented vasoconstriction is due largely to the amplifying effects of structural reductions in lumen diameter, as explained by the Law of Laplace, although angiotensin II responses appear to be enhanced independently of structural amplification. Vasoconstrictors such as endothelin and vasopressin have been reported to elicit diminished or normal responses in vessels from hypertensive rat models respectively. In vivo, circulating vasoconstrictor substances may be involved in maintaining the elevated blood pressure chronically, after the lumen diameter has been reduced. As mentioned above, except for angiotensin II, for which vascular responses appear to be enhanced in hypertensive patients, responses of small arteries to most vasoconstrictors are normal or diminished and only amplified by structural remodeling. Hyperinnervation of small arteries has also been suggested in young spontaneously hypertensive rats, but it is unknown whether this abnormality occurs in hypertensive patients. Increased sympathetic tone, which may be present in subsets of hypertensive subjects, may likewise increase peripheral resistance.

The ability of vessels to relax in response to endothelium-dependent stimuli is markedly impaired in hypertension, as evidenced by well-documented reductions in the vasodilation elicited by acetylcholine in rat and human vessels, particularly when blood pressure elevation is severe. The mechanism responsible for impaired endothelium-dependent relaxation is unclear. Deficient production of nitric oxide is one major possibility. However, it appears rather that nitric oxide deficiency may result from increased degradation of nitric oxide in hypertension. Enhanced oxidative stress and generation of free radicals present in the vascular wall in hypertension may accelerate nitric oxide degradation.[11] Alternatively, enhanced production of endothelial-derived constricting factors may impair vascular relaxation. The impairment of endothelium-dependent relaxation may be secondary to blood pressure elevation, since it is present to a greater extent in the more severe forms of hypertension, and in vascular disease associated with diabetes, hyperlipidemia and atherosclerosis, even in the absence of blood pressure elevation, and may be absent in very mild forms of hypertension. On the other hand, it may represent an important risk factor of complications of hypertension. Endothelium-independent relaxation, as that elicited by sodium nitroprusside, is usually conserved in experimental and in human hypertension.

Antihypertensive Therapy and Small Artery Function.
As with small artery structure, numerous studies have investigated the effects of antihypertensive therapy on small artery function. Angiotensin converting enzyme (ACE) inhibition restores endothelial function variably, as measured by acetylcholine-induced relaxation. Following 1 or 2-year treatment with the ACE inhibitor cilazapril, abnormal endothelium-dependent relaxation of small human arteries in vitro was normalized.[12] However, short-term treatment with cilazapril or enalapril failed to regress endothelial dysfunction measured in vivo.[13,14] Chronic calcium channel blockade also normalized endothelial function.[9] Interestingly, as with structural abnormalities, beta-adrenoceptor blockade with atenolol did not improve endothelial function.[7,8] These studies collectively show that in essential hypertension, normalization of endothelial function may depend specifically on the antihypertensive agent, rather than on the blood pressure-lowering effect of the drug.

ARTERIOLES

Arterioles with lumen diameters smaller than 100 µm are also an important site of vascular resistance.[3] As with small arteries, some arterioles undergo eutrophic remodeling in hypertension; for example, pial arterioles in stroke-prone spontaneously hypertensive rats, in which in fact this phenomenon was first described.[15] Arteriolar remodeling is not universal in hypertension, however, as it has been reported to be undetectable in arterioles of some vascular beds. Regression of remodeling toward normal, similar to that found in small arteries, has been reported to occur in arterioles of the brain in stroke-prone spontaneously hypertensive rats under antihypertensive therapy with ACE inhibitors.[15]

The contribution of very small arterioles to increased resistance may occur via an alternate mechanism that has been called rarefaction.[16] This phenomenon may be functional and reversible, or represent a permanent (anatomical) reduction of arteriolar density. It has been reported in several vascular beds of rat models of hypertension, including one kidney-one clip and spontaneously hypertensive rats, and in humans with hypertension. The extent to which rarefaction augments peripheral resistance has been estimated to represent between 15% and 20% of total peripheral resistance in some experimental models, but its definitive impact on blood pressure elevation remains to be established.

CONDUIT ARTERIES

Altered Compliance of Conduit Arteries in Hypertension

The large arterial network functions to deliver blood to the periphery with minimal loss of perfusion pressure and to convert pulsatile blood flow to a continuous flow, an effect termed the Windkessel effect. Systolic volume ejected by the heart has to be accommodated by large vessels as it flows to the periphery, and, accordingly, distensibility of conduit arteries, together with variations in the systolic volume ejected by the left ventricle, will play a major role as a determinant of systolic blood pressure. Pulse pressure is the result of interplay between effects of conduit arteries contributing to determine systolic pressure, and resistance arteries contributing to diastolic blood pressure. Resistance arteries, through reflected waves, may also participate in determination of systolic blood pressure at different levels of the vascular tree. Blunting of the Windkessel effect could have a significant role in the pathophysiology of hypertension. Vascular compliance is the ability to change the absolute diameter with changes in pressure, an absolute measure of blood buffering or storage capacity of blood vessels. It is greatest at the level of the proximal aorta, and decreases along the vascular tree towards the smaller, more distal arteries, since it is proportional to blood vessel volume. Distensibility is a relative term, the change in diameter relative to the resting diameter with changes in pressure, and is independent of the caliber or geometry of the vessel. It is the inverse of the elastic modulus, which is a measure of the stiffness of vessels, and depends on the components of the arterial wall. The nature of the arterial tree leads to generation of waves which are reflected in the periphery, and appear as secondary waves in diastole in normal vessels. These reflection waves may contribute to the level of systolic blood pressure if the reflection is premature, for example in individuals of short stature. The arterial stiffening occurring in the aorta in hypertension results in increases in wave velocity, and accordingly reflected waves in hypertension will appear in systole, contributing to raise systolic pressure.[17]

The ability of conduit arteries to modulate pulse pressure is affected by their stiffness. With aging, particularly in the presence of hypertension, decreased compliance of conduit arteries[17] may result in insufficient buffering of pulse pressure to continuous capillary flow. Thus, one of the effects of conduit artery disease in hypertension is excessive pulsatile pressure, which may contribute to small artery and end-organ damage. In fact, conduit artery abnormalities participate in the initiation of small artery remodeling as previously discussed, as well as in cardiac overload and hypertrophy.

Not all conduit arteries exhibit decreased compliance, at least early or in mild forms of high blood pressure.[18] Intermediate-sized muscular arteries such as the radial artery,[19] and other elastic vessels such as the carotid arteries, may not exhibit decreases in compliance, particularly when isobaric compliance is examined. In fact, in these vessels elastic modulus (stiffness) is not increased but decreased. As of yet, it is unclear whether decreases in conduit artery compliance, when and where they occur in hypertensive patients, represent a consequence of the elevated blood pressure, or instead are due to intrinsic modifications of the arterial wall. Certainly the structural components of the vessel wall play a preponderant role in determining wall stiffness. In particular, changes in the amounts and interactions of collagen and elastin (stiffer and elastic elements, respectively) are of importance with respect to compliance. It has been proposed that stiffness of the arterial wall in response to increasing blood pressure is biphasic; that is, at low pressures, elastin is the major determinant of stiffness whereas collagen influences compliance at high pressures. Other factors that probably affect conduit artery compliance include altered tone, remodeling, and extracellular matrix interactions with cellular elements. With aging, increasing stiffness of conduit arteries results in the well-known increase in systolic blood pressure unaccompanied by elevation of diastolic blood pressure; in fact the latter decreases, with increased pulse pressure. When this phenomenon is exaggerated, and systolic blood pressure is elevated beyond 160 mm Hg in the absence of elevation of diastolic blood pressure, we are faced with isolated systolic hypertension, which contributes significantly to cardiovascular morbidity in the elderly. This form of hypertension is essentially the result of changes in conduit artery compliance associated with extensive athero- and arteriosclerosis of the vascular wall.

Recently it has been suggested that there are genetic differences in the susceptibility of different populations to develop changes in the structure of the arterial wall.[19] In the same direction is the finding of an association between increased aortic stiffness and angiotensin type 1 receptor gene polymorphisms.[20] An interaction of genetic and environmental influences is implied as well by the greater reduction of aortic compliance and distensibility in salt-sensitive individuals.

Atherosclerosis and Arteriosclerosis. Atherosclerosis complicates the changes induced by aging and hypertension in the larger elastic conduit arteries such as aorta, carotid, femoral and in epicardial coronary vessels. These changes occur preferentially at sites of turbulent flow, such as bifurcations (carotid and terminal aorta, iliac arteries), small vessels arising from large ones (renal arteries), narrowing vessels (infrarenal aorta), and vessels subject to repetitive bending (coronary and femoral arteries). In hypertension, the intimal layer of the arterial wall undergoes increased endothelial permeability, macrophage and proteoglycan accumulation, smooth muscle cell and monocyte migration, and extracellular matrix deposition. In the conduit vessels, these intimal changes may advance to atherosclerotic plaque formation under the predisposing condition of hyperlipidemia. The atherosclerotic process affects the intima with formation of a plaque which may become unstable as the fibrous cap surrounding the lipid-rich core becomes thinner, leading to plaque instability, and eventually to fissure and plaque rupture followed by thrombus formation. The latter contributes to the atherothromboembolic complications of hypertension. In the presence of atherosclerotic risk factors, such as smoking, diabetes, hypertension and hyperlipidemia, upregulation of endothelial adhesion molecules (selectins, ICAMs, VCAMs) may favor adhesion and migration of monocytes into the intima, an early event in atherogenesis (Figure 4). Altered endothelial permeability in the presence of hyperlipidemia will contribute to the incorporation of low-density lipoproteins (LDL) into the vessel wall, where LDL becomes trapped and may become oxidized in response to increased superoxide formation (increased oxidative stress).[21] Minimally oxidized LDL induces production of monocyte chemotactic protein 1 (MCP-1), which together with injury of the endothelium produced by the oxidized LDL and upregulation of adhesion molecules, will stimulate the recruitment of monocytes to the vascular wall. Monocytes and platelets release growth factors and cytokines which stimulate the migration and proliferation of smooth muscle cells. Smooth muscle cells, monocytes and macrophages stimulate further peroxidation of LDL. Oxidized LDL is uptaken by scavenger receptors, and as macrophages and monocytes become loaded with oxidized LDL, they turn into foam cells (Figure 5). Proliferating smooth muscle cells and foam cells contribute to the formation of the fatty streak. Oxidized LDL is toxic for foam cells, leading to foam cell necrosis. The release of intracellular enzymes and necrotic debris contributes to the formation of the atherosclerotic plaque. Different stimuli including hypertension, oxidized LDL, endothelial injury associated with other risk factors, may activate production of endothelin-1 which stimulates smooth muscle migration and proliferation, and has chemotactic effects on circulating monocytes. At the same time, degradation of nitric oxide which antagonizes these effects is increased by the enhanced oxidative stress in the vascular wall, and accordingly the protective effects of nitric oxide, as antiadhesive, antithrombotic, vasorelaxant and antiproliferative, are impaired. Increased endothelin-1 formation could be one of the links between hypertension, diabetes, smoking (and other risk factors) and atherogenesis.

In the aorta and other vessels, atherosclerosis is associated with degeneration of the arterial media (arteriosclerosis), and both are accelerated by hypertension. It is the arteriosclerosis of the media that will be mostly responsible for the stiffness changes, as elastic laminae are fragmented and fibrous tissue deposition occurs, sometimes accompanied by mucoid degeneration which may lead to cystic medial necrosis, and the latter rarely to aortic dissection.

Antihypertensive Therapy and Conduit Artery Compliance. Antihypertensive therapy can affect arterial

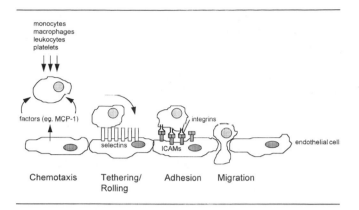

Figure 4. *Risk factors of cardiovascular disease induce endothelial injury and dysfunction, result in upregulation of adhesion molecules (selectins, ICAMs, VCAMs), and contribute to recruitment of monocytes, macrophages and smooth muscle cells, and progression of vascular disease.*

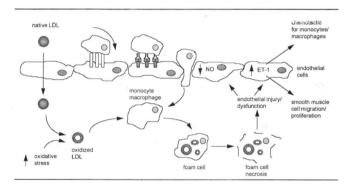

Figure 5. *Upregulation of endothelial adhesion molecules followed by migration of monocytes into the intima is an early event in atherogenesis as indicated in the preceding figure. Altered endothelial permeability in the presence of hyperlipidemia will contribute to the incorporation of LDL into the vessel wall, where LDL becomes oxidized in the presence of increased oxidative stress. Oxidized LDL is uptaken by scavenger receptors, and as macrophages and monocytes become loaded with oxidized LDL, they turn into foam cells. Oxidized LDL is toxic for foam cells, leading to foam cell necrosis, and increasing endothelial injury and dysfunction. Production of endothelin-1 (ET-1) may be activated, which further stimulates smooth muscle migration and proliferation, and has chemotactic effects on circulating monocytes. At the same time, degradation of nitric oxide (NO), which antagonizes these effects, is increased by the enhanced oxidative stress in the vascular wall, and accordingly the protective effects of nitric oxide, as antiadhesive, antithrombotic, vasorelaxant and antiproliferative, are impaired. Increased endothelin-1 formation may be a link between hypertension, diabetes, smoking (and other risk factors) and atherogenesis.*

compliance by two general mechanisms. First, simply by lowering blood pressure, antihypertensive agents produce a physiological shift to the more-compliant segment of a compliance-pressure curve, so that more elastin and less collagen is determining vascular compliance. Second, therapy could have direct effects on the vascular wall itself. The linking of collagen to smooth muscle cells and the degree to which the collagen jacket is tensed may play an important role, since collagen is less distensible than elastin. Its contribution is supposed to occur in the latter portion of the pressure curve, since collagen fibers may be coiled and not under tension until the smooth muscle cells in series and the elastin in parallel have been stretched. In the remodeled artery, with rearranged cellular and fibrillar components due to changes in the interaction of these structures, the collagen fibers may be recruited at higher distending pressures in some vessels which exhibit decreased stiffness, or collagen fibers may be increased in density in other vessels which exhibit increased stiffness such as the aorta. Calcium channel antagonists, angiotensin converting enzyme inhibitors, and nitrates may alter the mechanical properties of conduit arteries. The changes which occur may depend on the agent and dose used, the degree to which blood pressure is lowered, and the vascular bed examined. Whereas nitrates may increase compliance by vasodilation, angiotensin converting enzyme inhibitors and calcium antagonists may decrease stiffness (elastic modulus) without affecting arterial compliance.[22] Beta blockers appear not to result in changes in compliance or distensibility of large vessels. The latter is somewhat akin to what occurs in relation to the structure of small arteries.[7]

CONCLUSIONS

Changes in vascular structure and function play important roles in the pathophysiology of hypertension and, together with atherosclerosis, in the complications of hypertension. The limited improvement in cardiac-related clinical outcomes in randomized multicenter clinical trials by therapy aimed only at lowering blood pressure suggests that the goals of antihypertensive treatment should be broadened to include correction of the structural and functional abnormalities in blood vessels of essential hypertensive patients, since these changes could play a role in the pathogenesis of complications of high blood pressure. This hypothesis, although reasonable, requires proof in large randomized multicenter clinical trials demonstrating improvement of hard endpoints associated with correction of the surrogate vascular endpoints discussed in this chapter.

REFERENCES

1. Lund-Johansen, P. Haemodynamics in early essential hypertension—still an area of controversy. J. Hypertens 1983;1:209–213.

2. Bohlen, H.G. Localization of vascular resistance changes during hypertension. Hypertension 1986;8:181–183.

3. Schiffrin, E.L. Reactivity of small blood vessels in hypertension: Relation with structural changes. Hypertension 1992;19 (Suppl. II):II-1–II-9.

4. Korsgaard, N., Aalkjær, C., Heagerty, A.M., Izzard, A.S., and Mulvany, M.J. Histology of subcutaneous small arteries from patients with essential hypertension. Hypertension 1993;22:523–526.

5. Schiffrin, E.L., Deng, L.Y., and Larochelle, P. Morphology of resistance arteries and comparison of effects of vasoconstrictors in mild essential hypertensive patients. Clin. Invest. Med 1993;16:177–186.

6. Mulvany, M.J., Baumbach, G.L., Aalkjær, C., Heagerty, A.M., Korsgaard, N., Schiffrin, E.L., and Heistad, D.D. Vascular remodeling [letter]. Hypertension 1996;28:505–506.

7. Schiffrin, E.L., Deng, L.Y., and Larochelle, P. Progressive improvement in the structure of resistance arteries of hypertensive patients after 2 years of treatment with an angiotensin converting enzyme inhibitor. Comparison with effects of a beta blocker. Am. J. Hypertens1995;8:229–236.

8. Thybo, N.K., Stephens, N., Cooper, A., Aalkjær, C., Heagerty, A.M., and Mulvany, M.J. Effect of antihypertensive treatment on small arteries of patients with previously untreated essential hypertension. Hypertension 1995;25:474–481.

9. Schiffrin, E.L. and Deng, L.Y. Structure and function of resistance arteries of hypertensive patients treated with a beta-blocker or a calcium channel antagonist. J. Hypertens 1996;14:1247–1255.

10. Motz, W., Strauer, B.E. Improvement of coronary flow reserve after long-term therapy with enalapril. Hypertension 1996;27: 1031–1038.

11. Tschudi, M.R., Mesaros, S., Lüscher, T.F., and Malinski, T. Direct in situ measurement of nitric oxide in mesenteric resistance arteries. Hypertension 1996;27:32–35.

12. Schiffrin, E.L. and Deng, L.Y. Comparison of effects of angiotensin converting enzyme inhibition and beta blockade for 2 years on function of small arteries from hypertensive patients. Hypertension 1995;25:699–703.

13. Creager, M.A. and Roddy, M-A. Effect of captopril and enalapril on endothelial function in hypertensive patients. Hypertension 1994;24:499–505.

14. Kiowski, W., Linder, L., Nuesch, R., and Martina, B. Effects of cilazapril on vascular structure and function in essential hypertension. Hypertension 1996;27:371–376.

15. Baumbach, G.L. and Heistad, D.D. Remodeling of cerebral arterioles in chronic hypertension. Hypertension 1989;13:968–972.

16. Prasad, A., Dunnill, G.S., Mortimer, P.S., MacGregor, G.A. Capillary rarefaction in the forearm skin in essential hypertension. J Hypertens 1995;13:265–268.

17. O'Rourke, M. Mechanical principles in arterial disease. Hypertension 1995;26:2–9.

18. Hayoz, D., Rutschmann, B., Perret, F., Niederberger, M., Tardy, Y., Mooser, V., Nussberger, J., Waeber, B., Brunner, H.R. Conduit artery compliance and distensibility are not necessarily reduced in hypertension. Hypertension 1992;20:1–6.

19. Avolio, A. Genetic and environmental factors in the function and structure of the arterial wall. Hypertension 1995;26:34–37.

20. Safar, M.E., Frohlich, E.D. The arterial system in hypertension. Hypertension 1995;26:10–14.

21. Díaz, M.N., Frei, B., Vita, J.A., Keany, J.F. Antioxidants and atherosclerotic heart disease. New Engl J Med 1997;337:408–416.

22. Van Vortel, L.M., Kool, M.J., Boudier, H.A., Struijker Boudier, H.A. Effects of antihypertensive agents on local arterial distensibility and compliance. Hypertension 1995;26:531–534.

CHAPTER 5

Hypertensive Heart Disease

Roland E. Schmieder

In this chapter, hypertensive heart disease will be classified and recent data on left ventricular structure and function as well as coronary circulation in hypertensive heart disease will be highlighted.

PATHOPHYSIOLOGIC BACKGROUND OF LEFT VENTRICULAR HYPERTROPHY

In early stages of arterial hypertension, the development of left ventricular hypertrophy (LVH) represents a structural adaptation of the left ventricle to persistent pressure overload. The steadily increasing wall stress has been identified as the major trophic stimulus inducing hypertrophy in the myocardial cells. If arterial hypertension remains untreated and pressure overload persists, progressive myocardial hypertrophy and interstitial proliferation of connective tissue may occur. Excentric hypertrophy (i.e., dilation of the left ventricle) will result followed by a decrease in cardiac index and ejection fraction.

The development of LVH, however, cannot solely be linked to an increase in afterload or pressure load. In patients with mild-to-moderate essential hypertension, it has been reported that despite similar levels of afterload some hypertensives develop LVH and some do not. Constitutional factors, such as age and sex, as well as nutritive factors, such as obesity and sodium intake (Figure 1), and also different levels of stimulation of the sympathetic nervous system and the renin-angiotensin-aldosterone system appear to have modifying effects on the degree of LVH.[1] Accordingly, the degree of LVH depends not only on the extent of pressure elevation and duration of arterial hypertension but also on nonhemodynamic factors. The interaction of nonhemodynamic factors may also partially explain why a reduction of LVH sometimes does not occur despite arterial pressure control.[2]

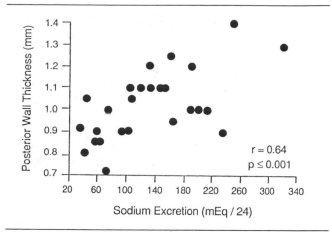

Figure 1. *Relation between sodium intake (estimated by 24-hour urine collection) and posterior wall thickness of the left ventricle. This relationship was independent of blood pressure level (r = 0.64, p <0.001), suggesting a direct trophic stimulus of high salt intake on myocardial hypertrophy.*

DIAGNOSIS OF LEFT VENTRICULAR HYPERTROPHY

The echocardiogram provides a more specific and sensitive assessment of anatomic LVH than either electrocardiogram (ECG) or chest x-ray. A typical pattern of LVH in a hypertensive patient can be visualized and quantified by 2-D guided M-mode echocardiography (Figure 2). Left ventricular mass measurements by echocardiography were found to correlate well with necropsy left ventricular mass, in particular in the pathologic range of left ventricular mass.[3] Consequently, echocardiography provides a very sensitive and specific tool for establishing the diagnosis LVH. Electrocardiography, in contrast, though specific for the detection of LVH, shows a lower sensitivity, although newer indices for LVH, such as the Cornell index [R in aVL + S in V_3] and its product with the QRS duration improved it clearly. Nevertheless the ECG represents the hallmark for evaluation of hypertensive macroangiopathy of the coronary arteries.

PREVALENCE AND INCIDENCE OF LEFT VENTRICULAR HYPERTROPHY

In an unselected population, such as the Framingham population, echocardiographic studies demonstrated a 16% prevalence of LVH in men and a 19% prevalence in women.[4] There is an independent increase in left ventricular mass with age from 8% in men under age 30 years to 33% in men age 70 or over. The corresponding rates in women range from 5% to 49%. In selected populations of hypertensive patients, up to 48% of the patients were reported to have echocardiographic LVH.

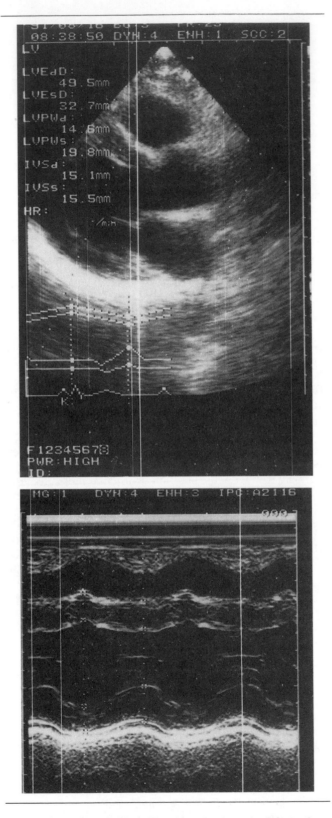

Figure 2. *Typical echocardiographic pattern demonstrating left ventricular hypertrophy in a hypertensive patient. LVEdD = diastolic diameter; LVEsD = systolic diameter; LVPWd = posterior wall thickness in diastole; IVSd = intraventricular septal wall thickness in diastole.*

PROGNOSTIC IMPLICATIONS OF LEFT VENTRICULAR HYPERTROPHY

Which prognostic implications can be linked with the detection of LVH in a hypertensive patient? Prospective data from the Framingham Heart Study showed that LVH, as evidenced by ECG and manifested by repolariziation abnormalities as well as increased voltage, was the lethal finding. Within five years, 33% of men and 21% of women were dead. ECG LVH seems to be associated with ventricular ectopy and the sudden death risk comparable to that of coronary heart disease or cardiac failure. ECG LVH was also associated with a three- to 15-fold increase in cardiovascular events, with greater risk ratios for cardiac failure and stroke. In the meantime, further echocardiographic studies confirmed these findings by revealing that cardiovascular events (sudden death, myocardial infarction, stroke) occurred significantly more frequently in patients with LVH than in patients without LVH.[5] Echocardiographic presence of LVH was associated with a twofold cardiovascular risk independent of blood pressure levels. These findings have been confirmed by further analyses from the Framingham study (Figure 3) as well as from prospective studies in the elderly from different European centers.

Compared to other cardiac risk factors, such as underlying coronary heart disease, left ventricular ejection fraction, sex, and age, LVH has been demonstrated to have its own prognostic value. In a study of 600 patients who all underwent cardiac catheterization and echocardiography, indices of LVH were identified as independent important predictors of survival. The relative risk associated with a 50% increase in mass was more than doubled, and only a 10% increase in posterior wall thickness was associated with an approximately sevenfold increase in the risk of dying.[6] The presence of LVH in patients with arterial hypertension therefore carries an increased risk for cardiovascular disease.

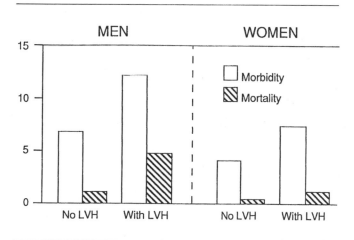

Figure 3. Four-year incidence of cardiovascular events in men and women in relation to the presence of left ventricular hypertrophy (LVH).

CARDIAC FAILURE DUE TO LEFT VENTRICULAR HYPERTROPHY

In the Framingham study, patients with arterial hypertension and LVH were characterized by a tenfold higher risk than normal for developing cardiac failure.[7] Seventy-five percent of all persons who developed cardiac failure during the course of the Framingham study were characterized by arterial hypertension as the underlying disease. From a pathogenetic point of view, the patients either had hypertension cardiac disease (i.e., LVH) or coronary heart disease with concomitant hypertension as a risk factor. Although systolic myocardial pump function at rest appeared to be maintained in early stages of LVH, with exercise a decrease of left ventricular pump function can be observed.[7] In addition, several studies using primarily noninvasive techniques have shown that hypertensive patients usually have alteration in left ventricular diastolic function before the appearance of impaired left ventricular systolic function and sometimes even before the development of LVH.[8] Abnormalities in left ventricular relaxation and filling increase with higher degrees of LVH.

SUDDEN DEATH

Data from the Framingham study have taught us that the course of LVH, especially when seen by ECG and when manifested by repolarization abnormalities as well as increased voltage, is an ominous portent of shortened life expectancy. After the first appearance of ECG LVH, mortality rates of 33% for men and 21% for women can be expected. ECG LVH is also associated with a threefold (positive Sokolow index) to fivefold (additional repolarization abnormalities) increased risk of sudden death.[9] Since the first observation at the Ochsner Clinic in 1981, more than a dozen studies have demonstrated that patients with LVH have a higher prevalence of ventricular arrhythmias than do normotensive or hypertensive patients without LVH. The pathogenetic link between LVH and sudden death might be found in the increased ventricular ectopy or myocardial ischemia that can be found in a subset of hypertensive patients. This is underlined by the data from many studies, which show that ventricular ectopy is more severe in hypertensive patients if LVH is present and vice versa (Figure 4). Increase in preload and hence cardiac sympathetic activity has been shown to induce ventricular arrhythmias at similar levels of LVH.[10]

CORONARY HEART DISEASE AND LEFT VENTRICULAR HYPERTROPHY

Various clinical studies have demonstrated that the extent of arteriosclerotic changes in the coronary blood vessels and of the echocardiographic-determined left ventricular mass independently predict a risk of cardiac death.[14] In addition,

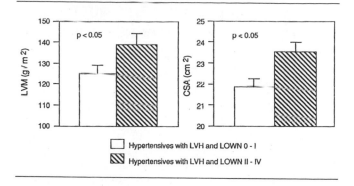

Figure 4. *Left ventricular hypertrophy (LVH) was more pronounced in patients with severe ventricular arrhythmias than in hypertensive patients. LVM = left ventricular mass; CSA = cross-sectional area.*

it has been reported that the extent of a myocardial infarction increases in the presence of LVH.[11] It has also been shown prospectively that hypertensive heart disease, if understood as LVH, doubles cardiovascular mortality for men and women. This relation was found to be independent of the influence of other classic risk factors such as age, smoking, arterial hypertension, antihypertensive therapy, increased cholesterol levels, and diabetes mellitus. Also, the risks of myocardial infarction and the incidence of angina pectoris increase with the presence of LVH. What, then, is the pathophysiologic link between LVH and coronary heart disease?

Coronary reserve is significantly depressed in hypertensives, even in the absence of coronary stenosis in normally shaped left ventricles without cardiac dilation and even in young patients (< 30 years of age).[12] Underlying causes for the observed reduction in coronary reserve have been attributed to the existence of coronary microangiopathy in hypertensive heart disease and the increase in systolic wall stress that is well known to accompany LVH. Morphometric analyses of myocardial biopsies in hypertensives with angiographically normal coronary arteries revealed thickening of all three layers of the vessel wall (i.e., of the intima and the media, and of the adventitial layer) in 70% to 80% of all patients. In all patients in whom pathologic blood vessels were present, the coronary reserve was clearly reduced whereas coronary resistance was only moderately reduced. Also, the number of capillary blood vessels does not increase parallel to the increase of left ventricular muscle mass, which finally leads, especially under conditions of stress, to a disproportionate relation between oxygen supply and demand.

Overall, the multifactorial origin of coronary heart disease in arterial hypertension and the various pathomechanisms and interactions between coronary heart disease in LVH lead to different therapeutic consequences. First, regression of LVH should be the main therapeutic goal in order to lower coronary risk. In the presence of arteriosclerotic changes in the coronary blood vessel, therapeutic intervention such as aortocoronary bypass or percutaneous transluminal coronary angioplasty should be considered in addition to antianginal therapy.

REDUCTION OF LEFT VENTRICULAR HYPERTROPHY AND PROGNOSTIC IMPLICATIONS

It is now generally accepted that reduction of LVH is the main therapeutic principle to reduce the risk associated with LVH. In an update of our previous meta-analysis,[13] we included all double-blind, randomized clinical studies in patients with primary hypertension published until December 1996. Although systolic and diastolic blood pressure was reduced to the same extent and duration of treatment and pretreatment LV mass were similar, reduction of LV mass was greater with ACE-inhibitors (12%) and calcium antagonists (11%) than with diuretics (8%) and β-blockers (5%) (Figure 5).

Reduction of left ventricular mass in hypertensive heart disease has been associated with a decrease in ventricular arrhythmias.[14] In addition, it was shown that diastolic functional abnormalities were reversed and systolic blood function improved.[15] Prospective examinations addressing the question of whether cardiovascular prognosis is improved with regression of LVH so far have been only preliminarily answered.[16] In the Framingham study, cardiovascular mortality was reduced after reduction of LVH. However, as LVH in the Framingham study was diagnosed via ECG, reduction of LVH also would implicate those who showed an improvement in cardiac failure and coronary heart disease. Prospective data from Eastern Europe showed, in a multicenter study of more than 500 hypertensive patients, that those who had echocardiographic evidence of decreased LVH with antihypertensive therapy demonstrated the lowest cardiovascular complication rate (15%) during the follow-up phase of five years, in contrast to a cardiovascular complication rate of 35% in patients who revealed a further increase of LVH.[17]

Additional supporting data come from the Cornell Medical Center in New York and from Brescia, Italy,[18] where reduction of LVH was also associated with a lower cardiovascular complication rate; i.e., myocardial infarction, sudden death, and stroke (Figure 5). Both studies also demon-

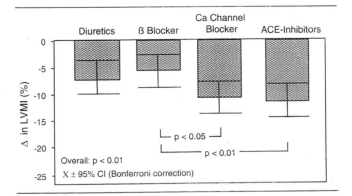

Figure 5. Changes in left ventricular mass.

strated that reduction of cardiovascular complications was independent of the improvement of other risk factors.

Thus, increasing evidence indicates that reduction of LVH is a promising therapeutic measure that may decrease cardiovascular risk associated with hypertensive heart disease.

REFERENCES

1. Schmieder RE, Messerli FH, Garavaglia GE, Nunez BD. Dietary salt intake: A determinant of cardiac involvement in essential hypertension. Circulation 1988;78:951–956.

2. Schmieder RE, Messerli FH, Garavaglia GE, Nunez BD, MacPhee AA, Re NR. Does the renin-angiotensin-aldosterone system modify cardiac structure or function in essential hypertension? Am J Med 1988; 84 (Suppl. 3A):136–139.

3. Devereux RB, Alonso DR, Lutas EM, et al. Echocardiographic assessment of left ventricular hypertrophy: Comparison to necropsy findings. Am J Cardiol 1986;57:450–458.

4. Levy D, Garrison RJ, Savage DD, Kannel WB, Castelli WP. Prognostic implications of echocardiographically determined left ventricular hypertrophy mass in the Framingham Heart Study. N Engl J Med 1990;322:1561–1566.

5. Koren MJ, Devereux RB, Casale PN, Savage DD, Laragh JH. Relation of left ventricular mass and geometry to morbidity and mortality in uncomplicated essential hypertension. Ann Intern Med 1991;114:345–352.

6. Cooper RS, Simmons BE, Castaner A, Santhanam V, Gahli J, Mar R. Left ventricular hypertrophy is associated with worse survival independent of ventricular function and the number of coronary arteries severely narrowed. Am J Cardiol 1990;65:441–445.

7. Tubau JF, Szlachcic J, Braun S, Massie BM. Impaired left ventricular function reserve in hypertensive patients with left ventricular hypertrophy. Hypertension 1989;14:1–8.

8. Fouad FM, Slominski JM, Tarazi RC. Left ventricular diastolic function in hypertension: Relation to left ventricular mass and systolic function. J Am Coll Cardiol 1984;3:1500–1506.

9. Kannel WB. Left ventricular hypertrophy as a risk factor: The Framingham experience. J Hypertens Suppl 1991;9(Suppl. 2):S3–S9.

10. Schmieder RE, Messerli FH. Determinants of ventricular ectopy in hypertensive cardiac hypertrophy. Am Heart J 1992;123:89–95.

11. Boden WE, Kleiger RE, Schechtman KB, et al. Clinical significance and prognostic importance of left ventricular hypertrophy in non-Q-wave acute myocardial infarction. Am J Cardiol 1988;62:1000–1004.

12. Strauer BE. Development of cardiac failure by coronary small vessel disease in hypertensive heart disease. J Hypertens 1991;9(Suppl. 2):S11–S20.

13. Schmieder RE, Martus P, Klingbeil A. Reversal of left ventricular hypertrophy in essential hypertension. A meta-analysis of randomized double-blind studies. JAMA 1996;275:1507–13.

14. Messerli FH, Nunez BD, Nunez MM, Garavaglia GE, Schmieder RE, Ventura HO. Hypertension and sudden death. Disparate effects of calcium entry blocker and diuretic therapy on cardiac dysrhythmias. Arch Intern Med 1989;149:1263–1267.

15. Schmieder R, Sturgill D, Garavaglia GE, Nunez BD, Messerli FH. Cardiac performance improves after regression of left ventricular hypertrophy Am J Med 1989;87:22–27.

16. Schmieder RE, Messerli FH. Reversal of left ventricular hypertrophy: A desirable therapeutic goal? J Cardiovasc Pharmacol 1990;16(Suppl. 6):16–22.

17. Yurenev AP, Dyakonova HG, Novikov ID, et al. Management of essential hypertension in patients with different degrees of left ventricular hypertrophy: Multicenter trial. Am J Hypertens 1992;5: 182S–189S.

18. Koren MJ, Savage DD, Casale PN, Laragh JH, Devereux RB. Changes in left ventricular mass predict risk in essential hypertension. Circulation 1990;82(Suppl. III):29 (abstract).

CHAPTER 6

The Kidney

George L. Bakris

Hypertension in the absences of diabetes is currently the second most common cause of end-stage renal disease in the United States.[1] Moreover, hypertension is a major contributor to many other disease processes that culminate in the development of end-stage renal disease. Bright first proposed the notion that development of hypertension is in some way connected with the kidney in 1841. This was based on autopsy examinations of patients dying with "dropsy." In these autopsies, Bright also noted that the left ventricular wall was hypertrophied and that the peripheral arteries were "hard."[2]

Other investigators such as Mahomed and later Bell described the kidney as normal in appearance prior to development of non-malignant essential hypertension. However, these investigators believed that vascular abnormalities in the renal bed primarily contributed to the genesis of hypertension. Regardless of the etiology it is clear, from all available data, that the level of blood pressure control as well as the choice of antihypertensive medications used to achieve this control is critical to preserve renal function.

To clarify and develop these issues, this chapter will discuss the role of hypertension in patients with and without coexisting renal or metabolic diseases. Second, it will focus on level of blood pressure control as a major determinate that preserves renal function. Lastly, there is a discussion of specific antihypertensive drug classes demonstrated to have "renoprotective" effects. The evidence for these "renoprotective" effects is discussed in the context of different levels of blood pressure control.

HYPERTENSION WITH NO COEXISTING DISEASES

It is clear that essential hypertension has a genetic base. This is evidenced by numerous recent studies charting populations of children as they get older and observing blood pressure patterns. These epidemiological studies revealed that a subgroup of patients with positive family histories for hypertension or cardiovascular disease have a higher predisposition for development of hypertension in adult life when compared to individuals without such a history.[3] These data coupled with recent advances in the area of molecular biology, point to the fact that hypertension is a vascular disease that involves abnormalities in endothelial regulatory mechanisms that may be genetically mediated.

In the natural history of essential hypertension and absence of other coexistent renal or metabolic diseases, renal failure, resulting in dialysis, is uncommon. This is contrary to the data that place hypertension second as a cause of end-stage renal disease (ESRD). This is primarily related to the fact that the United States Renal Data System accepts reports entered from forms compiled by practicing nephrologists that list hypertension as a primary etiology of ESRD. However, in the absence of a renal biopsy evidence to prove this diagnosis remains speculative. Moreover, cardiovascular complications such as stroke or myocardial infarction antecede development of renal failure in patients with hypertension. Finally, patients with essential hypertension that do develop ESRD do so primarily related to diabetes or other superimposed renal disease. Examples of such diseases include primary diseases of the kidney, such as focal glomerulosclerosis or coexistent metabolic diseases such as diabetes.

In patients with hypertension and no coexistent disease, aggressive control of blood pressure (discussed later in the chapter) will result in preservation of organ function. Commonly associated risk factors for cardiovascular disease such as microalbuminuria and left ventricular hypertrophy regress toward normal if blood pressure levels are adequately reduced and these reductions are sustained.[4] Moreover, the implications of microalbuminuria as a predictor of decline in renal function do not hold in uncomplicated hypertension the way they do in diabetes.[5]

The mechanism for the dissociation between microalbuminuria as a predictor of renal disease progression in diabetes versus hypertension primarily relates to the effect of glycated albumin on renal cells. Microalbuminuria results from increased "leakiness" of the glomerular capillary wall, a phenomenon related to elevations in intraglomerular pressure. If blood pressure is maintained at high levels over a period of time, the kidney loses its ability to autoregulate pressure. As a result, intraglomerular pressure increases and the glomerular capillary wall is stretched. This results in increased shunting of albumin through membrane pores and, hence, development of microalbuminuria.

Two fundamental pathophysiological differences separate diabetes from essential hypertension. First, intraglomerular pressure is increased early in diabetes. Second, and perhaps more importantly, albumin is glycated. This transforms albumin into an antigenic type molecule that now increases cytokine and matrix production by mesangial cells. This in turn leads to the development of diabetic nephropathy.[5,6] Hence, in uncomplicated essential hypertension, microalbuminuria is the *renal equivalent of the HbA₁c for glucose control.* It gives the physician an index of how long blood pressure has been poorly controlled. It correlates with cardiovascular but not renal mortality.[5]

HYPERTENSION WITH COEXISTING DISEASES

Presence of hypertension in patients with coexistent renal or metabolic diseases is extremely common. The most common medical cause of secondary hypertension is presence of primary renal disease. The primary renal diseases most commonly associated with hypertension, if diabetes is excluded, include focal glomerulosclerosis and glomerulonephritis from various causes including lupus erythematosis.

The most common cause of end-stage renal diseases in the United States is diabetes. One hundred percent of patients with diabetes that progress to dialysis have hypertension as defined as a blood pressure of > 135/85 mm Hg.[1] It is very clear that patients with diabetes whose arterial pressure is reduced to levels of ≤ 140/90 mm Hg have some preservation of renal function.[4,6] Moreover, this preservation of renal function is especially pronounced once renal insufficiency is present. There are now over five clinical trials with various types of antihypertensive medications, primarily angiotensin converting enzyme (ACE) inhibitors that demonstrate this fact.[4] Interestingly, both animal and clinical data support the concept that once renal insufficiency has developed, blood pressure control is a more powerful predictor for preservation of renal function than blood sugar control.[7,8] Thus, in order to maximally preserve renal function, blood pressure control should be diligently sought in all patients with hypertension that also have concomitant diseases affecting the kidney.

INTERVENTIONS THAT RESULT IN FAVORABLE RENAL OUTCOMES

Blood Pressure Control

Until recently blood pressure control has been predicated on the notion that blood pressure levels below 140/90 mm Hg are associated with reduced cardiovascular mortality. While this is correct, this level of control has not been challenged until recently to assess whether we can do better with regard to both reducing morbidity as well as mortality.

It is clear that one of the more important variables that predict preservation of renal function is the level of blood pressure control.[9] To date, however, only four clinical trials have assessed the question as to whether a lower level of blood pressure control truly reduces either cardiovascular or renal mortality e.g., need for dialysis. These trials and their results are listed in Table 1.

Based on these trials and other retrospective analysis, the recently published Joint National Committee report (JNC VI)

TABLE 1. CLINICAL TRIALS THAT RANDOMIZED TO DIFFERENT LEVELS OF BLOOD PRESSURE CONTROL WITH A.

Primary End-Point of Either Renal or Cardiovascular Morbidity or Mortality

Trial	1° End-Point	BP Control Levels	Outcome
AASK	Rate of decline in GFR	102-106;< 92 mmHg, MAP	To be completed in 2002
HDFP	Cardiovascular events	Usual control; diastolic < 90 mmHg	< 90, slower decline in serum Cr.
HOT	Cardiovascular events	Diastolic < 90, < 85, < 80 MMHG	Completed 1997, results not available
MDRD	Rate of decline in GFR	102-106, < 92 mmHg, MAP	< 92, slower decline in GFR*

ASSK—African American Study on the Progression of Kidney Disease; HDFP—Hypertension Detection and Follow-Up Program; HOt—Hypertension Optimal Treatment Trial; MDRD—Modification of Diet in Renal Disease Trial; GFR—glomerular filtratin rate as measureed by iothalamate clearance.

*Especially pronounced slowing in African Americans.

clearly states that certain populations must have their blood pressure lowered to levels of ≤ 130/85 mm Hg.[6] These populations include a) African Americans, b) those with diabetes, and c) those with renal insufficiency defined by a serum creatinine of ≥ 1.4 mg/dl and proteinuria of greater than one gram per day.

These recommendations are predicated primarily on retrospective data demonstrating that rates of decline in glomerular filtration rates are negligible when blood pressures are held in the range between 120 and 130 mm Hg systolic and 75 to 85 mm Hg diastolic. This is further solidified by data from the only completed randomized double blind placebo controls trial the Modification of Dietary Protein in Renal Disease (MDRD) trial.[10] This trial randomized patients with renal insufficiency to two different levels of blood pressure control, mean arterial pressure > 92 mm Hg and 102 to 106 mm Hg. Patients were followed for a period of three to four years. At this time, African Americans or those who had greater than one gram per day of proteinuria and randomized to the lower level of blood pressure control had greater preservation of renal function. However, since the number of African American patients in this study was small, the current African American Study of Kidney Disease trial (AASK trial) was designed to answer the question regarding level of blood pressure control and progression of renal disease. The results will be known in 2002.

A summary of retrospective data that plot the rate of decline in glomerular filtration rate versus the level of blood pressure control in patients with diabetic nephropathy is shown in Figure 1. It is clear from this work that the level of blood pressure control, regardless of antihypertensive medications used, is a very important factor in determining progression of renal disease.

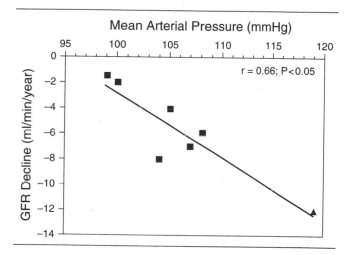

Figure 1. *A retrospective summary of clinical studies (> 2 years duration) in patients with either types I or II diabetic nephropahty that assess the impact of blood pressure level on nephropathy progression. Note the triangle represents no treatment of blood pressure over an average of two years in type I diabetic subjects.*

RENAL PRESERVATION AND SPECIFIC ANTIHYPERTENSIVE AGENTS

It is clear from all published studies that, given a reduction in blood pressure to levels approximating 140/90 mm Hg, ACE inhibitors clearly confer a benefit over other antihypertensive agents in regard to slowing progression of either diabetic or non-diabetic renal disease. Moreover, the JNC VI recommendation for treatment of hypertension in a patient with diabetes states that there are compelling indications for the use of ACE inhibitor as part of the "antihypertensive cocktail" to maximally slow progression of renal disease.

The reason for this benefit of ACE inhibitors lies in their ability to improve or ameliorate both hemodynamic and non-hemodynamic changes that occur in the kidney of a patient with diabetes (Table 2). This is the only class of antihypertensive agents, other than perhaps the angiotensin II receptor antagonists, that has these renal effects. It should be noted that the angiotensin II receptor antagonists have not been proven equivalent to ACE inhibitors in clinical trials as yet.[11] There are, however, three ongoing clinical trials with these agents in patients with diabetic renal disease. Thus, we must await the results of the clinical trials. It should be noted, however, that if the animal data are any indication of the outcome, as they were with ACE inhibitors, the results should be similar to ACE inhibitors.

Calcium channel antagonists (CCAs) have also had a role in slowing progression of renal disease. The non-dihydropyridine CCAs have been shown in multiple clinical and animal studies to consistently reduce proteinuria and slow progression of renal disease over the dihydropyridine CCAs.[12] Data from recent animal experiments demonstrate these differences are between the subclasses of CCAs (Table 3).

One of the major differences between subclasses of CCAs is their effect on renal autoregulation. This translates into differences in renal outcomes. Data from recent animal experiments compare the amount of glomerular scarring between four different CCAs at a level of 140 mm Hg systolic blood pressure (Figure 2). One can readily observe that, at similar levels of blood pressure control, non-dihydropyridine CCAs protect against increases in proteinuria and development of glomerular scarring when compared to commonly prescribed dihydropyridine agents. This distinction between CCAs, however, falls apart at systolic blood pressure levels of ≤ 110 mm Hg.[13] Unfortunately, it is not feasible clinically to take all patients to blood pressure levels this low in order to protect the kidneys.

Data derived from several large, randomized, double-blinded clinical trials demonstrate that diuretics also preserve renal function, given that blood pressure is controlled.[6,14] Moreover, in many patients with complicated hypertension one may never achieve blood pressure control without the use of a diuretic. Analyses of the SHEP trial as well as the HDFP Trial and data from a double-blind placebo controlled study in African Americans with

TABLE 2. HEMODYNAMIC AND NON-HEMODYNAMIC ALTERATIONS IN THE DIABETIC HYPERTENSIVE PATIENT WITH ASSOCIATED EFFECTS OF ANTIHYPERTENSIVE AGENTS.*

Pathophysiological alterations	Antihypertensive Effect on Alterations	
	Reverse or improve	Potentiate or worsen
Hemodynamic		
↑ Intraglomerular pressure	ARBs, ACEI, ?non-DHPCAs	None ?DHPCAs
↓ Autoregulation	None	DHPCAs (abolish)
↑ Glomerular capillary permeability	ACEI, ARBs, non-DHPCAs	DHPCAs (no effect) ?minoxidil, ?hydralazine
Non-Hemodynamic		
↑ Glomerular volume	?ARBs, ACEI, CAs	None
↑ Mesangial matrix	?ARBs, ACEI, non-DHPCAs	DHPCAs (no effect); α-blocker (no effect)
↓ ANP response	ACEI, CAs, diuretics	hydralazine/minoxidil, β-blockers

ACEI, angiotensin-converting enzyme inhibitor; ARB-angiotensin II receptor blockers, CAs, calcium channel blocker, Non-HDHPCAs, nondihropyridine calcium antagonists (verapamil, diltiazem), DHPCAs-dihydropyridine calcium antagonists (amlodipine-like agents), ANP-atrial natriuretic peptide.
*These effects occur in addition to blood pressure reduction, some of which may also be independent of blood pressure reduction. These agents generally do not reduce intraglomerular pressure, and only the dihydropyridine-type CAs do not have effects on permeability, because they have not effect on albuminuria.
↑ = Increase   ↓ = Decrease
Adapted from Bakris GL. Treatment of Hypertensive Patients with Diabetic Nephropathy. In Izzo J and Black HR (eds.) Am heart Assoc. *Hypertension Primer* 1993, Dallas, TX:357–360.

TABLE 3. POTENTIAL REASONS FOR DIFFERENCES IN RENOPROTECTION BETWEEN SUBCLASSES OF CALCIUM CHANNEL ANTAGONISTS

Variables	DHPCCAs	Non DHPCCAs
• ΔP	→	↓
• Mesangial matrix protein synthesis	→	↓
• Membrane permeability (mesangial cell exposure to glycated albumin)	→↑	↓
• Renal autoregulation	abolish	partially abolish
• Variable distribution of calcium channels on cells throughout body		

→ = no effect; ↓= decrease
DHPCCAs = dihydropyridine calcium channel antagonists
ΔP = differing pressure across glomerular capillary be

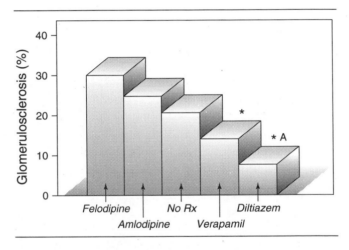

Figure 2. Differences in glomerulosclerosis development with a variety of calcium antagonists in a rat remnant kidney model. *P< 0.01 compared to either no treatment or amlodipine alone, #P < 0.05 compared to amlodipine alone. NT-no treatment, A-amlodipine, B-benazepril, A+B.

Adapted from Griffin K et al., Kidney Int., In Press.

diabetes all demonstrate that those randomized to a thiazide diuretic had a markedly slowed progression of renal disease. In this latter trial performed by WG Walter and colleagues, the diabetic patients randomized to ACE inhibitors failed to demonstrate a significantly greater benefit in renal preservation when compared to those given a thiazide diuretic.

Therefore, all classes of antihypertensive agents examined thus far in clinical studies demonstrate that controlling arterial pressure slows progression of renal disease. However, the three classes of antihypertensive agents shown to have favorable effects on renal outcome include the ACE inhibitors, non-dihydropyridine CCAs and diuretics. A summary of effects on surrogate markers of organ involvement from all classes of antihypertensive agents is show in Table 4.

TABLE 4. Effects of Antihypertensive Therapy on Metabolic, Cardiovascular, and Renal Markers Associated with Increased Morbidity and/or Mortality in the Patient with Diabetes and Hypertension.

	Central α agonists	α-Blockers	α, β-Blocker	Vasodilator	β-Blockers	ACEI	ARBs	CAs	Diuretics
Metabolic									
Cholesterol (LDL)	↑	↑	↑	↑	↑→*	↑	↑	↑	·↑→
Insulin resistance	↑	→	↑→	↑→	↑→	→	→	↑	↑→
Glucose control	↑	↑	↑	↑	↑→	↑→	↑	*↑↑	↑→
Cardiovascular									
Left ventricular hypertrophy	→	→	→	↑→	→	→	→	→	↑→
Renal									
Microalbuminuria	↑	↑	↓→	↑	↓→	→	→	**↓→↓	↓→

Note: This table summarized the general trends in the literature.
HDL, high-density lipoprotein; LDL, low-density lipoprotein; ACEI-ACE Inhibitor, ARB-Angiotensin II receptor antagonist.
→, no effect; ↑, increase; ↓, decrease.

* Only β-blockers with intrinsic symptopathomimetic activity; only when used in high doses (e.g., 480 mg/d diliazem, 480 mg/d verapamil, 90 mg/d nifedipine); **only non-dihydropyridine calcium antagonists (CAs, verapamil, diltiazem).

From Bakris, GL. Treatment of Hypertensive Patients with Diabetic Nephropathy. In Izzo J and Black HR (eds.) Am Heart Assoc. *Hypertension Primer* 1993. Dallas, TX:357–360.

AN APPROACH TO BLOOD PRESSURE MANAGEMENT IN PATIENTS WITH RENAL DISEASE

The general approach for treatment of hypertension in patients with concomitant diseases that affect the kidney should follow the outline of the JNC VI. Some general rules should be applied for the control of blood pressure in all patients with renal disease regardless of etiology.

1. All such patients have problems with *sodium handling*. Therefore, diuretics at least in low does should be used as part of the "antihypertensive cocktail" to lower blood pressure.

2. ACE inhibitor *should* be part of the "antihypertensive cocktail" unless renal function is poor, i.e. serum creatinine of < 3mg/dl, or hyperkalemia becomes a problem. It should be noted, however, that in many circumstances hyperkalemia might be eliminated by alterations in dietary ingestion of certain fruits and vegetables by the patient.

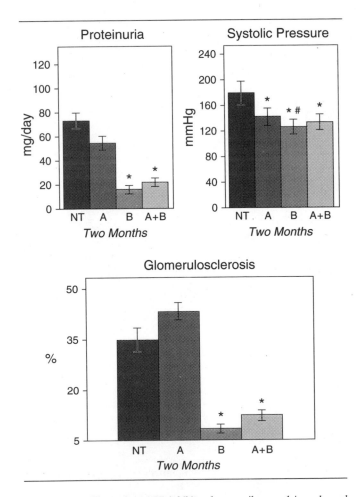

Figure 3. The effects of an ACE inhibitor, benazepril or a calcium channel antagonist, amlodipine, alone or combined on development of renal disease in a model of renal insufficiency at an average systolic pressure of 140 mmHg.

3. CCAs should also be a major part of the "antihypertensive cocktail" since they are very efficacious in reducing blood pressure. Non-dihydropyridine CCAs have additive effects on reducing proteinuria in the presence of an ACE inhibitor.[15] This is not true for dihydropyridine CCAs. Recent animal studies, however, demonstrate that ACE inhibitors tend to protect you from the lack of organ protection seen with dihydropyridine CCA alone (Figure 3).

Thus, it is clear that aggressive blood pressure control is important to preserve renal function in a person with hypertension. The correct approach is to use drugs in an "antihypertensive cocktail" that afford renal protection and at the same time alter major pathophysiologic mechanisms known to predispose to hypertension. In this way, blood pressure control can be affected and both renal as well as cardiovascular morbidity and mortality can be impacted.

REFERENCES

1. National High Blood Pressure Education Program Working Group. 1995 update of the working group reports on chronic renal failure and renovascular hypertension. Arch Intern Med 1996;156: 1938–1947.

2. Bright T. Tabular view of the morbid appearance in 100 cases connected with albuminous urine: With observations. Guy's Hosp Rep 1836;1:380–397.

3. Sadowski RH and Falkner B. Hypertension in pediatric patients. Am J Kidney Dis 1996;27:305–315.

4. Bakris GL, Mehler P, and Schrier R. Hypertension & Diabetes. In Schrier RW and Gottschalk CW (eds.) *Diseases of the Kidney*, 6th ed., Little Brown and Company, 1996: 1455–1464.

5. Bakris GL. Microalbuminuria: Prognostic Implications. Curr Opin in Nephrol and Hypertens 1996;5(3):219–233.

6. Joint National Committee Report on the Diagnosis and Treatment of Hypertension (JNC VI) Arch Intern Med 1997;157: 2413–2446.

7. Gaber, L, Walton C, Brown S, Bakris, GL. Effects of different antihypertensive treatments on morphologic progression of diabetic nephropathy in uninephrectomized dogs. Kidney Int 1994;46: 161–169.

8. Hebert LA, Bain RP, Verne D. For the Collaborative Study Group. Remission of nephrotic range proteinuria in type I diabetes. Kidney Int 1994;46:1688–1693.

9. Toto R, Mitchell HC, Smith RD, Lee HC, McIntire D, Pettinger WA. "Strict" blood pressure control and progression of renal disease in hypertensive nephrosclerosis. Kidney Int 1995;48:851–858.

10. Lazarus JM, Bourgoigne, JJ, Buckalew VM, Tom Greene, Levey AS, Milas NC, Paranandi L, Peterson JC, Porush JG, Rauch S, Soucie JIM, Stollar for the MDRD Group. Achievement and safety of a low blood pressure goal in chronic renal disease: The modification of diet in renal disease study group. Hypertension 1997;29:641–650.

11. Tarif N and Bakris GL. Angiotensin II receptor blockade and progression of renal disease in nondiabetic patients. Kidney Int 1997;52(Suppl 63):S-67-S-70.

12. Tarif N and Bakris GL. Preservation of renal function: the spectrum of effects by calcium channel blockers. Nephrol Dial Transpl 1997;12:2244–2250.

13. Griffin KA, Picken MM and Bidani AK. Deleterious effects of calcium channel blockage on pressure transmission and glomerular injury in rat remnant kidneys. J Clin Invest 1995;96:793–800.

14. Curb JD, Pressel SL, Cutler JA et.al., for the Systolic Hypertension in the Elderly Program Cooperative Research Group. Effect of diuretic-based antihypertensive treatment on cardiovascular disease risk in older diabetic patients with isolated systolic hypertension. JAMA 1996;276:1886–1892.

15. Bakris GL. Combination therapy for hypertension and renal disease in diabetes. In Mogensen CE (ed.) *The Kidney and Hypertension in Diabetes Melliltus*, 4th ed. Kluwer Academic, Boston, in press.

CHAPTER 7

Diuretics

Murray Epstein

Broadly speaking, the term diuretic refers to any agent that increases the flow of urine. In clinical practice, however, a diuretic is efficacious by virtue of its ability to induce a net negative balance of sodium from the body. Since the introduction into clinical medicine of organic mercurial diuretics over 50 years ago, many less toxic and more readily utilized diuretic compounds have been introduced. A wide variety of compounds are now available, and the differences in their action and degree of potency are currently exploited in a variety of clinical situations. Table 1 classifies the diuretics most commonly used in clinical practice according to primary site of action.

LOOP DIURETICS: OVERVIEW[1]

The loop diuretics (furosemide and bumetanide and torsemide) are so named because they act principally on the thick ascending limb of the loop of Henle. This nephron segment reabsorbs 20% to 30% of the filtered load of sodium chloride. By virtue of their ability to abolish a large portion of this loop function, loop diuretics are currently the most potent diuretics in clinical use. Because they have a very steep dose-response natriuresis curve, they have been termed high-ceiling diuretics.

Furosemide is readily absorbed from the gastrointestinal tract, binds avidly to plasma proteins, and is rapidly eliminated from the body. Furosemide is largely eliminated by renal excretion, primarily by proximal tubular secretion. About one third of the drug is excreted intact by the liver or metabolized before urinary or intestinal excretion. The onset of action may be anticipated 30 min to 60 min after oral administration or 2 min to 5 min after intravenous injection. The duration of action of a single orally administered tablet is about 6 hours, while a single intravenous injection lasts 3 hours.

Furosemide also affects renal water handling. Because of its principal action within the ascending limb, it usually

TABLE 1. SITE, MECHANISM, AND DURATION OF ACTION OF DIURETICS.

	Site of Action in Nephron	Mechanism of Action	Action (h)		
			Onset	Peak	Duration
Acetazolamide	1	Carbonic anhydrase inhibition	1 to 2	2	4 to 6
Thiazide and related drugs					
Moderate	3,1	Inhibit Na* reabsorption	1 to 2	4 to 6	12 to 24
Long acting	3,1	Inhibit Na reabsorption	2	6	24 to 36
Loop diuretics					
Ethacrynic acid	2	Inhibit NaCl‡ reabsorption	0.5 to 1	2 to 4	6 to 8
Furosemide	2,1	Inhibit NaCl reabsorption	0.5 to 1	2 to 4	6 to 8
Bumetanide	2,1	Inhibit NaCl reabsorption	0.5 to 1	2 to 3	4 to 6
Potassium-sparing agents					
Spironolactone	4	Competitive inhibition of aldosterone	8 to 24	24 to 48	48 to 72
Triamterene	4	Direct effect by reducing electrical potential between tubular cell and lumen	2 to 4	6 to 8	6 to 12
Amiloride	4	Direct effect by reducing electrical potential between tubular cell and lumen	2 to 4	4 to 6	6 to 12

*Na = sodium
‡NaCl = sodium cloride
Reproduced with permission from, Epstein M. Diuretic therapy in liver disease. In: Epstein M, ed. *The kidney in liver disease*, 4th ed. Philadelphia: Hanley & Belfus, 1996:447–458.

diminishes both free water clearance (C_{H_2O}) and the ability to concentrate urine.

THIAZIDE DIURETICS: OVERVIEW[2]

The thiazides and thiazide-like diuretics are very similar in their overall pharmacology and mechanism of action. There are, however, some differences that have important implications for clinical practice.

Common characteristics of this group of drugs are their low ceiling, flat dose-response curve, slow onset of effect, long duration of action, and tendency to reduce urine calcium. Low ceiling refers to the phenomenon whereby near maximum urinary sodium excretion is achieved at low doses of these diuretics and further increases in drug dose result in only small additional amounts of sodium excretion. In general, one should use the lowest dose possible in order to achieve the desired effect while minimizing adverse effects.

POTASSIUM-SPARING AGENTS

At present, there are three potassium-sparing agents, one an aldosterone antagonist (spironolactone), the other two inhibitors of tubular potassium secretion (amiloride and triamterene).

Spironolactone competitively blocks the uptake of aldosterone by its cytoplasmic receptor, thereby antagonizing its actions. It will reduce diuretic-induced potassium loss. However, its major use is in treatment of states of aldosterone excess, whether primary or secondary; for example, cirrhosis with ascites. As an aldosterone antagonist, spironolactone causes natriuresis and antikaluresis. Spironolactone does not cause magnesium wasting and can be used to replete magnesium deficits.

Both amiloride and triamterene block sodium transport in the collecting duct and are currently available for clinical use. Of the two, amiloride has been the more intensively studied and has been widely used as a pharmacologic probe to study sodium transport in a variety of tissues. Triamterene, although less well studied, seems (in general) to act by the same mechanism as amiloride but is less potent. Both have limited natriuretic effect but inhibit potassium secretion in the collecting duct.

Whereas the presence of mineralocorticoid is obligatory for the activity of spironolactone, it is not required in order for amiloride or triamterene to exert their actions. The effects of spironolactone and sodium channel blockers are additive because they act by distinct mechanisms. Triamterene is the potassium sparer contained in combination with 25 mg of hydrochlorothiazide and sold in the United States in several formulations, including Dyazide and Maxzide.

TREATMENT OF HYPERTENSION

Thiazide diuretics are utilized primarily as antihypertensive agents. These agents formed the foundation of the multicenter trials of the 1960s and 1970s and today remain among the few drug classes proven to have a favorable influence on noncardiac morbidity and mortality. In recent years, however, concern has centered in the "hidden" side effects of thiazides, including low-grade fatigue, impotence, and adverse biochemical effects such as hypokalemia, hyperuricemia, hyperglycemia, and dyslipidemia including hypercholesterolemia.[3-6] Consequently, their use as initial therapy of hypertension has declined to some extent in the recent past.

Although the recent practice of favoring newer classes of metabolically neutral agents such as angiotensin-converting enzyme (ACE) inhibitors and calcium antagonists is appropriate, the trend away from the use of diuretics probably constitutes an overreaction. The importance of abnormal salt excretion in the maintenance of sustained hypertension underscores the continuing role of diuretics in the antihypertensive armamentarium. The recent publication of Joint National Commission VI guidelines and the recommendation that diuretics and beta-blockers constitute step I agents may eventuate in wider usage of diuretics as antihypertensive agents.[7]

HOW DO DIURETICS LOWER BLOOD PRESSURE?

The basis for the antihypertensive action of diuretics is not completely established. Two possible mechanisms of action have been proposed: (1) that the hypotensive effect is a direct or indirect consequence of sodium (chloride) depletion, or (2) that diuretics act by direct or indirect vascular effects independent of the natriuresis.

The Importance of Salt Depletion

Multiple lines of evidence support the view that depletion of salt and extracellular volume underlies the hypotensive effect. A reduction of plasma volume by 10% to 15% accompanies the initial diuresis during the first week of therapy with thiazide-type diuretics at doses approximately half those producing maximal natriuretic effects. Over the short term, cardiac output falls and peripheral vascular resistance rises. With chronic administration, blood volume returns toward or to normal and peripheral resistance falls to below pretreatment levels.

The role of sustained volume depletion in the antihypertensive action of thiazides is emphasized by the demonstration that (1) upon cessation of diuretics, both body weight and plasma volume increase; and (2) by results from experiments with salt repletion during ongoing therapy demonstrating that ingestion of large amounts of salt can prevent or reverse the blood pressure lowering actions of diuretics.

Direct Vasodilator Effects of Diuretics

The observation that peripheral vascular resistance falls with diurectic therapy, coupled with the discovery of diazoxide (a benzothiadiazene that is a direct vasodilator without diuretic activity), has led to the suggestion that thiazides are direct vasodilators. Although several diuretics affect ion transport in vascular smooth muscle, it is clear that diuretics have minimal activity as direct vasodilators at plasma concentrations present during clinical use.

THIAZIDE-TYPE DIURETICS[2]

Doses

Thiazides have a fairly flat dose-response curve, so most of the antihypertensive effects are achieved with low doses. Although doses as high as 200 mg of hydrochlorothiazide per day have been used in the past, it is now readily apparent that as little as 25 mg given once a day will provide most of the blood pressure lowering effect and fewer of the metabolic side effects of larger doses. When added to other drugs, as little as 12.5 mg per day may be effective.

Despite having only a 12-hour to 16-hour duration of action, a single morning dose of hydrochlorothiazide will provide sustained antihypertensive effect.

Side Effects

A number of side effects accompany the use of thiazide diuretics. Allergic or idiosyncratic side effects, such as skin rash and pancreatitis, are relatively rare. Rather, one more commonly encounters a variety of biochemical changes as a consequence of the adjustments in tubular reabsortion that follow sustained diuretic administration (Table 2).[2-6] In essence, several of these complications arise as a consequence of contraction of the extracellular volume.

Hypokalemia

Urine potassium wastage is inevitable with diuretic therapy. By blocking reabsorption of sodium chloride in the distal tubule, the diuretic causes additional tubular fluid containing sodium to be delivered to the more distal portion of the nephron wherein potassium exchange for sodium occurs.

TABLE 2. METABOLIC SIDE EFFECTS OF CHRONIC DIURETIC THERAPY.

Azotemia

Hypokalemia

Hyperkalemia

Hyponatremia

Glucose intolerance

Dyslipidemia

Hyperuricemia

Hypermagnesemia

Metabolic alkalosis

Adapted from Epstein M, Materson BJ. Furosemide. In: Messerli FH, ed. *Cardiovascular drug therapy.* Philadelphia: W.B. Saunders, 2nd ed., 1996: 388–396.

The greatest amount of potassium wastage occurs initially while the diuresis is maximal.

The average fall in plasma potassium with continuous daily diuretic therapy for four weeks or longer is approximately 0.7 mmol/L to 0.8 mmol/L. Depending on the pretreatment potassium level, hypokalemia (serum $K^+ < 3.5$ mmol/L) may be observed in approximately one third of patients.

Diuretic-induced hypokalemia rarely causes symptoms, although muscular weakness and leg cramps may be noted. Nevertheless, an increase in ventricular ectopic activity has been observed.[5, 6] Furthermore, several investigators have demonstrated that the magnitude of hypokalemia correlates with the degree of ectopic activity. Furthermore, it has been proposed that diuretic-induced hypokalemia may be responsible for the excess rates of sudden death observed in some of the large clinical trials in which diuretic-induced hypokalemia was frequently noted and often not treated.

Hypokalemia may also be responsible for diuretic-induced glucose intolerance.

If diuretic therapy is to be continued, hypokalemia should be treated if it is symptomatic or severe or if patients are at high risk for cardiovascular disease.

There are several measures that the physician can undertake in order to minimize diuretic-induced hypokalemia.

- Use the smallest dose of diuretic possible.
- Use moderately long-acting diuretics, such as hydro-chlorothiazide, rather than longer acting agents.
- Reduce dietary sodium intake if possible to 2 g to 2.5 g (88 mmol to 132 mmol) per day.
- Increase dietary potassium intake.
- If more than two drugs are needed, attempt to select drugs that suppress the renin-angiotensin system; for example, converting enzyme inhibitors or beta-blockers. Because these drugs tend to diminish potassium excretion by the kidney, they will partially offset the tendency toward developing hypokalemia.

If these measures fail to correct or prevent hypokalemia, potassium supplementation should be undertaken with potassium chloride. Although generally safe, potassium chloride preparations may cause gastrointestinal irritation or ulceration. New microencapsulated preparations have excellent bioavailability and may decrease the incidence of this complication. Oral potassium in any form can cause diarrhea.

Hyperkalemia

Potassium-sparing diuretics predispose to hyperkalemia and, less often, to hyperchloremic acidosis. Generally, this complication assumes clinical importance only in patients with impaired ability to excrete potassium. This includes patients with renal insufficiency; diabetes with hyporeninemia or hypoaldosteronism; or those receiving beta-blockers, ACE inhibitors, or, of course, potassium chloride.

Hyponatremia

Both thiazide-type diuretics and loop diuretics block the ability of the kidney to generate free water. Consequently, a marked increase in water ingestion in patients receiving diuretics may result in hyponatremia. A typical scenario may include the following sequence of events. The physician may send the patient home on a diuretic regimen with the explanation that the drug may result in dehydration. The unwary patient may drink excessive amounts of water. Patients may also respond to thirst center stimulation mediated by antidiuretic hormone (ADH) and angiotensin II. Collectively, these events may lead to hyponatremia. The elderly are particularly vulnerable to hyponatremia, perhaps because of impairment in the ability to clear free water, which accompanies aging. It should be noted that furosemide induces dilutional hyponatremia much less frequently than do thiazide-type diuretics. This has been attributed to the differing effects of these two diuretics on the loop of Henle. Thus, whereas both diuretics impair renal diluting capacity, furosemide also produces an impairment of concentrating ability.

Glucose Intolerance

Glucose intolerance or frank non-insulin-dependent diabetes may develop or worsen during therapy. In prospective trials, the average level of fasting glucose, as well as the number of subjects who develop glucose intolerance, is higher among persons taking diuretics. The abnormality is often partially reversible upon cessation of diuretic therapy. The mechanism of diuretic-induced glucose intolerance is related to hypokalemia. Both impaired insulin release and impaired peripheral glucose uptake have been suggested as basis for the effect. In keeping with this observation, the effect on glucose metabolism can be ameliorated by potassium repletion. Furthermore, impaired glucose metabolism is not seen with potassium-sparing diuretics, which actually may improve glucose tolerance.

Hypercholesterolemia

Serum cholesterol levels increase during the initial 12 weeks of therapy with thiazide diuretics, with low-density lipoprotein cholesterol levels increasing by about 5% to 15%. These changes occur in men and postmenopausal women but not in premenopausal women.

The clinical significance of diuretic-induced elevation of cholesterol has not been established.

Hyperuricemia

Currently available diuretics elevate uric acid levels by decreasing uric acid excretion. Most diuretics, including the thiazides, are organic acids that may interfere with secretion of uric acid into the proximal tubule. This, however, is not the sole or even major mechanism of their effect on serum uric acid levels. The major effect has been attributed to a diuretic-induced volume contraction and resultant increased tubular reabsorption of uric acid. Diuretic-induced hyperuricemia need not be treated unless gout occurs.

LOOP DIURETICS

Loop diuretics (furosemide, bumetanide, torsemide) have no significant role as monotherapeutic agents in hypertension with normal renal function.[8] Their vasodilatory capacity is limited and they tend to activate strongly counter-regulatory vasoconstrictive mechanisms. They should, however, be pre-scribed in patients with reduced renal function (vide infra).

Although thiazide-type medications are the diuretic agents of choice for patients with hypertension and normal renal function, they may not be as effective in patients with creatinine clearances below 50 mL/min and are generally ineffective at creatinine clearances below 35 mL/min. In patients with such reduction in renal function, diuretic man-agement of hypertension should take the form of a loop diuretic, either as a sole agent or often in combination with other antihypertensive drugs.

Doses

Because both furosemide and bumetanide are short acting, they must be given two or three times daily to maintain contraction of plasma volume needed to maintain the blood pressure down.

Side Effects

In general, the metabolic side effects seen with loop diuretics are similar to those induced by thiazide-type diuretics. They may, however, differ with respect to magnitude.

Potassium Depletion

Urinary potassium excretion is increased because of inhibi-tion of potassium reabsorption in the ascending limb and enhanced potassium secretion in the distal nephron. However, the majority of patients receiving loop diuretics for antihypertensive therapy do not develop potassium depletion of significant magnitude.

Of note, although loop diuretics are more potent than distal diuretics, hypokalemia and potassium depletion are less marked in patients receiving loop diuretics. Although the mechanism has not been established, it has been postu-lated that the shorter duration of action of the loop diuretic is responsible for this phenomenon. The risk of diuretic-induced hypokalemia is increased in subjects with relatively large salt and water intakes.

Metabolic Alkalosis

Metabolic alkalosis, usually mild, is commonly associated with the used of loop-type diuretics. Its generation relates mainly to enhanced ammoniagenesis and, to a lesser extent, to the potential for a rapid loss of large amounts of bicar-bonate-poor fluids (contraction alkalosis).

CONGESTIVE HEART FAILURE

Whereas mild congestive heart failure may be treated with thiazide diuretics, loop diuretics such as furosemide must be utilized to manage patients with moderate-to-severe failure.[9] Chronic monotherapy with diuretics improves functional class in most patients, usually as a result of a reduction in left ventricular filling pressure with cardiac output relatively unchanged.

Much of the symptomatic improvement in congestive heart failure is due to reduction in pulmonary water, improvement in pulmonary compliance, reduction in resistance to airflow, and reduction in respiratory work. In experimental animals, normal subjects, and patients with congestive heart failure, a single intravenous dose of a loop diuretic reduces pulmonary vascular pressure with concomitant reductions in pulmonary wedge pressure, pulmonary artery pressure, and right atrial pressure.

The management of congestive heart failure is often complicated by an inability of orally administered furosemide to produce an effective diuresis. Patients with this diuretic resistance often require intravenous furosemide to achieve the desired clinical response. It has been suggested that the mechanism for this resistance is due to malabsorption of furosemide secondary to changes induced by congestive heart failure in the gastrointestinal tract, such as edema of the gut wall, delayed gastric emptying, decreased intestinal motility, or decreases in splanchnic blood flow.

In recent years, another specific use for furosemide in the setting of severe congestive heart failure is its administration in combination with captopril.[9] Newer treatment strategies have evolved utilizing the addition of an ACE inhibitor for afterload reduction. Whereas it has been shown that captopril can by itself improve survival in patients with Class III to Class IV congestive heart failure, the addition of furosemide is required to ensure concomitant natriuresis and correction of hyponatremia, if present.

REFERENCES

1. Epstein M, Materson BJ. Furosemide. In: Messerli FH, ed. Cardiovascular drug therapy, 2nd ed. Philadelphia: Saunders, 1996:388–396.

2. Materson BJ, Epstein M. Thaizide diuretics, chlorthalidone and metolazone. In: Messerli FH, ed. Cardiovascular drug therap, 2nd ed. Philadelphia: Saunders, 1996:412–420.

3. Daniels BS, Ferris TF. The use of diuretics in nonedematous disorders. Semin Nephrol 1988;8:342–353.

4. Tannen RL (principal discussant). Diuretic-induced hypokalemia. Kidney Int 1985;28:988–1000.

5. Kaplan NM. Our appropriate concern about hypokalemia. Am J Med 1984;77:1–4.

6. Weidmann P, Uehlinger DE, Gerber A. Antihypertensive treatment and serum lipoproteins (editorial review). J Hypertens 1985;3:297–306.

7. Joint National Committee on Detection, Evaluation and Treatment of High Blood Pressure: The Sixth Report of the Joint

National Committee on Detection, Evaluation, and Treatment of High Blood Pressure (JNCVI). Arch Intern Med 1997;157:2413–2446.

8. Epstein M. Diuretic therapy in liver disease. In: Epstein M, ed. The kidney in liver disease, 4th ed. Philadelphia: Hanely & Belfus, 1996:447–458.

9. Dzau VJ, Hollenberg NK. Renal response to captopril in severe heart failure: Role of furosemide in natriuresis and reversal of hyponatremia. Ann Intern Med 1984;100:777–782.

CHAPTER 8

Beta-Blockers

Lennart Hansson
Anders Svensson

In his classical 1948 paper Ahlquist defined the alpha- and beta-adrenoreceptors, respectively.[1] It then took ten years until the first description of pharmacologic blockade of a beta-receptor was described in 1958.[2] Clinically useful beta-blockers, such as pronethalol and propranolol, were introduced soon thereafter, and, in 1964, the first reports of an antihypertensive effect with these agents were published.[3,4] Since then, the developments in this field have been remarkably swift. Numerous studies have documented the usefulness of beta-blockers in the treatment of hypertension. It is beyond the scope of this chapter to cover this development in detail. Obviously, the inventor of the beta-blockers, Sir James W. Black, who was awarded the Nobel Prize in Medicine in 1988 for his discovery, should be mentioned, and the pioneering work of Prichard has already been alluded to. However, readers interested in a more detailed description of the development of beta-blockers for clinical practice in general and for the treatment of hypertension in particular are referred to β-*blockers in Clinical Practice* by Cruickshank and Prichard.[5]

In many countries, beta-blockers have attained the position of first-line therapy for hypertension. Their established position in this regard can be illustrated by early guidelines for antihypertensive therapy issued by the World Health Organization/the International Society of Hypertension in 1983[6] and the Joint National Committee from the United States in 1985.[7] Both groups listed beta-blockers as one of the two classes of agents considered suitable for first-line treatment of hypertension. In more recent recommendations from these two expert bodies, beta-blockers have maintained their first-line status.[8,9] It is, therefore, not surprising that beta-blockers are among the most widely prescribed antihypertensive agents worldwide and that a multitude of different agents within this group have been made clinically available.

It is the purpose of this chapter to briefly describe the clinical importance of beta-blocker treatment in hypertension, with special reference to the effects of beta-blocker treatment on morbidity and mortality. Some newer developments, especially studies dealing with "cardioprotection" and antiatherosclerotic effects, will also be discussed briefly.

EFFECT ON BLOOD PRESSURE: ADVERSE EFFECTS

Since Prichard's initial work in 1964,[3,4] numerous studies have confirmed the antihypertensive effect of beta-blockers (for full details, see reference 5). Because beta-blockers can be subdivided in numerous ways depending on their ancillary pharmacologic properties, it is interesting to note that both nonselective agents and $beta_1$-selective agents are effective in the treatment of hypertension (Table 1). The only clear-cut exception appears to be if $beta_1$-receptors are not blocked or if a potent $beta_1$-agonistic effect is present (Table 1). All other properties (for example, membrane stabilizing activity, the sympathomimetic effect, different degrees of water/lipid solubility, etc.) appear to play a minor role for the magnitude of the antihypertensive effect.[10] However, it is obvious that beta-blockers with the greatest degree of intrinsic sympathomimetic activity cause the smallest decrease in heart rate and have the least effect on atrioventricular conduction.[11] Moreover, a compound with marked agonistic activity down-regulates beta-receptors. Thus, when treatment is withdrawn, there is no post-beta-blockade hypersensitivity, which is in contrast to cessation of treatment with agents devoid of agonistic activity.[12] In practical terms, this means that abrupt cessation of treatment with a beta-blocker characterized by marked agonistic activity poses considerably less risk of tachycardia, palpitations, angina pectoris, or other complications than does cessation of treatment with an agent devoid of such activity.

The hemodynamic profile also seems linked to whether sympathomimetic activity is present. Most beta-blockers reduce arterial pressure through a reduction in cardiac output, whereas agents with marked agonistic activity lower blood pressure mainly through a reduction in vascular resistance, which is lowered below the initial baseline level.[13,14]

Efficacy

In some early studies with propranolol in hypertension, the claim was made that this treatment was at least as efficacious as treatment with sympatholytic agents such as guanethidine or bethanidine.[15] At the other extreme, a report based on a double-blind study in hypertensive Jamaicans found no antihypertensive effect whatsoever.[16] As is frequently the case, the truth appears to lie somewhere between these extremes. A number of comparative trials have reported that the magnitude of blood pressure reduction that can be obtained with beta-blocker treatment is similar to that caused by diuretics, for example, or other commonly used agents.[17,18]

From a practical standpoint, it is important to note that, despite their differences, most beta-blockers are effective in

TABLE 1. PHARMACOLOGIC ACTIONS OF SOME BETA-BLOCKERS.

Compound	Beta₁-Block	Beta₂-Block	MSA	Beta₁-Agonist	Beta₂-Agonist	Antihypertensive
Propranolol	+	+	+	-	-	+
Timolol	+	+	-	-	-	+
Oxprenolol	+	+	+	+	+	+
Pindolol	+	+	-	-	+	+
Atenolol	+	-	-	-	-	+
Metoprolol	+	-	-	-	-	+
Practolol	+	-	-	+	+	+
Epanolol	+	-	-	+	-	?
ICI 118,551	-	+	?	-	-	-
Labetalol	+	+	+	-	-	+
Carvedilol	+	+	-	-	-	+

MSA = membrane stabilizing activity (usually not clinically relevant at normal dosage)
+ = Exerts this effect.
- = No effect.
? = Data not available or contradictory.

hypertension when given once daily.[18] Thus, the duration of action is usually considerably longer than would be expected based on the plasma half-life.[19] It is also of some interest that some agents have an extremely long beta-blocking effect even after a single oral dose. Thus, the nonselective agent bopindolol, which has a clinically relevant degree of agonistic activity, has a demonstrable beta-blocking effect even 96 hours after a single oral dose.[20]

EFFECTS ON CARDIOVASCULAR HYPERTROPHY

A number of studies have addressed the effectiveness of beta-blockers in reversing left ventricular hypertrophy in hypertensive patients. Regretfully, many of these studies have been conducted in previously treated patients and without proper control groups. In a meta-analysis comprising 109 treatment studies in hypertensive patients, conducted up to December 1990, 31 studies have been conducted with beta-blockers.[21] In these studies, which altogether comprised 336 patients, left ventricular mass was reduced by an average of 9% during long-term treatment, and the fall in calculated left ventricular mass was 0.9 g/mm Hg reduction in mean arterial pressure.[21] The magnitude of this effect was of the same order as that seen with calcium antagonists and diuretics but only about half of the effect seen with angiotensin-converting enzyme inhibitors.[21] More recent meta-analyses of the effect of various antihypertensive agents have confirmed that ACE inhibitors and calcium antagonists are more effective in reversing LVH than diuretics and beta-blockers.[22,23] It is well established that left ventricular hypertrophy is a powerful risk indicator for cardiovascular disease.[24-26] Although it is logical to assume that reversal of left ventricular hypertrophy should lead to improved prognosis, so far only one study has suggested this.[27]

METABOLIC EFFECTS

Insulin resistance has been related to a number of diseases, such as non-insulin-dependent diabetes mellitus, obesity, hypertension, dyslipidemia, and atherosclerotic cardiovascular disease.[28] Insulin resistance can be defined as a relative reduction of glucose uptake, mainly in muscle tissue, or simply as decreased effectiveness of insulin on target tissues. This results in a compensatory increase of plasma insulin levels.

Some effects of insulin may be of importance in the development of hypertension: increased renal sodium reabsorption, activation of the sympathetic nervous system, and effects on ion exchange over cell membranes; insulin also acts by stimulating cell growth.[28]

Hypertensive patients often have metabolic disturbances related to insulin resistance, and hyperinsulinemia is a risk factor for future hypertension.[29,30] If the drugs used to treat hypertension increase insulin resistance or have other negative metabolic effects, the full potential benefit of the blood pressure reduction would not be attained.

In this regard, beta-blockers have some negative effects. Selective beta-blockers (e.g., atenolol, metoprolol) reduce insulin sensitivity by about 25%. With pindolol, which has marked intrinsic sympathomimetic activity (ISA), the reduction (17%) was about half of that seen with propranolol (30%), which is devoid of ISA.[31]

Obviously, beta-blockers decrease insulin sensitivity; however, there seem to be some differences among beta-antagonist compounds. These differences are perhaps more pronounced with regard to drug-induced changes in lipoprotein. Nonselective beta-blockers cause an increase of total serum triglycerides (averaging 32%) and a reduction of high-density lipoprotein cholesterol (16%), according to an editorial review by Weidmann et al.[32] These alterations are less pronounced with selective beta1-blockers and even more discrete with beta-blockers with ISA.[32]

PRIMARY PREVENTION

Are these negative metabolic changes of clinical relevance? No large prospective treatment studies have examined drug effects on lipoproteins and insulin sensitivity. However, persons with advanced, symptomatic cardiovascular disease (i.e., previous myocardial infarction) have clearly been shown to benefit from beta-blocker therapy in secondary preventive trials (Figure 1).[33-35] Patients with overt diabetes and myocardial infarction, who have both coronary heart disease and a deranged metabolism, seem to benefit the most from beta-blocker therapy.[36] This indicates that the positive effects of beta-blocker therapy outweigh the negative metabolic changes in patients with advanced disease. The hope that this positive effect on coronary heart disease can also be demonstrated in primary prevention, among patients without previous myocardial infarctions, has been the reason for several large studies. Some, such as the International Prospective Primary Preventive Study in Hypertension (IPPPSH) and Heart Attack Primary Prevention in Hypertension (HAPPHY) studies, have been designed to compare a diuretic and beta-blocker, but no difference between the drugs has been found.[37,38] Numerous studies on thousands of patients have clearly documented that beta-blockade in the post-myocardial infarction patient diminishes morbidity and mortality. In hypertensive patients who have had a myocardial infarction, beta-blockers can, therefore, be considered the drug of choice. No primary preventive effect on coronary heart disease was shown in the only placebo-controlled, randomized prospective study, the Medical Research Council (MRC) study.[39]

LIPID SOLUBILITY

Generally, beta-blockers are well tolerated. Symptoms, such as vivid dreams, sleep disturbances, fatigue, or reduced alertness are considered to be related to the central nervous system (CNS) and have been reported with all types of beta-blockers.[40] A difference between propranolol (nonselective,

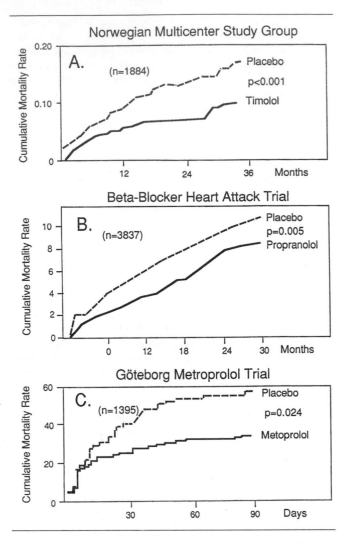

Figure 1. Three well-known intervention trials in post-myocardial infarction patients comparing placebo with the beta-blockers Timolol (A) in the Norwegian Timolol Study, Propranolol (B) in the American BHAT Study, and Metoprolol (C) in the Swedish Göteborg Metoprolol Trial. In all the studies, significantly lower death rates were seen in beta-blocker treatment.

lipophilic) and atenolol (selective, hydrophilic) has been reported in hypertensive men; atenolol was generally associated with improved well being; whereas, propranolol tended to cause minimal improvement or actual worsening.[41]

It has been suggested that hydrophilic beta-blockers may cause fewer CNS side effects than lipophilic substances because they do not easily pass the blood-brain barrier. However, the difference between beta-blockers may be more closely related to selectivity than to lipid solubility. Modern sustained-release formulations, which do not cause wide variations in plasma concentration, are better tolerated because CNS effects seem to be related to peak rather than to average plasma concentration.[40] Thus, in hypertensive patients, there were no differences between atenolol and metoprolol controlled-release formulations in terms of general well being and subjective symptoms.[42]

Beta-Blockers in Older Patients

In 1991 and 1992, three large studies of hypertension in elderly patients were published: The Systolic Hypertension in the Elderly Program (SHEP),[43] The Swedish Trial in Old Patients with Hypertension (STOP-Hypertension),[44] and the MRC trial of treatment in older adults.[45] In all three studies, beta-blockers and diuretics were used to treat elderly patients.

The SHEP study was designed to investigate antihypertensive treatment in patients over age 60 with isolated systolic hypertension. Initial treatment consisted of a diuretic, chlorthalidone, in low dosage; when needed, the beta-blocker atenolol was added in the actively treated group. The control group received a matching placebo. The number of study participants was 4,736, and the average follow-up was 4.5 years. The risk of stroke was reduced by 36% and the risk of myocardial infarction or coronary death was reduced by 27%. Treatment was generally well tolerated, with similar side effects in actively and placebo-treated groups.[43]

Older patients, aged 70 to 84 years, participated in the STOP-Hypertension study. A total of 1,627 patients were randomly assigned to active treatment or placebo. The active drug was either a beta-blocker (atenolol, metoprolol, or pindolol) or a diuretic (hydrochlorothiazide plus amiloride). The incidence of stroke was reduced by 47% and total mortality was reduced by 43%, both statistically highly significant. The treatment, which in two thirds of cases was a combined beta-blocker and diuretic, was well tolerated.[44]

The results of treatment in the MRC study were not quite so striking. Those of the 4,396 patients aged 65 to 74 who were treated with a beta-blocker (atenolol) or a diuretic (hydrochlorothiazide plus amiloride) had a 25% reduction in the incidence of stroke. The beta-blocker group showed no significant reduction, but 63% of patients stopped taking their randomized treatment or were lost to follow-up. Interpretation of this study is made even more difficult by the fact that a minority of the "placebo patients" remained on their randomized treatment and were followed up to the end of the study.[45] Thus, there is good reason to believe that the MRC study underestimated the beneficial effects of antihypertensive treatment.

In summary, these studies in elderly hypertensive patients without doubt demonstrate the value of antihypertensive treatment in this age group. Beta-blockers and diuretics were used, either alone or in combination, and were effective and well tolerated in patients up to and above 80 years of age.

New Developments

Although beta-blockers have been in clinical use for more than 35 years now, there are still some interesting new developments with these agents. Perhaps of greatest interest is the demonstration that these agents, in selected case, may be useful in the treatment of congestive heart failure (CHF), a condition that usually is regarded as a contraindication to the use of beta-blockers. The first observations that beta-blockers could be used successfully in the treatment of congestive cardiomyopathy were published already in 1975.[46]

More recently the non-selective beta-blocker carvedilol, which has a vasodilating effect due to alpha-adrenergic blocking property,[47] has been shown in a large prospective intervention trial to significantly improve survival in CHF.[48] It is interesting to note that carvedilol also exerts a dramatic effect in experimental myocardial infarction. In several animal models this compound reduced infarct size not only more effectively than placebo, it was also significantly better in this regard than other beta-blockers.[49-51]

It is conceivable that the cardioprotective effects of carvedilol to a certain extent may depend on its antioxidant activity. This emanates from the carbazole moiety which is unique to carvedilol as compared to other beta-blockers in clinical use.[52]

CONCLUSIONS

Beta-blockers have been in general used for more than three decades, are well tolerated, and are associated with generally mild side effects. Beta-blockers, when used in several large studies, have demonstrated a reduction in morbidity and mortality. Beta-blockers are cost-effective[53] and will undoubtedly remain a cornerstone in the treatment of hypertension.

REFERENCES

1. Ahlquist RP. A study of the adrenotropic receptors. Am J Physiol 1948;153:586–600.

2. Powell CE, Slater IH. Blocking of inhibitory adrenergic receptors by a dichloroanalogue of isoproterenol. J Pharmacol 1958;122: 480–488.

3. Prichard BNC. Hypotensive action of pronethalol. Br Med J 1964;I:1227.

4. Prichard BNC, Gillam PMS. Use of propranolol (Inderal) in treatment of hypertension. Br Med J 1964;2:725–727.

5. Cruickshank JM, Prichard BNC. Beta-blockers in clinical practice. Edinburgh: Churchill-Livingstone, 1987.

6. WHO/ISH Third Mild Hypertension Conference. Guidelines for the treatment of mild hypertension: Memorandum from a WHO/ISH meeting. Bull World Health Organ 1983;61:53–56.

7. Subcommittee on Definition and Prevalence of the 1984 Joint National Committee. Hypertension prevalence and the status of awareness, treatment, and control in the United States: Final report of the Subcommittee on Definition and Prevalence of the 1984 Joint National Committee. Hypertension 1985;7:457–468.

8. WHO/ISH Expert Committee. 1989 guidelines for the management of hypertension: Memorandum from a WHO/ISH meeting. J Hypertens 1989;7:689–693.

9. 1988 Joint National Committee on Prevention, Detection, Evaluation, and Treatment of High Blood Pressure. The Sixth report of the Joint National Committee on Prevention, Detection, Evaluation, and Treatment of High Blood Pressure. Arch Intern Med 1997;157:2413–2446.

10. Hansson L. Beta-blockers and related drugs for the treatment of hypertension. Curr Opinion Cardiol 1988;3:692–701.

11. Taylor SH. Role of cardioselectivity and intrinsic sympath-omimetic activity in beta-blocking drugs in cardiovascular disease. Am J Cardiol 1987;59:18F–20F.

12. Prichard BNC. Pharmacologic aspects of intrinsic sympath-omimetic activity in beta-blocking drugs. Am J Cardiol 1987;59:13F–17F.

13. Man in't Veld AJ, Schalekamp MADH. Effects on 10 different b-adrenoceptor antagonists on hemodynamics, plasma renin activity, and plasma norepinephrine in hypertension: The key role of vascular resistance changes in relation to partial agonist activity. J Cardiovasc Pharmacol 1983;5:(Suppl. 1)S30–S45.

14. Hansson L, Svensson A, Gudbrandsson T, Sivertsson R. Treatment of hypertension with beta-blockers with and without intrinsic sympathomimetic activity. J Cardiovasc Pharmacol 1983;5(Suppl. 7):S26–S29.

15. Prichard BNC, Gillam PMS. Treatment of hypertension with pro-pranolol. Br Med J 1969;1:7–16.

16. Humphreys GS, Delvin DG. Ineffectiveness of propranolol in hypertensive Jamaicans. Br Med J 1968;2:601–603.

17. Paterson JW, Dollery CT. Effect of propranolol in mild hyperten-sion. Lancet 1966;2:1148–1150.

18. Wilcox RG. Randomised study of six beta-blockers and a thiazide diuretic in essential hypertension. Br Med J 1978;2:383–385.

19. Carruthers SG, Kelly JG, McDevitt DG, et al. Duration of action of beta-blocking drugs. Br Med J 1973;2:177.

20. Platzer R, Galeazzi RL, Niederberger W, Rosenthaler J. Simultaneous modeling of bopindolol kinetics and dynamics. Clin Pharmacol Ther 1984;36:5–13.

21. Dahlöf B, Pennert K, Hansson L. Reversal of left ventricular hypertrophy in hypertensive patients. A metaanalysis of 109 treat-ment studies. Am J Hypertens 1992;5:95–110.

22. Schmieder RE, Martus P, Klingbeil A. Reversal of left ventricular hypertrophy in essential hypertension. A meta-analysis of random-ized double-blind studies. JAMA 1996;275:1507–1513.

23. Jennings GL, Wong J. Reversibility of left ventricular hypertrophy and malfunction by antihypertensive treatment. In: Handbook of Hypertension, Vol 18, Assessment of Hypertensive Organ Damage. Eds.: Hansson L, Birkenhäger WH. Elsevier, Rotterdam 1997;184–223.

24. Levy D. Left ventricular hypertrophy. Epidemiological insights from the Framingham Heart Study. Drugs 1988;35(Suppl. 5):1–5.

25. Levy D., Garrison RJ, Savage DD, Kannel WB, Castelli WP. Prognostic implications of echocardiographically determined left ventricular mass in the Framingham Heart Study. N Engl J Med 1990;322:1561 1566.

26. Messerli FH, Ventura HO, Elizardi DJ, et al. Hypertension and sudden death: Increased ventricular ectopic activity in left ventricu-lar hypertrophy. Am J Med 1984;77:18–22.

27. Muiesan ML, Salvett M, Rizzone D, Castellano M, Donato F, Agabiti-Rosei E. Association of change in left ventricular mass with prognosis during long-term antihypertensive treatment. J Hypertens 1995;13:1091–1095.

28. DeFronzo RA, Ferranini E. Insulin resistance: A multifaceted syn-drome responsible for NIDDM, obesity, hypertension, dyslipi-daemia and atherosclerotic cardiovascular disease. Diabetes Care 1991;14:173–194.

29. Pollare T, Lithell H, Berne C. Insulin resistance is a characteristic feature of primary hypertension independent of obesity. Metabolism 1990;39:167–174.

30. Skarfors ET, Lithell HO, Selinus I. Risk factors for the development of hypertension: A 10 year longitudinal study in middle aged men. J Hypertens 1991;9:217–223.

31. Lithell HOL. Effect of antihypertensive drugs on insulin, glucose and lipid metabolism. Diabetes Care 1991;14:203–209.

32. Weidmann P, Wehlinger DE, Gerber A. Editorial review. Antihypertensive treatment and serum lipoproteins. J Hypertens 1985;3:297–306.

33. Hjalmarson Å, Elmfeldt D, Herlitz J, et al. Effect on mortality of metoprolol in acute myocardial infarction. Lancet 1981;2:823–827.

34. Norwegian Multicentre Study Group. Timolol-induced reduction in mortality and reinfarction surviving acute myocardial infarction. N Engl J Med 1981;304:801–807.

35. β-blocker Heart Attack Trial Research Group. 1. Mortality results 1982. A randomized trial of propranolol in patients with acute myocardial infarction. JAMA 1982;247:1707–1714.

36. Kjekshus J, Gilpin E, Cali G, et al. Diabetic patients and beta-blockers after acute myocardial infarction. Eur Heart J 1990;11:43–50.

37. The IPPPSH Collaborative Group. Cardiovascular risk and risk factors in a randomized trial of treatment based on the beta-blocker oxprenolol: The International Prospective Primary Prevention Study in Hypertension (IPPPSH). J Hypertens 1985;3:379–392.

38. Wilhelmsen L, Berglund G, Elmfeldt D, et al. Beta-blockers versus diuretics in hypertensive men: Main results from the HAPPHY trial. J Hypertens 1987;5:561–572.

39. Medical Research Council Working Party. MRC trial of treatment of mild hypertension: Principal results. Br Med J 1985;291:97–104.

40. Dahlöf C, Dimenäs E, Kendall M, Wiklund I. Quality of life in cardiovascular diseases. Emphasis on b-blocker treatment. Circulation 1991;84(Suppl.VI):VI-108–VI-118.

41. Steiner SS, Friedhoff AJ, Wilson BL, et al. Antihypertensive therapy and quality of life: A comparison of atenolol, captopril, enalapril and propranolol. J Hum Hypertens 1990;4:217–225.

42. Dimenäs E, Östergren J, Lindvall K, et al. Comparison of CNS-related subjective symptoms in hypertensive patients treated with either a new controlled release (CR/ZOC) formulation of metoprolol or atenolol. J Clin Pharmacol 1990;30:S82–S90.

43. SHEP Cooperative Research Group. Prevention of stroke by antihypertensive drug treatment in older persons with isolated systolic hypertension. Final results of the Systolic Hypertension in the Elderly Program (SHEP). JAMA 1991;265:3255–3264.

44. Dahlöf B, Lindholm LH, Hansson L, et al. Morbidity and mortality in the Swedish Trial in Old Patients with Hypertension (STOP-Hypertension). Lancet 1991;338:1281–1285.

45. MRC Working Party. Medical Research Council trial of treatment of hypertension in older adults: Principal results. Br Med J 1992;304:405–412.

46. Waagstein F, Hjalmarson Å, Varnauskas E, Wallentin I. Effect of chronic beta-adrenergic receptor blockade in congestive cardiomyopathy. Br Heart J 1975;37:1022–1036.

47. McTavish D, Campoli-Richards D, Sorkin Em. Carvedilol. A review of its pharmacodynamic and pharmacokinetic properties, and therapeutic efficacy. Drugs 1993;45:232–258.

48. Packer M, Bristow MR, Cohn JN, Colucci WS, Fowler MB, Gilbert EM, Shusterman NH, for the US Carvedilol Heart Failure Study Group. The effect of carvedilol on morbidity and mortality in patients with chronic heart failure. N Engl J Med 1996;334:1349–1355.

49. Bri A, Slivjak M, DiMartino MJ, Feuerstein GZ, Linee P, Poyser RH, Ruffolo RR Jr, Smith EF III. Cardioprotective effects of carvedilol, a novel beta-adrenoceptor antagonist with vasodilating properties, in anaesthetised minipigs: comparison with propranolol. Cardiovasc Res 1992;26:518–525.

50. Feuerstein GZ, Hamburger SA, Smith EF III, Bril A, Ruffolo RR Jr. Myocardial protection with carvedilol. J Cardiovasc Pharmacol 1992;19(Suppl 1):S138–S141.

51. Hamburger SA, Barone FC, Feuerstein GZ, Ruffolo RR Jr. Carvedilol (Kredex®) reduces infarct size in a canine model of acute myocardial infarction. Pharmacol 1991;43:113–130.

52. Yue TL, Lysko PG, Barone FC, Gu JL, Ruffolo RR Jr. Carvedilol, a new antihypertensive drug with unique antioxidant activity: potential role in cerebroprotection. Ann NY Acad Sci 1994;738:230–242.

53. Edelson JT, Weinsten MC, Tostesson A, et al. Long-term cost-effectiveness of various initial monotherapies for mild to moderate hypertension. JAMA 1990;263:408–413.

Beta-Blockers with Vasodilating Activity: Focus on Carvedilol

Marvin Moser
William H. Frishman

β-Blockers have been recommended as one of the initial medications for the treatment of hypertension by the Fifth and Sixth Joint National Committees on Detection, Evaluation, and Treatment of High Blood Pressure.[1,2] They are one of only two classes of drugs that have been shown to reduce hypertension-related cardiovascular and cerebrovascular morbidity and mortality in long-term clinical trials.[3,4] β-Blockers also have been shown to prevent recurrence of myocardial infarction in patients with ischemic heart disease.[5]

Although β-blockers are effective antihypertensive drugs, their use may result in an increase in peripheral resistance, at least initially, and a reduction in cardiac output. This latter effect may explain the occurrence of symptoms of fatigue and lack of energy experienced by some patients. However, some more recently developed β-blockers have vasodilating activity (Table 1).[6] The α_1-receptor blocking action of carvedilol that results in vasodilation tends to counteract some of the physiologic effects of a β-blocker. Placebo-controlled and comparative studies have established that carvedilol is an effective antihypertensive drug that is well tolerated.[7-13]

EFFECTS ON BLOOD PRESSURE

Placebo Comparisons

In double-blind, placebo-controlled trials, the use of 6.25 to 50 mg daily of carvedilol (given either once or twice daily) resulted in a statistically significant reduction in blood pressure over that achieved by placebo (Table 2). A mean decrease in sitting systolic blood pressure (SBP) of 7.2 mm Hg and 10.9 mm Hg was achieved with once daily and twice

This chapter was adapted in part from Moser M, Frishman W. Results of therapy with carvedilol, a β-blocker vasodilator with antioxidant properties, in hypertensive patients. Am J Hypertens 1998;11:15S-22S, with permission.

TABLE 1. COMPARATIVE PHARMACOLOGICAL PROPERTIES OF VARIOUS β-ADRENOCEPTOR ANTAGONIST DRUGS HAVING VASODILATORY ACTIVITY

	β-Adrenoceptor Antagonist Potency*	β_1-Adrenergic Selectivity	ISA at β-Receptors	α-Adrenoceptor Antagonist Activity	Direct Vasodilator Action
Bucindolol	1.0	No	No	No	Yes
Carvedilol**	2.4	No	No	Yes	No
Labetalol	0.3	No	Yes	Yes	No
Pindolol	6.0	No	Yes	No	No

*Relative to propranolol (+1.0)
** In addition, carvedilol has antioxidant and antiproliferative properties, and weak calcium-entry blocking action in experimental animals
ISA = intrinsic sympathomimetic activity
From Frishman WH[28] with permission.

TABLE 2. CHANGES IN SITTING SYSTOLIC AND DIASTOLIC BLOOD PRESSURES WITH CARVEDILOL AND PLACEBO

Time	Placebo		50 mg Carvedilol once daily		25 mg Carvedilol twice daily	
	N	mmHg	N	mmHg	N	mmHg
Baseline	93	154/101.9	90	153/101.6	96	152/100.8
End of study*	93	-4.1/-3.4	90	-7.2/-8.7	96	-10.9/-10.6

*4 weeks maintenance of carvedilol after 8 to 10 week titration phase.
Data on File, SmithKline Beecham Pharmaceuticals 1996.
Reproduced from Moser M, Frishman W: Results of therapy with carvedilol: a β-blocker vasodilator with antioxidant properties, in hypertensive patients. Am J Hypertens 1998; 11: 16S.

daily carvedilol, respectively, compared with a 4.1 mm Hg decrease with placebo. A mean reduction of 10.6 mm Hg in sitting diastolic blood pressure (DBP) was noted with twice daily carvedilol therapy compared with −3.4 mm Hg with placebo. Nineteen percent of placebo-treated patients experienced a reduction in DBP to < 90 mm Hg, whereas 66% of patients taking twice daily carvedilol and 56% taking once daily carvedilol achieved this degree of blood pressure response (data on file, SmithKline Beecham Pharmaceuticals, 1996).

Twenty-four hour ambulatory monitoring has demonstrated a consistent reduction of blood pressure with a trough-to-peak ratio of 76.9% in patients taking once daily therapy and 90.1% in patients taking twice daily therapy (i.e., about 90% of the blood pressure-lowering effect is still noted at the time of next dose) (Figure 1).[14] Blood pressure and heart rate responses to exercise are blunted with this medication when compared with placebo.[9]

Although once daily administration of carvedilol is effective, twice daily administration produces a greater decrease in blood pressure, a higher percentage of responders, and a higher trough-to-peak response rate without a significant increase in symptoms.

Effects on Standing Blood Pressure and Postural Changes

In a comparative study of carvedilol and placebo, changes in standing blood pressure (after three minutes) were greater with once daily and twice daily carvedilol than with placebo (−6.5/−7.6, −11.3/−9.9, and −3.2/−2.3 mm Hg respectively) but symptoms of postural hypotension were not frequent (data on file, SmithKline Beecham Pharmaceuticals 1996). Mean standing blood pressure on carvedilol decreased from a baseline of 153/103 mm Hg to 140.7/93.1 mm Hg at the end of a four-week study.

Comparative Studies with Other Antihypertensive Drugs

In a short-term comparative study with another β-blocker (propranolol), carvedilol 50 mg significantly decreased total peripheral resistance, whereas resistance increased with propranolol 40 mg.[12] This finding is not unexpected in view of the vasodilating properties of carvedilol. Compared with other β-blockers, heart rate is not decreased to as great an extent with carvedilol either at rest or after exercise, the increase in post-exercise SBP and DBP is less with carvedilol, and cardiac output in hypertensive patients is maintained or slightly increased by carvedilol in contrast to at least an initial decrease after therapy with other β-blockers[12,15-17]).

In comparative studies with other β-blockers (atenolol[7,13] and acebutolol [data on file, SmithKline Beecham Pharmaceuticals 1996]), an angiotensin converting enzyme (ACE) inhibitor (captopril[8]), a long-acting calcium channel blocker (slow-release nifedipine[7]) and hydrochlorothiazide[10], equivalent blood pressure-lowering has been noted with carvedilol in doses of 25 to 50 mg once daily (Tables 3 and 4).

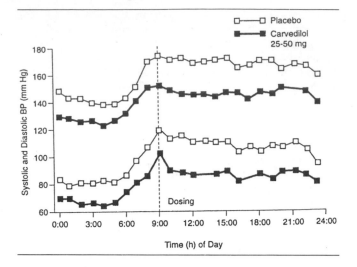

Figure 1. 24 hour blood pressure readings after carvedilol (25 or 50 mg once daily) or placebo in 15 patients (modified from Lund-Johansen et al.[14] with permission).

The results of these studies have been summarized elsewhere.[11] Although the percentage of responders in these studies is slightly greater with acebutolol and slow-release nifedipine than with carvedilol, the differences between the drugs were not significant.

In the approximately 35% of patients who may have an inadequate response to carvedilol, the addition of 25 mg hydrochlorothiazide per day results in additional blood pressure reduction. Forty percent of patients who have an inadequate response to carvedilol alone achieve goal blood pressures (DBP < 90 mm Hg) with combination treatment. The addition of carvedilol in poor responders to hydrochlorothiazide also results in a decrease in blood pressure. Thus, the use of a diuretic with carvedilol in patients who have an inadequate response to monotherapy increases the response rate.[10,13]

An additional blood pressure decrease has also been reported in nonresponders to a calcium channel blocker when carvedilol was added (data on file, SmithKline Beecham Pharmaceuticals 1996).[18]

EFFECT ON METABOLIC PARAMETERS

The use of beta-blockers, especially those without intrinsic sympathomimetic activity (ISA), may increase triglycerides and decrease high-density lipoprotein (HDL) cholesterol levels.[19]

Lipids

Several studies with carvedilol 6.25 to 25 mg twice daily report essentially no change in total cholesterol, HDL cholesterol or low density lipoprotein (LDL) cholesterol.[8,20,21] Decreases of 3 to 4 mg/dL in total and LDL cholesterol concentrations, an increase of 7 mg/dL in triglycerides, and a decrease of 2 to 3 md/dL in HDL cholesterol concentrations

TABLE 3. COMPARATIVE ANTIHYPERTENSIVE EFFICACY OF CARVEDILOL AND SELECTED β-BLOCKERS

Regimen	N	Mean Change from Baseline		Response Rate (%) (DBP ≤ 90 mmHg)
		BP (mmHg)	HR (beats/min)	
Carvedilol* (25-50 mg once daily)	161	-19/-15	-6	66
Atenolol (50-100 mg once daily)	164	-17/-14	-8	63
Carvedilol* (25-50 mg once daily)	105	-20/-13	-12	67
Acebutolol (200-400 mg twice daily)	112	-22/-15	-11	75

*Therapy initiated at 12.5 mg daily for 2 days.
BP = blood pressure; HR = heart rate; DBP = diastolic blood pressure.
Reproduced from Moser[11] with permission

TABLE 4. ANTIHYPERTENSIVE EFFICACY OF CARVEDILOL COMPARED WITH CAPTOPRIL, SLOW-RELEASE NIFEDIPINE OR HYDROCHLOROTHIAZIDE

Regimen	N	Mean Change from Baseline		Response Rate (%) (DBP ≤ 90 mmHg)
		BP (mmHg)	HR (beats/min)	
Carvedilol* (25–50 mg once daily)	147	-17/-16	-7	66
Captopril (25–50 mg twice daily)	151	-17/-13	-1	60
Carvedilol (25–50 mg once daily)	103	-19/-14	-5	63
Slow-release Nifedipine (20–40 mg twice daily)	102	-20/-16	-1	75
Carvedilol (25–50 mg once daily)	100	-21/-15	-5	65
Hydrochlorothiazide (25–50 mg once daily)	100	-23/16	-2	73

*Therapy initiated at 12.5 mg daily for 2 days.
BP = blood pressure; HR = heart rate; DBP = diastolic blood pressure.
Reproduced from Moser[11] with permission.

were noted, however, with higher doses of carvedilol (data on file, SmithKline Beecham Pharmaceuticals 1996). None of these changes was statistically significant.

No differences in changes in total, HDL or LDL cholesterol levels were noted between drugs in a six-month study that compared carvedilol 25 to 50 mg daily with captopril 25 to 50 mg daily (Figure 2).[8]

Glucose Metabolism

Fasting serum glucose concentrations were essentially unchanged in trials in which carvedilol 6.25 to 25 mg twice daily was compared with placebo.[19,22,23] In one study of 49 patients with non-insulin-dependent diabetes mellitus, adjustments to oral hypoglycemic therapy were not required with either carvedilol or metoprolol.[19] Blood pressure responses in non-insulin- and insulin-dependent diabetics were equivalent with carvedilol 25 to 50 mg twice daily and metoprolol 50 to 100 mg twice daily. In another study that compared carvedilol and nifedipine in patients with essential hypertension and non-insulin-dependent diabetes mellitus, similar reductions in blood pressure were observed. After four weeks of treatment, no significant changes from baseline chemistries were seen in either group.[22] These data and others[23] suggest that carvedilol can be used as an antihypertensive agent in patients with Type II diabetes mellitus.

Effects on Renal Function

A decrease in microalbuminuria has been reported in patients treated with carvedilol 25 to 50 mg daily or 25 mg plus 25 mg hydrochlorothiazide.[10] In comparative studies with an ACE inhibitor, beta-blocker, diuretic or calcium channel blocker, carvedilol was shown to decrease microalbuminuria to a greater extent than the other agents tested (Figure 3).[24] Data also indicate that glomerular filtration rate

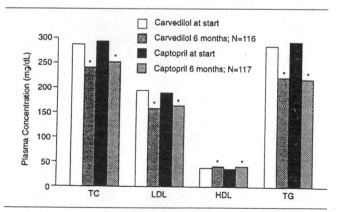

Figure 2. *Changes in serum lipids in a 6 month double-blind study of 220 hypertensive patients receiving either carvedilol (25 to 50 mg/day) or captopril (25 to 50 mg/day). *P <.0001 vs baseline. start = end of 4-week placebo washout phase; HDL = high-density lipoprotein; LDL = low-density lipoprotein; TC = total cholesterol; TG = triglyceride. Data from Hauf-Zachariou et al.[8]*

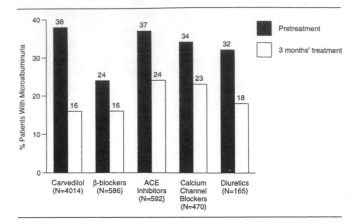

Figure 3. *Percentage of patients with reduction or increase in urinary albumin level with carvedilol compared to other antihypertensive agents (from Marchi & Ciriello[24] with permission).*

and renal blood flow are not significantly changed and renovascular resistance is decreased following chronic use of this medication in patients with essential hypertension.[25]

COMPARISON WITH LABETALOL

Labetalol is another β-blocker with α-receptor blocking activities. The relative efficacies of this agent and carvedilol have been determined in a one-year trial comparing twice daily carvedilol 25 to 50 mg daily with twice daily labetalol 100 to 400 mg daily (data on file, SmithKline Beecham Pharmaceuticals 1996). At 1 year, blood pressure reduction was similar (carvedilol –11/–9 mm Hg, labetalol –9/–9 mm Hg) and no differences in heart rate were noted between the groups. Fifty three percent of patients on carvedilol achieved a goal DBP of < 90 mm Hg or a decrease of 10 mm Hg; 45% of nonresponders on carvedilol responded when hydrochlorothiazide was added. Sixty-three percent of patients on labetalol achieved a goal DBP of < 90 mm Hg; 36% of nonresponders experienced a blood pressure reduction when the diuretic was added.

Metabolic Effects of Labetalol and Carvedilol

Labetalol increased total cholesterol concentrations by 5 mg/dL from 217 to 222 mg/dL in this one-year study, whereas total cholesterol concentrations remained essentially unchanged at 230 to 228 mg/dL in patients taking carvedilol. LDL cholesterol concentrations did not change significantly (carvedilol 148 to 144 mg/dL, labetalol 139 to 142 mg/dL), but triglyceride concentrations increased by 17 mg/dL with both drugs. There were no significant differences in fasting serum glucose concentrations (carvedilol 109 to 115 mg/dL, labetalol 108 to 112 mg/dL).

These long-term trial data indicate that when carvedilol is compared with labetalol, a medication with similar physiologic effects on blood pressures, blood pressure is reduced to an equivalent degree with minimal effects on lipid or glucose parameters.

EFFECTS IN OLDER PATIENTS AND BLACK PATIENTS

Carvedilol appears to be as effective in elderly hypertensive subjects as in younger patients.[26] Similar numbers of patients older than 65 years of age with DBP < 90 mm Hg responded to carvedilol as compared with other beta-blockers, captopril, calcium channel blockers and hydrochlorothiazide.

Unlike other β-blockers or ACE inhibitors which do not appear to lower blood pressure equally in black and white subjects, there are no reported differences in response rates with carvedilol.

SIDE EFFECTS

Side effects that were noted in more than 2% of subjects on carvedilol in placebo-controlled trials are summarized in Table 5. Dizziness, asthenia and postural hypotension appear to occur more frequently with higher doses of carvedilol (i.e., > 50 mg daily) than with placebo (data on file, SmithKline Beecham Pharmaceuticals 1996). The type and frequency of adverse events or withdrawals as a result of side effects were not significantly different in patients who received once- or twice-daily carvedilol therapy or placebo. Withdrawal rates were 5% (twice daily carvedilol), 3% (once daily carvedilol) and 1% (placebo).

Comparative data with carvedilol and other beta-blockers, ACE inhibitors, or calcium channel blockers show little difference in the number of adverse reactions that occurred in >2% of subjects (Table 6).

Orthostatic blood pressure changes are not significantly different between carvedilol and other antihypertensive agents and occurred in <2% of patients. Dizziness, however,

TABLE 5. SIDE EFFECTS NOTED IN >2% OF SUBJECTS ON CARVEDILOL

Event	Placebo (n=2275)	Carvedilol* 25 mg (n=469)	Carvedilol* 50 mg (n=794)
Headache	11.0	6.8	6.2
Dizziness	2.9	3.7	9.4
Asthenia	2.5	3.5	5.1
Postural hypotension	1.8	0.7	3.2
Nausea	1.4	2.1	2.2
Dyspnea	0.6	2.8	2.2

* One or two doses daily; data collected cumulatively over 2 months.
Modified from data on file, SmithKline Beecham Pharmaceuticals 1996.
Reproduced from Moser M, Frishman W: Results of therapy with carvedilol: a β-blocker vasodilator with antioxidant properties, in hypertensive patients. Am J Hypertens 1998;11:19S.

Table 6. Incidence (%) of Adverse Events Reported in >2% of Patients Participating in 8-Week Comparative Studies with Carvedilol and Other Antihypertensive Medications

Event	Carvedilol 5-50 mg QD* (n=616)	Atenolol 50-100 mg QD (n=164)	Acebutolol 200-400 mg BID (n=112)	Captopril 20-50 mg BID (n=151)	SR-Nifedipine 25-40 QD (n=102)	HCTZ 25-50 mg QD (n=100)
Dizziness	4.9	4.3	-	2.0	4.9	4.0
Headache	4.4	1.2	3.6	4.6	3.9	3.0
GI symptoms	4.4	3.0	7.1	4.0	5.9	2.0
Somnolence	1.9	1.8	-	-	2.0	1.0
Fatigue	1.5	2.4	1.8	-	3.9	1.0
Asthenia	1.5	1.8	2.7	-	1.0	-
Vertigo	1.1	-	2.7	-	-	-
Edema	-	1.8	-	-	7.8	1.0
Paresthesia	-	-	-	-	2.9	-
Rhinitis	-	-	2.7	-	-	1.0
Cough/bronchospasm	-	-	2.7	1.3	-	-
Flushing	-	-	-	7.8	-	-
Abnormal dreaming	-	-	-	-	2.0	-

*Treatment initiated with 12.5 mg daily for 2 days in 413 patients. SR = slow release; HCTZ = hydrochlorothiazide; GI = gastrointestinal
Adapted from Moser[11] with permission.

occurred more frequently in patients over 65 years of age (11.4%) than in younger patients (3.2%) (Table 7).

DISCUSSION

Numerous studies in patients with hypertension have shown that carvedilol is an effective antihypertensive drug that reduces peripheral resistance without altering cardiac output or renal function. Long-term data demonstrate that blood pressure lowering is maintained in a high percentage of patients, and is similar to effects noted with ACE inhibitors, calcium channel blockers, other β-blockers and diuretics. A majority of patients who do not respond to carvedilol monotherapy experience a decrease in blood pressure when small doses of a diuretic (12.5 to 25 mg of hydrochlorothiazide or its equivalent) are added to treatment. Long-term therapy with carvedilol does not appear to adversely affect serum lipids or glucose metabolism. Based on available data, carvedilol should probably be started at doses of 6.25 mg twice daily with an increase to 25 mg twice daily if normotensive blood pressures are not achieved. Some patients will respond to once daily therapy.

Where, then, might this beta-blocker vasodilator fit into the treatment algorithm for hypertensive patients? Are there any data to suggest that its use provides an advantage over other presently available conventional beta-blockers or other antihypertensive drugs? Some of the properties that may distinguish carve-dilol from other agents are reviewed elsewhere[27,28] and are summarized in Table 8).

A significant reduction in mortality and morbidity has been demonstrated in patients with congestive heart failure who are given carvedilol in addition to standard triple drug therapy (i.e., ACE inhibitor, diuretic and digitalis).[29-33] These results cannot be attributed completely to vasodilation or reduction in preload and afterload. Part of the effect might be related to the reduction in myocardial oxygen demand and cardiac work as a result of β-blocker action, but the potent antioxidant effects of carvedilol and effects on cardiac remodeling might also be responsible for the beneficial outcome.[34,35] In animal myocardial infarction models, the use of

TABLE 7. INCIDENCE (%) OF ADVERSE EVENTS REPORTED IN >2% OF PATIENTS WITH 25-50 MG CARVEDILOL ONCE DAILY* IN HYPERTENSIVE PATIENTS OLDER OR YOUNGER THAN 64 YEARS OF AGE

Event	> 64 Years (n=123)	≤ 64 Years (n=493)
Dizziness	11.4	3.2
GI Symptoms	6.5	3.9
Headache	3.3	4.7
Vertigo	3.3	0.6
Somnolence	2.4	1.8

*Carvedilol initiated at 12.5 mg daily for 2 days in 413 patients.
GI = gastrointestinal
Adapted from Moser (11) with permission.

TABLE 8. PROPERTIES OF CARVEDILOL

1. Lowers blood pressure in both younger and older black and white patients.

2. Reduces peripheral resistance.

3. Does not reduce cardiac output or renal function in long-term studies.

4. Has a neutral effect on lipids and glucose.

5. Is well tolerated by most patients.

6. Possesses antioxidant effects in pharmacologic studies (inhibits oxygen-free radicals. This action may be important in slowing down the process of atherogenesis and protecting against brain tissue injury).

7. Reduces morbidity and mortality in patients with congestive heart failure who are already being treated with angiotensin converting enzyme inhibitors, diuretics and digitalis (reduces pre-load and afterload).

8. Reduces infarct size to a significant degree in animal models, and improves survival (effect not demonstrated with other β-blockers).

9. Has antiproliferative effects on smooth muscle cells (in response to angiotensin-II, platelet-derived growth factor, etc.).

From Moser M, Frishman W: Results of therapy with carvedilol: a β-blocker vasodilator with antioxidant properties, in hypertensive patients. Am J Hypertens 1998; 11: 21S.

carvedilol reduces the degree of cardiac muscle damage.[36,37] These findings suggest that carvedilol might have specific advantages in the management of hypertensive patients at high risk for heart disease or in those with ischemic heart disease or congestive heart failure. Preliminary data suggest that carvedilol may also produce some beneficial effects in subjects with nephropathy.

In addition, carvedilol reduces oxidation of LDL cholesterol and smooth muscle proliferation, several of the initiating factors in the atherogenic process.[38] These effects do not appear to be present to any great extent in other β-blockers. Further studies are necessary to determine the clinical significance of these observations.

Based on presently available animal and human data, carvedilol appears to be not only an effective antihypertensive agent, but a medication with additional properties that may help to reduce the risk of cardiovascular disease by affecting the process of atherogenesis and remodeling.

REFERENCES

1. Joint National Committee on Detection, Evaluation and Treatment of High Blood Pressure: The Fifth Report of the Joint National Committee on Detection, Evaluation and Treatment of High Blood Pressure (JNC V). Arch Intern Med 1993;153:154–183.

2. The Sixth Report of the Joint National Committee on Prevention, Detection, Evaluation and Treatment of High Blood Pressure (JNC VI). Arch Intern Med 1997;157:2413–2446.

3. Hebert PR, Moser M, Mayer J, et al. Recent evidence on drug therapy of mild to moderate hypertension and decreased risk of coronary heart disease. Arch Intern Med 1993;153:578–581.

4. Staessen J, Fagard R, for the European Trial on ISH in the Elderly: Recent studies with nitrendipine, a moderate long acting dihydropyridine, that reduces strokes in elderly subjects primarily with isolated systolic hypertension. Lancet 1997;350:757–764.

5. Yusuf S, Peto R, Lewis J, et al: Beta blockade during and after myocardial infarction: an overview of the randomized trials. Prog Cardiovasc Dis 1985;27:335–371.

6. Eggertsen R, Sivertsson R, Andren I., et al: Acute and long-term hemodynamic effects of carvedilol, a combined β-adrenoceptor blocking and precapillary vasodilating agent, in hypertensive patients. J Cardiovasc Pharmacol 1987;10(Suppl. 11):S97–100.

7. Hall S, Prescott RI, Hallman RJ, et al. A comparative study of carvedilol, slow-release nifedipine, and atenolol in the management of essential hypertension. J Cardiovasc Pharmacol 1991;18 (Suppl. 4):S35–38.

8. Hauf-Zachariou U, Widmann L, Zulsdorf B, et al. A double-blind comparison of the effects of carvedilol and captopril on serum lipid concentrations in patients with mild to moderate essential hypertension and dyslipidaemia. Eur J Clin Pharmacol 1993;45:95–100.

9. Heber ME, Brigden GS, Caruana MP, et al. Carvedilol for systemic hypertension. Am J Cardiol 1987;59:400–405.

10. Langdon CG, Baxter GA, Young PH: A multicenter comparison of carvedilol with hydrochlorothiazide in the treatment of mild-to-moderate essential hypertension. J Cardiovasc Pharmacol 1991;18(Suppl. 4):S51–56.

11. Moser M: Clinical experience with carvedilol. J Human Hypertens 1993;7(Suppl. 1):S16–20.

12. Wendt T, van der Does R, Schrader R, et al. Acute hemodynamic effects of the vasodilating and β-blocking agent carvedilol in comparison to propranolol. J Cardiovasc Pharmacol 1987;10(Suppl. 11):S147–150.

13. Widmann L, van der Does R, Horrmann M, Machwirth M: Safety and antihypertensive efficacy of carvedilol and atenolol alone and in combination with hydrochlorothiazide. Eur J Clin Pharmacol 1990;38:S143–146.

14. Lund-Johansen P, Omvik P, Nordrehaug JE, et al: Carvedilol in hypertension: effects on hemodynamics and 24 hour blood pressure. J Cardiovasc Pharmacol 1992;19(Suppl. 1):S27–34.

15. Franz I-W, Agrawal B, Wiewel D, et al: Comparison of the antihypertensive effects of carvedilol and metoprolol on resting and exercise blood pressure. Clin Invest 1992;70:S53–57.

16. Lund-Johansen P, Omvik P: Chronic haemodynamic effects of carvedilol in essential hypertension at rest and during exercise. Eur Heart J 1992;13:281–286.

17. Morgan TO, Snowden R, Butcher L: Effect of carvedilol and metoprolol on blood pressure, blood flow and vascular resistance. J Cardiovasc Pharmacol 1987;10(Suppl. 11):S124–129.

18. Takabatake T, Ohta H, Yamamoto Y, et al. Combination therapy with carvedilol and nicardipine in essential hypertension: an open study. Drugs 1988;36(Suppl 6):124–128.

19. Ehmer B, van der Does R, Rudorf J: Influence of carvedilol on blood glucose and glycohemoglobin A1 in noninsulin-dependent diabetics. Drugs 1988;36(Suppl. 6):136–140.

20. Goto Y, Tamachi H, Fusegawa Y, et al: Effects of carvedilol on serum lipids in patients with essential hypertension. J Cardiovasc Pharmacol 1991;18(Suppl. 4):S45–50.

21. Seguchi H, Nakamura H, Aosaki N, et al: Effects of carvedilol on serum lipids in hypertensive and normotensive subjects. Eur J Clin Pharmacol 1990;38:S139–142.

22. Albergati F, Paterno E, Venuti RP, et al. Comparison of the effects of carvedilol and nifedipine in patients with essential hypertension and noninsulin-dependent diabetes mellitus. J Cardiovasc Pharmacol 1992;19(Suppl. 1):S86–89.

23. Giugliano D, Acampora R, Marfella R, et al: Metabolic and cardiovascular effects of carvedilol and atenolol in non-insulin-dependent diabetes mellitus and hypertension. Ann Intern Med 1997;126:955–959.

24. Marchi F, Ciriello C: Efficacy of carvedilol in mild to moderate essential hypertension and effects on microalbuminuria: a multicenter, randomized, open-label, controlled study versus atenolol. Adv Ther 1995;12:212–221.

25. Dupont AG, Van der Niepen P, Taeymans Y, et al: Effect of carvedilol on ambulatory blood pressure, renal hemodynamics and cardiac function in essential hypertension. J Cardiovasc Pharmacol 1987;10(Suppl. 11):S130–136.

26. Morgan TO, Anderson A, Cripps J, et al. The use of carvedilol in elderly hypertensive patients. Eur J Clin Pharmacol 1990;38:S129–133.

27. Ruffolo RR Jr., Boyle DA, Venuti RP, et al: Preclinical and clinical pharmacology of carvedilol. J Human Hypertens 1993;7(Suppl. 1):S2–15.

28. Frishman WH: Carvedilol. N Engl J Med 1998;339:1759–1765.

29. Bristow MR, Gilbert EM, Abraham WT, et al for the MOCHA Investigators: Multicenter Oral Carvedilol Heart Failure Assessment (MOCHA): a six-month dose-response evaluation in class II-IV patients (abst). Circulation 1995;92(Suppl. 1):I–142.

30. Colucci WS, Packer M, Bristow MR, et al. Carvedilol inhibits clinical progression in patients with mild heart failure (abst). Circulation 1995;92(Suppl. 1):I–395.

31. Das Gupta P, Broadhurst P, Raftery EB, et al. Value of carvedilol in congestive heart failure secondary to coronary artery disease. Am J Cardiol 1990;66:1118–1123.

32. Packer M, Colucci WS, Sackner-Bernstein J, et al for the PRECISE Study Group: Prospective, randomized evaluation of carvedilol on symptoms and exercise tolerance in chronic heart failure: results of the PRECISE trial (abst). Circulation 1995;92(Suppl. 1):I–143.

33. Packer M, Bristow MR, Cohn JN, et al: The effect of carvedilol on morbidity and mortality in patients with chronic heart failure. N Engl J Med 1996;334:1349–1355.

34. Yue T-L, McKenna PJ, Lysko PG, et al. Carvedilol, a new antihypertensive, prevents oxidation of human low-density lipoprotein by macrophages and copper. Atherosclerosis 1992;97:209–216.

35. Yue T-L, Cheng Y-Y, Lysko PG, et al. Carvedilol, a new vasodilator and beta adrenoceptor antagonist, is an antioxidant and free radical scavenger. J Pharmacol Exp Ther 1992;263:92–98.

36. Bril A, Slivjak M, DiMartino MJ, et al. Cardioprotective effects of carvedilol, a novel (-adrenoceptor antagonist with vasodilating properties, in anaesthetized minipigs: comparison with propranolol. Cardiovasc Res 1992;26:518–525.

37. Hamburger SA, Barone FC, Feuerstein GZ, et al: Carvedilol (Kredex®) reduces infarct size in a canine model of acute myocardial infarction. Pharmacology 1991;43:113–120.

38. Sung C-P, Arleth AJ, Ohlstein EH: Carvedilol inhibits vascular smooth muscle cell proliferation. J Cardiovasc Pharmacol 1993;21:221–227.

CHAPTER 10

Centrally Acting Antihypertensive Drugs

Thomas D. Giles

Centrally acting antihypertensive drugs achieve their therapeutic effect primarily by acting on sites in the central nervous system to decrease sympathetic activity and increase parasympathetic activity. Drugs in use in current practice or under clinical development act variably as agonists on α_2-adrenoceptors or imidazoline (I), of the I_1 subclass receptors. Moxonidine and rilmenidine act on I_1 receptors, with less effect on α_2-adrenoceptors (~35:1), while clonidine acts equally on the α_2 and I_1 receptors; α-methyldopa, guanabenz, and guanfacine act primarily on the α-adrenoceptor (Figure 1).[1]

SELECTIVE IMIDAZOLINE RECEPTOR (SIRA) AGONISTS[2,3,4,5,6,7]

The antihypertensive drugs that utilize primarily the I_1 receptor to achieve their antihypertensive effect are moxonidine and rilmenidine. A principal site for the antihypertensive action of the I-receptor drugs is the reticular formation of the rostral ventrolateral medulla. In response to stimulation of these neurons, sympathetic nerve activity is reduced, resulting in systemic vasodilation, slowing of the heart rate, and reduction in the secretion of catecholamines from the adrenal medulla and, indirectly, renin from the kidney. These drugs also increase parasympathetic outflow, which contributes to the slowing of the heart rate, and have potentially favorable effects on the cardiac ventricular fibrillation threshold. Since these drugs have low affinity for the α_2-adrenoceptors in the locus ceruleus and higher sympathetic nuclei, fewer side effects associated with stimulation of those areas, such as sedation and dry mouth, occur.

Moxonidine

Moxonidine is approved and available throughout Europe and Latin America as a film-coated tablet containing 0.2 mg/0.3 mg/0.4 mg of moxonidine.

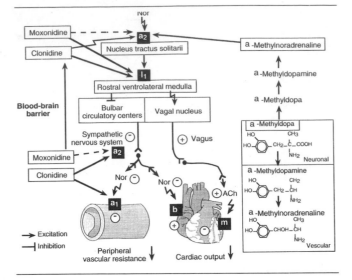

Figure 1. *The sites of action of the major centrally acting antihypertensive drugs are illustrated. Drugs such as moxonidine (and rilmenidine) have their primary action on imidazoline (I_1) receptors in the rostral ventrolateral medulla, with less effect on α_2-adrenoceptors in the nucleus tractus solitarii and the locus ceruleus (not shown). Clonidine has balanced effects on both I_1, and α_2-adrenoceptors, while α-methyladrenaline (the metabolite of α-methyldopa) chiefly exerts an effect on the α_2-adrenoceptors (From Palm D, Hellenbrecht D, Quiring K. Pharmakologie noradrenerger und adrenerger systeme. In: Forth W, Henschler D, Rummel W, Starke K, eds.: Allemeine und Spezielle Pharmacologie und Toxikologie. Manheim, Germany: BI Wissenschaftsverlag, 1992: 148–199.*

Following oral administration, moxonidine is rapidly (t-max around 1 hour) and almost completely absorbed from the gastrointestinal tract. the absolute bioavailability of the oral dosage form is approximately 88%.[6] The metabolites are not pharmacologically active. The drug passes into maternal milk and is excreted mainly by the kidney. About 60%–80% of the orally administered moxonidine dose is excreted as unchanged drug into the urine. Renal impairment reduces the renal clearance of moxonidine, resulting in increased AUC and C_{max} values. Moxonidine absorption is not affected by ingestion of food and does not interact with hydrochlorothiazide, digoxin or moclobemide. An interaction with lorazepam was observed in that co-administration showed impairment of cognitive function greater than had been predicted when the two compounds were considered separately.

Onset of moxonidine's action is gradual. Moxonidine decreases blood pressure in a dose-dependent fashion, with the greatest reductions seen after four hours and lasting up to seven hours after dosing. Moxonidine reduces plasma norepinephrine and epinephrine and plasma renin activity at rest and with exercise. It also reduces peripheral vascular resistance, and cardiac output remains unaffected or shows a slight increase.

At present, the recommended initial dose of moxonidine in patients with stages 1 and 2 hypertension is 0.2 mg once daily, and the maximum recommended daily dose is 0.6 mg. The drug is usually titrated according to individual response.

Rilmenidine

Rilmenidine[7,8] acts via the central nervous system and interacts preferentially with imidazoline receptors. Its pharmacological profile is similar to that of moxonidine, and it is administered daily in 1- or 2-mg doses.

Clonidine

Clonidine, an imidazoline compound, acts on both the I_1 receptor (30%) and the α_2-adrenoceptor (70%) in the central nervous system. The initial dose of clonidine is 0.1 mg twice daily, and therapeutic doses have generally ranged from 0.2 mg to 0.6 mg daily.

α-methyldopa

α-methyldopa is initially dosed at 250 mg once or twice daily, with a recommended maximum of 2 g daily. Although α-methyldopa is an effective antihypertensive, the drug is no longer recommended as a basic treatment because of the frequency of side effects, which include sedation (20% to 30%), fatigue, mouth dryness, and nasal congestion (10% to 75%), depression, dizziness, dyspnea, orthostatic hypotension, and diarrhea.

Treatment of Hypertension

The use of centrally acting drugs to treat patients with primary systemic arterial hypertension has great appeal due to evidence that supports the role of the autonomic nervous system in the pathogenesis and maintenance of the disease. Moreover, increased activity of the sympathetic nervous system increases the kidneys' production of renin, the rate-limiting enzyme for the renin-angiotensin-aldosterone system, which also plays a role in the development and maintenance of hypertension.

The centrally acting antihypertensives currently available in the United States, i.e., α-methyldopa and clonidine, are recommended only as supplemental antihypertensive agents for more severe hypertension, primarily because of the side effects of sedation and dry mouth, which while not dangerous, adversely influence the patient's quality of life.[9] Additionally, the adverse effect of so-called "rebound" hypertension upon withdrawal, particularly of clonidine, has been a major limiting factor for many physicians. Thus, the following discussion will deal primarily with the newer antihypertensive drugs, moxonidine and rilmenidine, which have far fewer side effects and are currently more likely to achieve greater widespread usage than have clonidine and α-methyldopa (Figure 2).[10]

Although not yet approved for use in the United States, moxonidine has been shown to be effective in reducing systemic arterial blood pressure in hypertensive subjects in both placebo-controlled and comparative clinical trials. Moxonidine has a similar effect on 24-hour blood pressure, whether administered as 0.4 mg once daily or 0.2 mg bid. Importantly, moxonidine attenuates the morning rise in blood

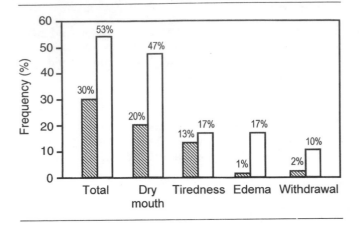

Figure 2. *A comparison of adverse events during therapy with moxonidine (black column) and clonidine (white column) are shown. The significantly lower frequency of adverse effects with moxonidine are reflective of the preponderance of action at the imidazoline receptors rather than the α_2-adrenoceptors.*

pressure and lowers blood pressure by decreasing peripheral vascular resistance. A 26% to 33.5% reduction in plasma norepinephrine and a 23% to 35.5% reduction in plasma renin activity occurred 4 to 6 hours after single oral doses of moxonidine. Compared with clonidine, moxonidine lowered blood pressure to a similar degree but with fewer adverse side effects, i.e., dry mouth and fatigue. Importantly, discontinuation of moxonidine therapy was not associated with an "overshoot" of blood pressure and heart rate during the withdrawal period. The antihypertensive efficacy of moxonidine was similar to that observed for diuretics (hydrochlorothiazide), β-adrenoceptor antagonists (atenolol), calcium channel blockers (nifedipine), angiotensin I-converting enzyme (ACE) inhibitors (enalapril, captopril) or α-adrenoceptor antagonists (prazosin). Moxonidine therapy reduces standing blood pressure to levels similar to those of supine or sitting blood pressure and attenuates the blood pressure increase associated with physical exercise. Data from uncontrolled studies suggest that moxonidine has no adverse effects on lipid or glucose metabolism and, in fact, may lower plasma glucose in patients with diabetes mellitus.

Regression of left ventricular hypertrophy in hypertensives following treatment with moxonidine after 6 months of treatment and interventricular septal thickness, measured by magnetic resonance imaging, decreased by 15%.[11]

Rilmenidine has been shown to lower blood pressure as effectively as clonidine, beta-blockers, and hydrochlorothiazide; it does not produce orthostatic hypotension, and the incidence of dry mouth, drowsiness, and constipation with rilmenidine use is two- to threefold lower than it is with the other 3 drugs. The 1- and 2-mg doses of rilmenidine are equivalent to the 0.15 mg and 0.3 mg doses of clonidine and, at equipotent doses, side effects were fewer with rilmenidine than with clonidine. Rilmenidine therapy is not associated with changes in blood glucose, urea, potassium, uric acid, or creatinine, and cholesterol and triglycerides exhibited a mild decrease in elderly patients and patients with diabetes or dyslipidemia. Rilmenidine has been found to decrease left ventricular hypertrophy and to increase arterial compliance.

TREATMENT OF HEART FAILURE

The use of clonidine in the treatment of heart failure has been reported to produce favorable hemodynamic changes attributed to the drug's ability to decrease sympathetic outflow, decrease parasympathetic nervous system activity, and decrease activity of the renin-angiotensin system.[12] These effects occur up acute administration and continue throughout long-term use.[13] Moxonidine also has favorable hemodynamic and neurohumoral effects in patients with heart failure[14] and is now being evaluated for use in treating heart failure; a large-scale mortality and morbidity trial of Moxcon was initiated in mid-1998.

CONCLUSION

It has long been suspected that abnormalities of autonomic nervous system activity might play a pivotal role in the pathogenesis of hypertension and other cardiovascular conditions, e.g., heart failure. The pioneering use of centrally acting drugs such as clonidine and methyldopa provided encouraging data that lent much credence to the concept of centrally mediated abnormalities in hypertension. Unfortunately, these early drugs were associated with adverse side effects that, while not totally excluding them from use, clearly reduced enthusiasm for their widespread application.

The exciting pharmacological discovery of the new generation of drugs that are selective for the imidazoline group of receptors and are associated with fewer side effects has rekindled enthusiasm for incorporating these drugs into the therapeutic armamentarium as first-line treatments for hypertension and perhaps eventually for the treatment of heart failure.

REFERENCES

1. Schrader J, Schoel G, Gundlach K, Scholz M, Scheler F. Antihypertensive Wirkdauer und morgendlicher Blutdruckanstieg unter Moxonidin in der ambulanten 24-Stunden-Blutdruck-messung. Nieren-und Hochdruckkrankheiten 1992;21: 531–533.

2. Reis DJ. The rostral ventrolateral medulla: a target of therapy for hypertension. In: Julius S, Philipp Th, eds. Sympathetic overstimulation and hypertension: imidazoline receptor agonists. Berlin: Saned, 1994;19–31.

3. Ernsberger P, Friedman JE, Koletsky RJ. The I_1-imidazoline receptor: from binding site to therapeutic target in cardiovascular disease. J Hypertens 1997;15(Suppl. 1):S9–S23.

4. Schafers RF, Philipp T. Moxonidine in hypertension treatment: a clinical summary. In: Julius S, Philipp Th, eds. Sympathetic over-stimulation and hypertension: imidazoline receptor agonists. Berlin: Saned, 1994;77–95.

5. Prichard BNC, Graham BR. The use of moxonidine in the treatment of hypertension. J Hypertens 1997;15(Suppl. 1):S47–S55.

6. Yu A, Frishman WH. Imidazoline receptor agonist drugs: a new approach to the treatment of systemic hypertension. J Clin Pharmacol 1996;36:98–111.

7. Reid JL, Panfiloz V, MacPhee G, Elliott HL. Clinical pharmacology of drugs acting on imidazoline and adrenergic receptors. Studies with clonidine, moxonidine, rilmenidine, and atenolol. Ann New York Acad Sci 763:1995;673–678.

8. Verbeuren TJA, Xuan TD, Konig-Berard, Viton P. Rilmenidine. Cardiovasc Drug Rev. 1990;8:56–70.

9. The Sixth Report of the Joint National Committee on Prevention, Detection, Evaluation, and Treatment of High Blood Pressure. Arch Intern Med 1997;157:2413–2446.

10. Planitz V. Comparison of moxonidine and clonidine HCI in treating patients with hypertension. J Clin Pharmacol 1987;27:446–451.

11. Eichstädt H, Richter W. Bäder W, et al. Demonstration of hypertrophy regression with magnetic resonance imaging under the new adrenergic inhibitor moxonidine (abstract). Cardiovasc Drug Ther 1989;3(Suppl. 2): 583.

12. Giles TD, Iteld BJ, Mautner RK, Rognoni PA, Dillenkoffer RL. Short-term effects of intravenous clonidine in congestive heart failure. Clin Pharmacol Ther 1981;30:724–728.

13. Manolis AJ, Olympios C, Sifaki M, Handanis S, Bresnahan M, Gavras I, Gavras H. Suppressing sympathetic activation in congestive heart failure: a new therapeutic strategy. Hypertension 1995;26: 719–724.

14. Mitrovic W, Neutzner J, Huthing J, Thormann J, Schlepper M. Hemodynamic and neurohumoral effects of alpha-2 agonist moxonidine in patients with dilated cardiomyopathy. Revue Europeene de Biotechnologie Medicale 1990;12(abstract):159.

CHAPTER 11

Alpha₁-Blockers

Norman M. Kaplan

The Sixth Joint National Committee Report includes alpha-blockers as appropriate choices for initial therapy of patients with a variety of concomitant conditions including dyslipidemia and prostatism.[1] In addition, their ability to increase insulin sensitivity makes them attractive for treatment of patients with non-insulin dependent diabetes mellitus.[2]

MECHANISM OF ACTION

Alpha₁-blockers are vasodilators, acting both on arterioles and veins.[3] The specificity for alpha-adrenoreceptors induces relaxation of vascular smooth muscle with little reflex stimulation of cardiac output because cathecholamine release is modulated via nonblocked alpha₂-receptors (Figure 1).[5] As a result, peripheral resistance falls during rest and during various cardiovascular stresses, while cardiac output remains unchanged or slightly increased and cardiovascular reflex-control mechanisms are well maintained.[4] These favorable hemodynamic effects have been well demonstrated during exercise, when they particularly contrast with the effects of beta-adrenergic receptor blockers,[5] which often are poorly tolerated by athletes.

As stated in a review of peripheral adrenergic receptors in hypertension, "considerable evidence suggests that altered postjunctional sensitivity to adrenergic stimulation contributes to the overall increase in sympathoadrenal activity in the hypertensive state"(p.108).[6] Because alpha-blockers inhibit the postsynaptic receptor response to catecholamines, they may lower blood pressure by modulating a basic mechanism involved in the pathogenesis of hypertension. This makes these agents particularly attractive in patients characterized by an increased vascular resistance due to enhanced

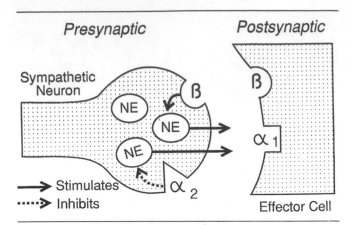

Figure 1. Schematic view of the action of prazosin as a postsynaptic alpha-blocker. By blocking the alpha₁-adrenergic receptor on the vascular smooth muscle, catecholamine-induced vasoconstriction is inhibited. The alpha₂-receptor on the neuronal membrane is not blocked; therefore, inhibition of additional norepinephrine release by the short feedback mechanism is maintained. Adapted from Kaplan NM. Clinical hypertension, 7th ed. Baltimore: Williams & Wilkins, 1998.

smooth muscle tone, before distinct structural changes in the arterioles have taken place.

PHARMACOLOGICAL PROPERTIES

The antihypertensive actions of various alpha-blockers differ according to their pharmacokinetic and pharmacodynamic properties.[7] These properties have been examined for prazosin, the first and only member of this class available for over 10 years; terazosin, introduced in 1987; and doxazosin, which became available in 1991.

Terazosin and doxazosin are less lipid-soluble and have half or less of the affinity for alpha₁-receptors than does prazosin. For these and other reasons, they induce a less rapid and less profound initial fall in blood pressure, particularly after standing, than does prazosin. This may translate into differences in the propensity for first-dose and subsequent hypotensive symptoms and certainly provides for a longer duration of action for the second-generation alpha₁-blockers. Whereas sustained, 24-hour reduction in blood pressure has been shown only with two daily doses of prazosin 12 hours apart,[8] once-daily doses of either terazosin[9] or doxazosin[10] provide 24-hour antihypertensive action.

ANTIHYPERTENSIVE EFFICACY

All agents approved by the U.S. Food and Drug Administration for the treatment of hypertension must be both "safe and efficacious." At present, efficacy is judged solely by assessing the surrogate endpoint; that is, the fall in blood pressure by millimeters of mercury. However, this relative efficacy of alpha-blockers versus other approved antihypertensive agents has been questioned.[3] Therefore, we have critically reviewed the available literature with a particular focus on the effectiveness of alpha₁-blockers as monotherapy in mild-to-moderate essential hypertension in placebo-controlled, randomized, double-blind trials, mostly involving fairly large numbers of patients.

Prazosin

Previously published reviews[11] have amply documented the efficacy of prazosin monotherapy in the treatment of mild-to-moderate hypertension since it was introduced in 1976. Data from four trials[12–15] are provided in Table 1. In addition, multiple comparative studies have shown that, in variable doses, prazosin has an antihypertensive effect that is virtually equal to the effects of various other antihypertensive agents.[2]

Of additional interest are two interrelated issues: the propensity for fluid retention and the maintenance of the antihypertensive effect. In studies of small groups of patients with mild-to-moderate hypertension, relatively small increases in plasma and extracellular fluid volumes have been observed in patients receiving prazosin for 8 to 24 weeks.[13,16] Despite these increases, the antihypertensive efficacy was generally well maintained, although a lesser overall fall in blood pressure occurred in those patients with greater increases in fluid volume. Addition of a diuretic will enhance the antihypertensive efficacy of prazosin.[17]

The antihypertensive effect has been found to persist over periods of one to seven years in retrospective, uncontrolled studies reported from New Zealand[18] and Australia.[19] In these analyses, the majority of patients given prazosin alone or in combination with other drugs had little loss of efficacy with constant doses of the drugs.

In summary, prazosin has generally been found to be effective, equal to other agents, and rarely accompanied by a loss of efficacy. Moreover, when used as a third agent in patients whose hypertension was controlled by a diuretic and a beta-blocker, prazosin has been equal in efficacy and overall patient acceptance to hydralazine or nifedipine.[20] In this and in many other studies, the final dose of prazosin has been 10 mg or more, considerably more than many physicians have prescribed, so the perception of lesser effectiveness may reflect the use of submaximal doses.

Terazosin

The efficacy of terazosin monotherapy versus placebo is comparable to that reported in other studies with prazosin[21,31] (Table 2).

Doxazosin

This long-acting alpha₁-blocker has been found to lower both systolic and diastolic blood pressure approximately 10 mm Hg in multiple groups of patients with mild-to-moderate hypertension[10,23–25] (Table 2). In the multicenter trial reported by Cox et al.,[23] the drug was equally effective in patients over age 65 and in younger patients, as well as in both black and nonblack patients.

TABLE 1. ANTIHYPERTENSIVE EFFICACY OF PRAZOSIN VS PLACEBO.

Source, year	Agent	No. of Patients	Follow-up, week	Dose, mg/d	Baseline Supine BP,* mm Hg	Reduction in BP at End of Study
Mroczek et al. 1974[12]	Prazosin	21	12	16[†]	156/101	-16/-9
	Placebo	18	12	16	155/99	+1/+1
Mulvihil-Wilson et al. 1979[13]	Prazosin	11[‡]	4	1 to 15	118[§]	-11
	Placebo	11	4	1 to 15	121	+5
McNair et al. 1980[14]	Prazosin	12[‡]	4	1 to 20	176/108	-10/-7
	Placebo	12	4	1 to 20	172/107	-4/-1
Torvik and Madsbu. 1986[15]	Prazosin	57	4	0.5 to 10	161/103	-10/-9
	Placebo	57	4	0.5 to 10	158/103	-3/-4

* BP indicates blood pressure.
† Mean dose
‡ Cross-over study where patients were their own controls
§ Mean arterial pressure
From Khoury AF, Kaplan NM. Alpha-blocker therapy of hypertension: An unfulfilled promise. JAMA 1991;266:394–398.

TABLE 2. ANTIHYPERTENSIVE EFFICACY OF TERAZOSIN OR DOXAZOSIN VS PLACEBO.

Source, year	Agent	No. of Patients	Follow-up, week	Dose, mg/d	Baseline Supine BP,* mm Hg	Reduction in BP at End of Study
Dauer. 1986[21]	Terazosin	38	4	1 to 40	152/101	-9/-9
	Placebo	26	4	1 to 40	147/99	-3/-5
Luther et al. 1990[22] (black patients)	Terazosin	168	4 to 13	2 to 40	153/102	-6/-6
	Placebo	99	4 to 13	2 to 40	153/101	-1/-3
Luther et al. 1990[22] (white patients)	Terazosin	290	4 to 13	2 to 40	152/100	-8/-8
	Placebo	194	4 to 13	2 to 40	154/100	-2/-3
Cox et al. 1986[23]	Doxazosin	378	9 to 24	1 to 16	159/101	-10/-9
	Placebo	172	9 to 24	1 to 16	155/101	-1/-3
Smyth et al. 1988[10]	Doxazosin	20	9	1 to 16	163/102	-10/-10
	Placebo	18	9	1 to 16	168/103	-1/-2
Scott et al. 1988[24]	Doxazosin	26	10	1 to 16	181/105	-6/-10
	Placebo	26	10	1 to 16	181/105	0/-4.8
Ames and Kiyasu. 1989[25]	Doxazosin	73	10	1 to 16	157/100	-9/-6
	Placebo	74	10	1 to 16	154/101	0/-2
Neaton et al. 1993[27]	Doxazosin	134	208	2 to 4	141/91	-14/-12
	Placebo	234	208	2 to 4	141/91	-9/-9

*BP indicates blood pressure.
From Khoury AF, Kaplan NM. α-blocker therapy of hypertension: An unfulfilled promise. JAMA 1991; 266:394-398.

No tolerance to the antihypertensive effect of doxazosin was found over 5 years in patients in an open, long-term extension of a one year randomized, double-blind, parallel comparison to atenolol.[26] The average reductions in blood pressure at 5 years were –16/–17 mm Hg on a mean dose of 62.5 mg per day of atenolol and –14/–14 mm Hg on a mean dose of 5.1 mg of doxazosin. Adverse effects and withdrawals from therapy were similar for those two agents. The Treatment of Mild Hypertension Study (TOMHS) has demonstrated in a 4-year followup that doxazosin lowered arterial pressure to the same extent as antihypertensive agents from other drug classes.[27] In contrast to the other agents, however, doxazosin exerted a statistically significant favorable effect on lipoproteins.[28]

Comparison between agents

In two double-blind studies, two of the three agents have been compared against each other and a placebo.[9,15] Both of the newer agents, terazosin and doxazosin, given once daily, were slightly more effective than was prazosin given twice daily, providing about a 2 mm Hg greater fall in supine and standing blood pressures.

Side Effects

The side effects of the three are similar in type, but the most bothersome side effects, first-dose hypotension and syncope, are less common with terazosin and doxazosin than with prazosin, probably because they are slower in onset of action and, therefore, do not induce abrupt falls in blood pressure.[11] Overall, postural syncope has been reported in fewer than 2% of patients given either of these agents.[11] Nonetheless, standing blood pressures should be monitored, particularly if postural symptoms are experienced.

First-dose hypotension was rather frequently seen when prazosin was initially started at a dose of 2 mg, particularly when added to a diuretic or to a low-sodium diet.[29] In the clinical trials with doxazosin involving over 1,500 patients, no syncopal episodes occurred at the starting dose of 1 mg.[11]

Beyond orthostatic dizziness, the most commonly reported side effects are fatigue, headache, palpitations, and nausea, each reported in about 5% of patients. Most of these symptoms are fairly mild and tend to diminish in severity with continued use of the drugs. Withdrawal rates from both terazosin and doxazosin are between 5% and 10%.[11] Compared to other classes of antihypertensive agents, rates of withdrawal from therapy because of side effects have been fairly close.[23]

Moreover, in the only randomized, placebo-controlled study of a representative agent from all five major classes of antihypertensive drugs, the alpha-blocker doxazosin was the only one which was associated with less sexual dysfunction than placebo.[30]

Despite the propensity to postural hypotension, the hemodynamic effects of alpha-blockade do not interfere with the rise in cardiac output during exercise, and there is no interference with exercise ability.[5]

EFFECTS ON SERUM LIPIDS

All three alpha-blockers have been repeatedly and almost uniformly shown to significantly lower serum total and low-density lipoprotein cholesterol and triglyceride levels and raise high-density lipoprotein cholesterol levels all by about 2% to 5%, resulting in a 5% to 10% decrease in the ratio of total cholesterol to high-density lipoprotein cholesterol.[28,31] The mechanisms for these virtually unique favorable effects on lipids among antihypertensive agents remain undefined, but numerous possibilities have been offered including (1) an increase in low-density lipoprotein receptor activity, as seen in cultured skin fibroblasts;[32] (2) an increase in lipoprotein lipase activity;[33] and (3) a decrease in the fractional catabolic rate of high-density lipoprotein cholesterol.[34]

In whatever manner they occur, these favorable influences on serum lipids are one of the major advantages of this class of drugs, in contradiction to the adverse effects noted with diuretics and most beta-blockers.[28,30]

EFFECTS ON PLATELET AGGREGATION

Doxazosin has been shown to inhibit platelet aggregation and favorably affect fibrinolysis.[35] Whether these effects are of clinical significance has not been determined.

EFFECTS ON INSULIN SENSITIVITY

A significant increase in insulin sensitivity measured by the euglycemic insulin clamp technique was found in 12 moderately obese normoglycemic hypertensive patients given prazosin for 12 weeks in an average daily dose of 5.3 mg with an attendant 14/9 mm Hg fall in standing blood pressure.[36] Similar findings have been demonstrated for doxazosin.[31]

USE IN PATIENTS WITH CONCOMITANT DISEASE

These generally favorable effects of lipid and glucose metabolism have been translated into clinical evidence that alpha$_1$-blockers may improve both diabetic control and dyslipidemias.[31,37-39] For example, in a double-blind, randomized, parallel study of doxazosin and hydrochlorothiazide in 107 patients, favorable effects on plasma lipids were seen with the alpha-blocker, whereas triglycerides increased and HDL-lipoprotein levels fell with HCTZ (Table 3).[38] The recent study by Ferrara et al.[39] clearly showed that even when compared with an ACE inhibitor, doxazosin had a more favorable effect on lipoproteins (Table 4).

Besides hypertensive patients with diabetes or dyslipidemia, alpha-blockers may be used safely in patients with bronchospasm or peripheral vascular disease, two other conditions in which the use of beta-blockers may be a problem.

TABLE 3. EFFECTS ON PLASMA LIPIDS OF DOXAZOSIN AND HYDROCHLOROTHIAZIDE (HCTZ).

Change (mg/dl)	Doxazosin (n = 50)	HCTZ (n = 48)
Total cholesterol (TC)	−8.4*	+1.3
High-density lipoprotein (HDL)	−1.3	−4.0‡
Low-density lipoprotein (LDL)	−5.4	+0.3
Triglycerides	−3.6	+22.8
HDL/TC ratio	+.004†	−.05

*p < .05; †p = .01; ‡p < .001

Modified from Grimm, RH, et al., reference 38.

TABLE 4. EFFECTS ON PLASMA LIPIDS OF LIPID PARAMETERS IN DOXAZOSIN AND CAPTOPRIL GROUPS.

	Doxazosin	Captopril
	Geometric Mean	Geometric Mean
Cholesterol (mg/dL)	223	233
Triglycerides (mg/dL)	111	120
HDL†-cholesterol (mg/dl)	36*	34
LDL‡-cholesterol (mg/dL)	159	168
HDL†-total cholesterol	0.16*	0.15*

*p < 0.08
† HDL indicates high-density lipoprotein.
‡ LDL indicates low-density lipoprotein.
Modified from Ferrara LA, Di Marino L., Russo O, et al. Doxazosin and captopril in mildly hypercholesterolemic hypertensive patients: The Doxazosin-Captopril in Hypercholesterolemic Hypertensives Study. Hypertension 1993;21:97–104.

No adverse effects on kidney function have been noted in patients with renal insufficiency who were given alpha-blockers,[40] but there are no long-term studies on the effect these agents may have on the progression of renal disease.

EFFECTS ON LEFT VENTRICULAR HYPERTROPHY

Left ventricular hypertrophy frequently occurs in untreated hypertensive patients and has been associated with a higher incidence of various cardiovascular complications. Regression of left ventricular hypertrophy has been documented with most antihypertensive agents, including the alpha-blockers prazosin,[41] terazosin,[42] and doxazosin.[27,43]

EFFECTS ON PROSTATIC OBSTRUCTION

Both terazosin[44] and doxazosin[45] provide excellent relief from the destructive symptoms of benign prostatic hypertrophy (BPH) and these agents are now generally the initial medical therapy for such patients. In those who are also hypertensive, the expected fall in blood pressure is noted;

whereas in those who are normotensive, little effect on blood pressure is seen.[45]

COMMENT

With prior concerns that the treatment of hypertension with diuretics and beta-blocker-based therapies had not provided the expected primary protection against coronary disease, the use of other classes of antihypertensive agents has been widely encouraged. The 1997 Joint National Committee Report[1] includes alpha-blockers as recommended choices for initial monotherapy, and the multiple advantages that these agents provide—particularly in their unique ability to improve other cardiovascular risk factors—lead us to conclude that they should be used more widely.

Their major drawback, postural hypotension, can be minimized by use of small initial doses of the slower-acting, newer agents, terazosin and doxazosin. A few patients may be unable to tolerate this or other side effects, although the total percentage of patients who cannot tolerate alpha-blockers is probably little different from that seen with other classes of drugs. The availability of second-generation alpha-blockers will likely lead to greater use of these agents in the treatment of hypertension in a manner that will maximally reduce overall cardiovascular risks while having favorable influences on concomitant conditions.

REFERENCES

1. The Sixth Report of the Joint National Committee on Prevention, Detection, Evaluation, and Treatment of High Blood Pressure. Arch Intern med 1997; 157:2413–2446.

2. Kaplan NM. Chapter 7: Primary hypertension:drugs. Treatment in clinical Hypertension, 7th ed. Williams & Wilkins, Baltimore, 1998.

3. Julius S. Are different hemodynamic patterns of antihypertensive drugs clinically important? Eur J Clin Pharmacol 1990;38(Suppl. 2):S125–S128.

4. Schäfers RF, Reid JL. Alpha blockers. In: Kaplan NM, Brenner BM, Laragh JH, eds. New therapeutic strategies in hypertension. New York: Raven, 1989: 51–69.

5. Thompson PD, Cullinane EM, Nugent AM, et al. Effect of atenolol or prazosin on maximal exercise performance in hypertensive joggers. Am J Med 1989;86(Suppl. 1B):104–109.

6. Michel MC, Brodde O-E, Insel PA. Peripheral adrenergic receptors in hypertension. Hypertension 1990;16:107–120.

7. Meredith PA, Elliott HL, Kelman AW, et al. Application of pharmacokinetic-pharmacodynamic modelling for the comparison of quinazoline a-adrenoceptor agonists in normotensive volunteers. J Cardiovasc Pharmacol 1985;7:532–537.

8. Weber MA, Tonkon MJ, Klein RC. Effect of antihypertensive therapy on the circadian blood pressure pattern. Am J Med 1987;82(Suppl. 1A):50–52.

9. Deter G, Cutler RE, Dietz AJ, et al. Comparison of the safety and efficacy of once-daily terazosin versus twice-daily prazosin for the

treatment of mild to moderate hypertension. Am J Med 1986;80(Suppl. 5B):62–67.

10. Smyth P, Pringle S, Jackson G, et al. 24-hour control of blood pressure by once daily doxazosin: A multicentre double-blind comparison with placebo. Eur J Clin Pharmacol 1988;34:613–618.

11. Humphreys JE, Waite MA. Alpha-1 blockers: A new generation of antihypertensive agents. J Clin Pharmacol Ther 1989;14:263–283.

12. Mroczek WJ, Fotiu S, Davidov ME, et al. Prazosin in hypertension: A double-blind evaluation with methyldopa and placebo. Curr Ther Res 1974;16:769–777.

13. Mulvihill-Wilson J, Graham RM, Pettinger W, et al. Comparative effects of prazosin and phenoxybenzamine on arterial blood pressure, heart rate, and plasma catecholamines in essential hypertension. J Cardiovasc Pharmacol 1979;1(Suppl. 6):S1–S7.

14. McNair A, Rasmussen S, Nielsen PE, et al. The antihypertensive effect of prazosin on mild to moderate hypertension, changes in plasma volume, extracellular volume and glomerular filtration rate. Acta Med Scand 1980;207:413–416.

15. Torvik D, Madsbu H-P. Multicentre 12-week double-blind comparison of doxazosin, prazosin and placebo in patients with mild to moderate essential hypertension. Br J Clin Pharmacol 1986;21: 69S–75S.

16. Bauer JH, Jones LB, Gaddy P. Effects of prazosin therapy on BP, renal function, and body fluid composition. Arch Intern Med 1984;144:1196–1200.

17. Colucci WS. Alpha-adrenergic receptor blockade with prazosin. Ann Intern Med 1982;97:67–77.

18. New Zealand Hypertension Study Group. Four- to seven-year follow-up of patients on prazosin. N Z Med J 1980;92:341–342.

19. Walker RG, Whitworth JA, Saines D, et al. Long-term treatment of moderate and severe hypertension and lack of 'tolerance.' Med J Aust 1981;2:146–147.

20. Ramsay LE, Parnell L, Waller PC. Comparison of nifedipine, prazosin, and hydralazine added to treatment of hypertensive patients uncontrolled by thiazide diuretic plus beta-blocker. Postgrad Med J 1987;63:99–103.

21. Dauer AD. Terazosin: an effective once-daily monotherapy for the treatment of hypertension. Am J Med 1986;80(Suppl.5B): 29–34.

22. Luther RR, Klepper MJ, Maurath CJ, et al. Effects of terazosin on serum lipid levels in hypertensive blacks. J Hum Hypertens 1990;4:154–156.

23. Cox DA, Leader JP, Milson JA, et al. The antihypertensive effects of doxazosin: A clinical overview. Br J Clin Pharmacol 1986;21: 83S–90S.

24. Scott PJ, Hosie J, Scott MG. A double-blind and cross-over comparison of once daily doxazosin and placebo with steady-state pharmacokinetics in elderly hypertensive patients. Eur J Clin Pharmacol 1988;34:119–123.

25. Ames RP, Kiyasu JY. Alpha-1 adrenoceptor blockade with doxazosin in hypertension: Effects on blood pressure and lipoproteins. J Clin Pharmacol 1989;29:123–127.

26. Daae LNW, Westlie L. A 5-year comparison of doxazosin and atenolol in patients with mild-to-moderate hypertension. Blood Pressure 1998;7:39–45.

27. Neaton JD, Grimm RH Jr, Prineas RJ, et al. for the Treatment of Mild Hypertension Study Research Group: Treatment of mild hypertension study. JAMA 1993;270:713–724.

28. Grimm RH Jr, Flack JM, Grandits GA, et al. Long-term effects on plasma lipids of diet and drugs to treat hypertension. Treatment of Mild Hypertension Study (TOMHS) Research Group. JAMA 1996; 275:1549–1556.

29. Stokes GS, Graham RM, Gain JM, et al. Influence of dosage and dietary sodium on the first-dose effects of prazosin. Br Med J 1977;1:1507–1508.

30. Grimm RH Jr, Grandits GA, Cutler JA, et al. Relationships of quality-of-life measures to long-term lifestyle and drug treatment in the Treatment of Mild Hypertension Study. Arch Intern Med 1997;157:633–648.

31. Andersson P-E, Lithell H. Metabolic effects of doxazosin and enalapril in hypertriglyceridemic, hypertensive men. Am J Hypertens 1996;9:323–333.

32. Leren TP. Doxazosin increases low density lipoprotein receptor activity. Acta Pharmacol Toxicol 1985;56:269–272.

33. Rubba P, De Simone B, Marotta T, et al. Adrenergic blocking agents and lipoprotein lipase activity. J Endocrinol Invest 1989;12:119–122.

34. Sheu WH, Swislocki AL, Hoffman BB, et al. Effect of prazosin treatment on HDL kinetics in patients with hypertension. Am J Hypertens 1990;3:761–768.

35. Jeng J-R, Sheulo H-H, Jeng C-Y, et al. Effect of doxazosin on fibrinolysis in hypertensive patients with and without insulin resistance. Am Heart J 1996;132:783–789.

36. Pollare T, Lithell H, Selinus I, et al. Application of prazosin is associated with an increase of insulin sensitivity in obese patients with hypertension. Diabetologia 1988;31:415–420.

37. Feher MD, Henderson AD, Wadsworth J, et al. Alpha-blocker therapy; a possible advance in the treatment of diabetic hypertension—results of a cross-over study of doxazosin and atenolol monotherapy in hypertensive non-insulin dependent diabetic subjects. J Hum Hypertens 1990;4:571–577.

38. Grimm RH, Flack JM, Schoenberger J, Gonzalez NM, Liebson P, et al. Alpha blockade and thiazide treatment of hypertension: A double-blind randomized comparison of doxazosin and hydrochlorothiazide. Am J Hypertens 1996;9:445–454.

39. Ferrara LA, Di Marino L, Russo O, et al. Doxazosin and captopril in mildly hypercholesterolemic hypertensive patients: The Doxazosin-Captopril in Hypercholesterolemia Hypertensive Study. Hypertension 1993;21:97–104.

40. Anderton JL, Notghi A. An evaluation of the efficacy and safety of doxazosin in the treatment of hypertension associated with renal insufficiency. J Hum Hypertens 1990;4(Suppl. 3):52–57.

41. Ram CV, Gonzalez D, Kulkarni P, et al. Regression of left ventricular hypertrophy in hypertension. Effects of prazosin therapy. Am J Med 1989;86(Suppl. 1B):66–69.

42. Yasumoto K, Takata M, Yoshida K, et al. Reversal of left ventricular hypertrophy by terazosin in hypertensive patients. J Hum Hypertens 1990;4:13–18.

43. Corral JL, López NC, Pecorelli A, et al. Doxazosin in the treatment of mild or moderate essential hypertension: An echocardiographic study. Am Heart J 1991;121(1 Pt. 2):352–356.

44. Lepor H, Williford WO, Barry MJ, et al. The efficacy of terazosin, finasteride, or both in benign prostatic hypertrophy. N Engl J Med 1996;335:533–539.

45. Lepor H, Kaplan SA, Klinberg I, Mobley DF, et al. Doxazosin for benign prostatic hyperplasma: long-term efficacy and safety in hypertensive and normotensive patients. J Urol 1997;157:525–530.

CHAPTER 12

Angiotensin-Converting Enzyme Inhibitors

Ehud Grossman
Yehonatan Sharabi

Angiotensin-converting enzyme (ACE) inhibitors were approved for the treatment of hypertension in the 1980s. These agents inhibit the generation of angiotensin II (A II) and thereby block the renin angiotensin system. Since their introduction they have become very popular and their use has increased dramatically because they are effective in lowering blood pressure; have a favorable hemodynamic and metabolic profile; protect the vascular tree, the heart, and the kidney; and are tolerated well with relatively few side effects. This chapter summarizes the clinical experience accumulated with ACE inhibitors in the management of hypertension and other cardiovascular disorders.

THE ROLE OF THE RENIN-ANGIOTENSIN-ALDOSTERONE (RAAS) SYSTEM IN THE PATHOGENESIS OF HYPERTENSION AND END ORGAN DAMAGE

The renin-angiotensin-aldosterone system (RAAS) participates in the regulation of blood pressure and fluid and electrolyte balance. This system responds mainly to low pressure in the afferent arterioles and sodium concentration in the macula densa; and also to beta adrenergic excitation and use of diuretics and vasodilating substances. Activation of this system leads to the formation of renin in the juxta glomerular apparatus that converts angiotensinogen, a protein derived from the liver, to the inactive peptide angiotensin I (A I). ACE converts A I to A II, and inactivates the potent vasodilator bradykinin that can induce cough and may stimulate the release of both vasodilating prostaglandins and nitric oxide.[1] ACE is produced predominantly in lung tissue, but it has been found in nearly all mammalian tissues.[1] There are 2 alleles—insertion/deletion (I/D)—of the ACE gene. The homozygous DD (deletion) genotype of the ACE gene has been associated with increased circulating levels of ACE. The D allele of the ACE gene is associated with microalbuminuria as well as with retinopathy and left ventricular hypertrophy, and seems to be an independent risk factor for target organ damage in essential hypertension.[2] The deletion polymorphism in the ACE gene reduces the long term beneficial effect of ACE inhibition on the progression of diabetic nephropathy in patients with insulin dependent diabetes.[3]

Enzymatic pathways independent of ACE which may contribute to the generation of A II have been described in many tissues including blood vessels and the heart.[4] The effects of A II at the type I (AT_1) receptor produces physiological consequences critical to the cardiovascular homeostasis, including vasoconstriction, sodium and fluid retention, augmentation of the sympathetic activity, cellular growth, and positive inotropic effect. The RAAS has been show to participate in the pathophysiology of systemic hypertension, congestive heart failure (CHF) and diabetic nephropathy.[5,6] There is evidence that activation of the RAAS may increase the risk of cardiovascular morbidity and mortality. Alderman et al.[7] showed that hypertensive patients with high renin levels exhibit a higher rate of cardiovascular morbidity and mortality. Therefore, blocking this system may lower blood pressure, improve heart failure, hinder deterioration of renal function in patients with diabetic nephropathy, and may also reduce cardiovascular morbidity and mortality.

PHARMACOLOGY

ACE inhibitors are a group of drugs that by binding to the ACE's zinc site inhibit its action (Table 1). The various drugs differ in the chemical group serving as the binding ligand to the enzyme's zinc site: sulphydryl carboxyl, and phosphoryl. They also differ in the pharmacokinetics, duration of action, prodrug activity, and tissue bioavailability. The clinical significance of the differences between the chemical classes has not been established.[8]

Most drugs (except captopril and lisinopril) are lipid-soluble prodrugs requiring hydrolysis after absorption to form the active ACE inhibitor. Peak serum concentration of the active compound is achieved for most drugs within 1 to 4 hours after oral administration. Captopril, an active drug, reaches a peak blood level within 30 to 60 minutes after oral ingestion and therefore became useful in the treatment of hypertensive urgency. Most drugs, except fosinopril and spirapril, are eliminated mainly through the kidney and therefore the dose should be reduced in patients with renal failure. Fosinopril has a balanced renal-hepatic excretion with increasing the proportion of hepatic excretion when renal impairment occurs, so that no decrease in dose is needed in the presence of renal impairment.[8] The drugs also differ in their ability to penetrate and bind to tissue ACE with quinapril, benazepril, and ramipril having the highest potency of binding to tissue ACE.[9] Evidence suggests that increased potency of binding to tissue ACE may provide a protective effect in local tissues, because structural changes

TABLE 1. VARIOUS ACE INHIBITORS.

Drug	Residue	Dosage* (min-max)	Adminis-tration	Elimi-nation
Benazepril	Carboxylic	5–40	o.d.	Renal
Captopril	Sulphydryl	12.5–150	t.i.d.	Renal
Cilazapril	Carboxylic	1–10	o.d.	Renal
Enalapril	Carboxylic	5–40	b.i.d.	Renal
Fosinopril	Phosphoryl	10–40	o.d.	Renal & Hepatic
Lisinopril	Carboxylic	5–40	o.d.	Renal
Moexipril	Carboxylic	7.5–30	o.d.	Renal
Perindopril	Carboxylic	1–16	o.d.	Renal
Quinapril	Carboxylic	5–80	o.d.	Renal
Ramipril	Carboxylic	1.25–20	o.d.	Renal
Trandolapril	Carboxylic	1–4	o.d.	Renal
Spirapril	Carboxylic	12.5–50	o.d.	Hepatic

*Dosage in mg.

occurring during the chronic state of hypertension, such as cardiovascular hypertrophy, are possibly mediated by activation of tissue ACE.

HYPOTENSIVE EFFECT OF ACE INHIBITION

ACE inhibitors reduce blood pressure by several mechanisms. The most clear one is the reduction of circulating levels of A II, thereby removing the direct vasoconstriction induced by this peptide. The reduction of circulating A II levels also decreases aldosterone secretion and blunts the increase in sympathetic activity thereby contributing to the antihypertensive effect of ACE inhibitors.[10] ACE inhibitors may also lower blood pressure by direct inhibiting vascular hypertrophy[11] and enhancing endothelium dependent relaxation.[12] In addition, they inhibit the degradation of bradykinin—a vasodilatatory and weak antiagregant peptide and enhance the synthesis of the vasodilatory prostaglandins.[13,14] These substances enhance the vasodilatation induced by ACE inhibitors but may also be responsible to the frequent cough and rare angioneurotic edema seen with ACE inhibitors use.

Essential Hypertension

Clinical studies demonstrated the efficacy of ACE inhibitors in lowering blood pressure.[15–18] They are more effective in patients with high-renin forms of hypertension, and may induce a dramatic fall in blood pressure in patients who are volume depleted by prior dietary sodium restriction or diuretic use.[19] Several studies showed that blacks, with lower renin levels as a group, respond less well to ACE inhibitors than do white hypertensives.[20] However, elderly hypertensive patients who also tend to have low renin levels respond well to ACE inhibitors.[17] The currently available ACE inhibitors seem comparable in their antihypertensive potency, although direct comparisons have not been made between them. Clinical studies point to comparable efficacy of ACE inhibitors with other antihypertensive agents.[17,21]

Renovascular Hypertension

In patients with renovascular hypertension, correction of the stenosis is the treatment of choice. However, in those who cannot undergo reconstructive surgery or angioplasty, ACE inhibitors may be effective since hypertension is induced by increased plasma renin activity. ACE inhibitors may impair function of the kidney behind the stenosis, since the glomerular filtration pressure in the affected kidney depends on the A-II-mediated vasoconstriction of the efferent arteriole. Therefore, in patients with bilateral renal artery stenosis or renal artery stenosis of a single kidney, ACE inhibitors may induce a deterioration in renal function. This phenomenon may be used to diagnose renal artery stenosis. The reduction in glomerular filtration rate (GFR) induced by ACE in-hibitors in the post-stenotic kidney results in an increase in plasma renin activity. Documenting exaggerated increase in plasma renin activity following captopril or an abnormal captopril renoscan suggest renal artery stenosis. A decrease in renal function following ACE inhibitors suggest bilateral artery stenosis or renal artery stenosis of a single kidney. Therefore, ACE inhibitors are contraindicated in patients with bilateral renal artery stenosis or renal artery stenosis of a single kidney. Rare cases of renin producing tumor and pheochromocytoma may respond well to treatment with ACE inhibitors.

Hypertensive Crisis

ACE inhibitors can be used in hypertensive urgency or emergency. The rapidly acting captopril is preferable to the other ACE inhibitors, and may be given either by the usual oral route or sublingually.[22-25] Sublingual captopril is well tolerated and effective in reducing blood pressure, the onset of action occurs within 5–10 minutes, reaching a maximum within 30 minutes and lasting for at least 2 hours. Following oral administration of captopril on an empty stomach, maximal blood pressure reduction is observed within 30–90 minutes.[22] The hypotensive response is usually not excessive unless the patient is volume depleted. Comparative trials have observed fewer side effects with captopril than with nifedipine administration,[26-31] and most studies concluded that captopril should be considered as a first line therapy in the acute management of hypertensive urgency.[26-31] However, no outcome data are available attesting to benefits of captopril in this clinical situation. Enalaprilat is the only available ACE inhibitor that can be administered intravenously. Enalaprilat rapidly lowers blood pressure within minutes in patients with severe hypertension, without causing excessive hypertension or adverse reactions. The initial recommended dose for enalaprilat is 0.625 to 1.25 mg administered over 5 minutes. The maximal single dose should not exceed 5 mg for patients receiving diuretics and 1.25 mg for patients with renal impairment.[32] The initial dose can be repeated after 1 hour if clinical response is inadequate. The total daily dose should not exceed 20 mg. In patients with severe renal insufficiency, the dose should be decreased because the compound is excreted primarily by the kidney. In patients with hypertensive emergency, the response rate is about 65%, with a higher rate of response in patients with high-renin forms of hypertension. Enalaprilat may be an alternative treatment for hypertensive emergency in patients with congestive heart failure. The most common adverse effect is hypotension. The risk for hypotension increases in patients with evidence of renal hypertension, volume depleted patients, and patients with prior use of diuretics. Enalaprilat can be easily replaced by oral enalaril for long-term maintenance therapy.

METABOLIC EFFECTS

Unlike diuretics and beta blockers, ACE inhibitors do not adversely affect lipid profile and insulin sensitivity in non-diabetic patients with hypertension.[33] In some small studies, ACE inhibitors even improved lipid profile and insulin sensitivity. Some evidence suggests that serum apolipoproteins A-I and A-II, major apolipoproteins of the high density lipoprotein fraction, are increased by ACE inhibition.[34] Interestingly, ACE inhibitors may actually prevent diuretic-induced hyperlipidemia and hyperglycemia.[35,36] ACE inhibitors do not stimulate the sympathetic nervous system, as heart rate does not increase and the plasma levels of adrenaline and noradrenaline do not increase or even decreased during treatment.[37] The inhibition of A II mediated aldosterone secretion by ACE inhibitors may lead to hyperkalemia, particularly in patients with underlying renal insufficiency who are given potassium sparing agents or potassium supplements.[38]

CARDIAC EFFECTS

Reduction of Left Ventricular Mass

Left ventricular hypertrophy (LVH) is a consequence of long-standing hypertension and is considered to be an independent risk factor for cardiovascular morbidity and mortality.[39] Whether reduction of LVH improves morbidity and mortality has to be documented, but indirect evidence suggests that it may be beneficial.[40] Antihypertensive agents are capable to regress LVH but not all agents are equipotent in this regard.[41] A II and aldosterone accelerate myocardial hypertrophy and fibrosis[42] and therefore blocking the RAAS should be the ultimate way to reduce left ventricular mass. Indeed, in a recent study, Gottdiener et al.[43] showed that diuretics and ACE inhibitors are both equipotent in reducing left ventricular mass (LVM). However, the investigators used as an ACE inhibitor captopril twice daily; that does not control blood pressure throughout the day and even so, only captopril reduced LVM significantly. Dahlof et al.[44] studied by meta-analysis the effect of antihypertensive pharmacological therapy on LVM. The absolute reductions in ventricular mass were 44.7 grams for ACE inhibitors, 26.9 grams for calcium antagonists, 22.8 grams for beta-blockers, and 21.4 grams for diuretics. A recent meta-analysis, reviewing 39 double blind clinical studies done until July 1995, showed clearly that ACE inhibitors reduce LVM more than all other antihypertensive agents.[45]

Congestive Heart Failure

Congestive heart failure (CHF) is one of the sequela of long standing hypertension. There is good evidence that increased levels of A II and aldosterone with vasoconstriction and sodium retention have negative effects in CHF. Therefore, blocking the RAAS with ACE inhibitors would be beneficial. Several studies have shown that patients with CHF especially due to systolic dysfunction, either symptomatic or asymptomatic, and an ejection fraction of less than 35% who received an ACE inhibitor showed a statistically significant reduction in mortality compared with patients who did not receive an ACE inhibitor.[46–48]

In the SAVE study, patients with a myocardial infarction and ejection fraction less than 40% in the postinfarction period benefited significantly when an ACE inhibitor was given in addition to routine therapy.[46] Deaths from cardiovascular causes, recurrent myocardial infarction, and CHF were reduced. The reduction in total mortality is dependent on pretreatment ejection fraction.[48] A meta-analysis of 16 randomized trials showed that a significant reduction in total mortality was observed only in patients with an ejection fraction of less than 25%.[48]

RENAL EFFECTS

The natural course of essential hypertension and hypertension associated with advanced renal parenchymal disease, is characterized by a progressive deterioration of renal function.[49] Hypertension can accelerate renal deterioration in diabetic patients. Reduction of arterial pressure was shown to reduce urinary excretion of albumin and to attenuate renal deterioration in diabetic patients.[50] Recent studies demonstrated that ACE inhibitors have beneficial effects on renal function above and beyond those simply due to blood pressure control.[51–56] Ravid et al.[51] showed that enalapril may attenuate renal deterioration in normotensive patients with non-insulin-dependent diabetes mellitus and microalbuminuria. Viberti et al.[53] showed that captopril treatment impedes progression to clinical proteinuria and prevents the increase in albumin excretion rate in nonhypertensive patients with insulin-dependent diabetes mellitus and persistent microalbuminuria.

Recently it was shown that the ACE inhibitor lisinopril slows the progression of renal disease in normotensive insulin-dependent diabetic patients, even if they have no albuminuria.[54] Lewis et al.[52] showed that in normotensive or hypertensive patients with insulin-dependent diabetes mellitus and nephropathy, treatment with the ACE inhibitor, captopril, reduced the risk of doubling the serum creatinine concentration by 48%. Captopril treatment was also associated with a 50% reduction in the risk of the combined end points of death, dialysis, and transplantation. The reduction in risk was the greatest in a subgroup of patients with elevated baseline serum creatinine. In a meta-analysis of 100 studies providing data on renal function, proteinuria, or both—before and after treatment with an antihypertensive agent—Kasiske et al.[55] showed that ACE inhibitors decreased proteinuria independent of changes in blood pressure, treatment duration, and the type of diabetes or stage of nephropathy. In comparison with other antihypertensive agents, ACE inhibitors had an additional favorable effect on GFR that was independent of blood pressure changes. The renoprotective effects of ACE inhibitors in diabetic nephropathy are related to a selective vasodilation of the efferent arteriole that reduce the capillary intraglomerular pressure. Recently it has been shown that ACE inhibitors may provide protection against the progression of renal insufficiency in patients with nondiabetic renal disease.[57-59]

In a prospective, double-blind, randomized study, Maschio et al.[57] showed that in patients with various underlying renal diseases the ACE inhibitor benazapril reduced the doubling of the baseline serum creatinine concentration or the need for dialysis by 53%. In another study, it has been shown that the ACE inhibitor, ramipril, can reduce proteinuria and the rate of GFR decline in patients with nondiabetic proteinuric nephropathy with proteinuria of 3 g or more per 24 hours.[58] In a recent meta-analysis including 1,594 patients in 10 studies, Giatras et al.[59] showed that ACE inhibitors are more effective than other antihypertensive agents in reducing the development of end-stage nondiabetic renal disease (pooled relative risk was 0.70). Thus, it seems that blocking the RAAS by inhibition of the ACE produces a renoprotective effect in diabetic nephropathy and in proteinuric nondiabetic glomerulopathy.

TOLERABILITY AND PROFILE OF SIDE EFFECTS

ACE inhibitors are safe and well tolerated with relatively low rate of adverse events. Monane et al.[60] showed recently that elderly hypertensive patients comply better with ACE inhibitors than with other antihypertensive agents. The overall rate of side effects with ACE inhibitors is about 10% to 20% with dry, nonproductive cough, that may occur in 5–20%, as the most frequent and troublesome one.[61] Angionurotic edema is less common and was reported in 1–2% of the treated patients.[62] First-dose hypotension may occur with ACE inhibitors particularly in patients who are volume depleted.[19] Other side effects include elevation of serum potassium particularly in patients with underlying renal insufficiency who are treated with potassium supplements or potassium sparing agents.[38] Deterioration of renal function may occur mainly in patients with renal artery stenoses, either bilateral or in a solitary kidney.[62] Some specific side effects such as taste disturbances, rash, and leukopenia, have been reported, but are infrequent. Rare side effects are pancreatitis and other gastrointestinal effects, hypoglycemia, and central nervous system abnormalities. Nonspecific side effects such as headache, dizziness, fatigue, diarrhea, and nausea are listed but usually do not cause a problem. ACE inhibitors are contraindicated in pregnancy because they cause fetal injury and death,[63] but it appears relatively safe in lactating mothers with nursing infants.[64] The relative incidence of side effects is fairly close among the various ACE inhibitors. However, in one meticulous study, captopril was superior to enalapril in quality life measure.[65]

COMBINATION WITH OTHER ANTIHYPERTENSIVE AGENTS

Less than 50% of hypertensive patients will achieve goal blood pressure (< 140/90 mm Hg) with ACE inhibitors as monotherapy.[17,66] Most of these patients will require addition of other agents.[66] Combination of hydrochlorothiazide and ACE inhibitors should produce an additive hypotensive effect, because the two classes of drugs have complementary and different pharmacologic mechanisms of action.[67] Diuretics stimulate the renin-angiotensin system and blocking this system is more effective when the system is activated. ACE inhibitors attenuate the decrease in serum potassium observed with hydrochlorothiazide alone, and may offset the diuretic-induced insulin resistance.[68] Combination of ACE inhibitors and calcium antagonists may better protect the kidney in diabetic patients, and may reduce the rate of calcium antagonists-induced leg edema.[69] ACE inhibitors were also combined successfully with beta or alpha blockers. The combination with beta blockers seems to be less effective in reducing blood pressure since these agents suppress the renin-angiotensin system. However, this combination is recommended in patients after myocardial infarction and in patients with congestive heart failure wherein low dose beta blockers therapy has shown promise.

DRUG INTERACTION

Nonsterioidal anti-inflammatory drugs (NSAID) may abolish the hypotensive effect of ACE inhibitors, because some of the ACE inhibitors' effects are mediated through prostaglandins synthesis. The combination of NSAID and ACE inhibitors may be particularly nephrotoxic because they dilate afferent and efferent arterioles, respectively, thereby reducing the GFR. Antacids may also decrease efficacy of ACE inhibitors.[70] Concomitant treatment of ACE inhibitors with potassium-sparing agents, potassium supplements, or cyclosporin increase the risk of hyperkalemia, particularly in diabetic patients and in patients with renal insufficiency.[70]

ACE inhibitors may increase plasma lithium levels and may precipitate lithium toxicity.

PRACTICAL CLINICAL USE

ACE inhibitors can be used for initiating antihypertensive therapy. In subgroups of patients with congestive heart failure, post-myocardial infarction, left ventricular hypertrophy, diabetic nephropathy, and nondiabetic renal failure, ACE inhibitors should be considered as the first drug of choice. Treatment should be initiated with the lowest recommended dose, particularly in elderly patients, patients treated with diuretics, and patients with renal failure. The hypotensive effect may sometimes be observed only after 2 to 4 weeks and therefore the dose should be increased gradually in 2 to 4 week intervals. Renal function and serum potassium levels should be monitored in the first week of treatment and then twice a year. Mild hyperkalemia is common in medical outpatients using ACE inhibitors, especially in those with renal insufficiency or congestive heart failure. However, once hyperkalemia is identified during the use of ACE inhibitors, subsequent severe hyperkalemia is uncommon in patients younger than 70 years with normal renal function.[71] A close follow-up is required in patients with hyperkalemia. The expected response rate is less than 50% and a combination with diuretics or calcium antagonists is recommended when blood pressure is not well controlled on the maximal tolerated dose. For those patients who respond well to ACE inhibitors but do not tolerate the drug because of dry cough angiotensin II receptor antagonist seems to be an ideal substitute.

SUMMARY

ACE inhibitors are safe and effective in lowering blood pressure. In addition, these drugs have a favorable hemodynamic and metabolic profile and protect the vascular tree. The various drugs differ in their pharmacokinetics, duration of action, prodrug activity, and tissue bioavailability. The overall rate of side effects with ACE inhibitors is low, with dry, nonproductive cough that may occur in 5–20%, as the most frequent and troublesome one. Indeed there are no prospective studies showing that this class of drugs reduce morbidity and mortality in hypertensive patients. However, there is compelling evidence that ACE inhibitors are beneficial in subgroups of patients with congestive heart failure, post-myocardial infarction, diabetic nephropathy, and nondiabetic renal failure. Use of ACE inhibitors as the first drug of choice in these patients seems to be justified.

REFERENCES

1. Rosendorff C. The renin-angiotensin system and vascular hypertrophy. J Am Coll Cardiol 1996;28:803–812.

2. Pontremoli R, Sofia A, Tirotta A, Ravera M, Nicolella C, Viazzi F, Bezante GP, Borgia L, Bobola N, Ravazzolo R, Sacchi G, Deferrari G.

The deletion polymorphism of the angiotensin I-converting enzyme gene is associated with target organ damage in essential hypertension. J Am Soc Nephrol 1996;7;2550–2558.

3. Parving HH, Jacobsen P, Tarnow L, et al. Effect of deletion polymorphism of angiotensin converting enzyme gene on progression of diabetic nephropathy during inhibition of angiotensin converting enzyme. BMJ 1996;313:591–594.

4. Urata H, Nishimura H, Ganten D, Arakawa K. Angiotensin-converting enzyme-independent pathways of angiotensin II formation in human tissues and cardiovascular diseases. Blood Press (Suppl.)1996;2:22–28.

5. Laragh JH, Baer L, Brunner HR, et al. Renin, angiotensin and aldosterone system in pathogenesis and management of hypertensive vascular disease. Am J Med 1972;52:633–652.

6. Curtiss C, Cohn JN, Vrobel T, Franciosa JA. Role of the renin-angiotensin system in the systemic vasoconstriction of chronic congestive heart failure. Circulation 1978;58:763–770.

7. Alderman MH, Madhavan S, Ooi WL, Cohen H, Sealey JE, Laragh JH. Association of the renin-sodium profile with the risk of myocardial infarction in patients with hypertension. N Engl J Med 1991;324:1098–1104.

8. Kaplan NM. Treatment of hypertension. In Kaplan NM (ed.) Clinical Hypertension. Williams & Wilkins. 1994;191–280.

9. Johnston CI, Fabris B, Yamada H, et al. Comparative studies of tissue inhibition by angiotensin converting enzyme inhibitors. J Hypertens 1990;7(Suppl. 5):S11–S16.

10. van den Meiracker AH, Man in't Veld AJ, Admiraal PJJ, et al. Partial escape of angiotensin converting enzyme (ACE) inhibition during prolonged ACE inhibitor treatment. J Hypertens 1992;10: 803–812.

11. Wang D-H, Prewitt RL. Captopril reduces aortic and microvascular growth in hypertensive and normotensive rats. Hypertension 1990;15:68–77.

12. Mombouli J-V, Nephtali M, Vanhoutte PM. Effects of the converting enzyme inhibitor cilazapril on endothelium-dependent responses. Hypertension 1991;18(Suppl. 4):II22–II29.

13. Gavras I. Bradykinin-mediated effects of ACE inhibition. Kidney Int 1992;42:1020–1029.

14. Quilley J. Duchin KL, Hudes EM, McGiff JC. The antihypertensive effect of captopril in essential hypertension: relationship to prostaglandins and the kallikrein-kinin system. J Hypertens 1987;5:121–128.

15. Grimm RH Jr, Flack JM, Grandits GA, et al. Long-term effects on plasma lipids of diet and drugs to treat hypertension. JAMA 1996;275:1549–1556.

16. Oren S, Messerli FH, Grossman E, Garavaglia GE, Frohlich ED. Immediate and short-term cardiovascular effects of fosinopril, a new angiotensin-converting enzyme inhibitor, in patients with essential hypertension. J Am Coll Cardiol 1991;17:1183–1187.

17. Materson BJ, Reda DJ, Cushman WC, et al. Single-drug therapy for hypertension in men. A comparison of six antihypertensive agents with placebo. N Engl J Med 1993;328:914–921.

18. Dunn FG, Oigman W, Ventura HO, Messerli FH, Kobrin I, Frohlich ED. Enalapril improves systemic and renal hemodynamics and allows regression of left ventribular mass in essential hypertension. Am J Cardiol 1984;53(1):105–108.

19. Postma CT, Dennesen PJW, de Boo T, Thien T. First dose hypotension after captopril; can it be predicted? A study of 240 patients. J Hum Hypertens 1992;6:205–209.

20. Saunders E, Weir MR, Kong BW, et al. A comparison of the efficacy and safety of a beta-blocker, a calcium channel blocker, and a converting enzyme inhibitor in hypertensive blacks. Arch Intern Med 1990;150:1707–1713.

21. Shapiro DA, Liss CL, Walker JF, et al. Enalapril and hydrochlorothiazide as antihypertensive agents in the elderly. J Cardiovasc Pharmacol 1987;10(Suppl. 7):S160–S162.

22. Gales MA. Oral antihypertensives for hypertensive urgencies. Annals of Pharmacotherapy 1994;28:352–358.

23. Biollaz J, Waeber B, Brunner HR. Hypertensive crisis treated with orally administered captopril. Eur J Clin Pharmacol 1983;25:145–149.

24. Case DB, Atlas SA, Sullivan PA, et al. Acute and chronic treatment of severe and malignant hypertension with the oral angiotensin-converting enzyme inhibitor captopril. Circulation 1981;64:765–771.

25. Tschollar W, Belz GG. Sublingual captopril in hypertensive crisis. Lancet 1985;1:34–35.

26. Di Veroli C, Pastorelli R. Orally dissolved captopril compared with captopril in standard oral administration in the treatment of hypertensive emergencies and urgencies in the elderly. Current Therapeutic Research 1991;50:586–590.

27. Komsuoglu B, Sengun B, Bayram A, Komsuoglu SS. Treatment of hypertensive urgencies with oral nifedipine, nicardipine, and captopril. Angiology 1991;42:447–454.

28. Pascale C, Zampaglione B, Marchisiti M. Management of hypertensive crisis: nifedipine in comparison with captopril, clonidine, and furosemide. Current Therapeutic Research 1992;51:9-18.

29. Pastorelli R, Ferri C, Santucci A. New therapeutic possibilities in hypertensive emergencies. Current Therapeutic Research 1991;50:857–868.

30. Ceyhan B, Karaaslan Y, Caymaz O, et al. Comparison of sublingual captopril and sublingual nifedipine in hypertensive emergencies. Japanese Journal of Pharmacology 1990;52:189–193.

31. Karachalios GN, Chrisikos N, Kintziou H, et al. Treatment of hypertensive crisis with sublingual captopril. Current Therapeutic Research 1990;48:5–9.

32. Gavras H. The role of angiotensin converting enzyme inhibitors in the management of urgent hypertensive situations: a review. Cardiovascular Drug Reviews 1992;10:117–124.

33. Matthews DM, et al. The Effect of captopril on blood pressure and glucose tolerance in hypertensive non-insulin dependent diabetics. Postgrad Med J 1986;62:73–75.

34. Sasaki J, Arakawa K. Effect of captopril on serum lipids, lipoproteins, and apolipoproteins in patients with mild essential hypertension. Curr Ther Res;1986;40:898.

35. Weinberger MH. Blood pressure and metabolic responses to hydrochlorothiazide, captopril and the combination in black and white mild-to-moderate hypertensive patients. J Cardiovasc Pharmacol 1987;7(Suppl. I);S52–S55.

36. Malini PL, Strochi E, Ambrosioni E, et al. Long-term antihypertensive metabolic and cellular effects of enalapril. J Hypertens (Suppl.)1984;2:S101–S105.

37. Grossman E, Messerli Fh, Oren S, Soria F, Schmieder RE. Disparate cardiovascular responses to stress tests during isradipine and fosinopril therapy. Am J. Cardiol 1993;72:574–579.

38. Rimmer JM, Horn JF, Gennari FJ. Hyperkalemia as a complication of drug therapy. Arch Intern Med 1987;147:867–869.

39. Levy D, Garrison RJ, Savage DD, et al. Prognostic implications of echocardiographically determined left ventricular mass in the Framingham Heart Study. N Engl J Med 1990;322:1561–1566.

40. Messerli FH, Soria F. Does a reduction in left ventricular hypertrophy reduce cardiovascular morbidity and mortality? Drugs 1992;44(Suppl. 1):141–146.

41. Messerli FH, Oren S, Grossman E. Left ventricular hypertrophy and antihypertensive therapy. Drugs 1988;35(Suppl. 5):27–33.

42. Sun Y, Ramires FJ, Weber KT. Fibrosis of atria and great vessels in response to angiotensin II or aldosterone infusion. Cardiovasc Res 1997;35:138–147.

43. Gottdiener JS, Reda DJ, Massie BM, et al. for VA Coop. Study Group on Antihypertensive Agents. Effect of single-drug therapy on reduction of left ventricular mass in mild to moderate hypertension: comparison of six antihypertensive agents with placebo. Circulation 1997;95:2007–2014.

44. Dahlof B, Pennart K, Hansson L. Regression of left ventricular hypertrophy—a meta-analysis. Clin-Exp-Hypertens-A. 1992;14: 173–180.

45. Schmieder RE, Martus P, Kingbeil A. Reversal of left ventricular hypertrophy in essential hypertension: A meta-analysis of randomized double-blind studies. JAMA 1996;275:1507–1513.

46. Pfeffer MA, Braunwald E, Moye LA, et al. for the SAVE Investigators. Effect of captopril on mortality and morbidity in patients with left ventricular dysfunction after myocardial infarction. N Engl J Med 1992;327:669–677.

47. SOLVD Investigators. Effects of enalapril on survival in patients with reduced left ventricular ejection fractions and congestive heart failure. N Engl J Med 1991;325:293–302.

48. Garg R, Yusuf S. for the Collaborative Group of ACE Inhibitor Trials. Overview of randomized trials of angiotensin-converting enzyme inhibitors on mortality and morbidity in patients with heart failure. JAMA 1995;273:1450–1456.

49. Klag MJ, Whelton PK, Randall BL, Neaton JD, Brancati FL, Ford CE, Shulman NB, Stamler J. Blood pressure and end-stage renal disease in men. N Engl J Med 1996;334:13–18.

50. Parving HH, Andersen AR, Smidt UM, Svendsen PA. Early aggressive antihypertensive treatment reduces rate of decline in kidney function in diabetic nephropathy. Lancet 1983;1:1175–1179.

51. Ravid M, Savin H, Jutrin I, et al. Long-term stabilizing effect of angiotensin-converting enzyme inhibition on plasma creatinine and on proteinuria in normotensive type II diabetic patients. Ann Intern Med 1993;118:577–581.

52. Lewis EJ, Hunsicker LG, Bain RP, et al. The effect of angiotensin-converting-enzyme inhibition on diabetic nephropathy. N Engl J Med 1993;329:1456–1462.

53. Viberti G, Mogensen CE, Groop LC, et al. Effect of captopril on progression to clinical proteinuria in patients with insulin dependent diabetes mellitus and microalbuminuria. European Muroalbuminuria Captopril Study Group. JAMA 1994;271:275–279.

54. The EUCLID Study Group. Randomised placebo controlled trial of lisinopril in normotensive patients with insulin-dependent diabetes and normoalbuminuria or microablbuminuria. Lancet 1997;349:1787–1792.

55. Kasiske BL, Kalil RS, Ma JZ, Liao M, Keane WF. Effect of antihypertensive therapy on the kidney in patients with diabetes: a meta-regression analysis. Ann Intern Med 1993;118:129–138.

56. Maki DD, Ma JZ, Louis TA, Kasiske BL. Long-term effects of anti-hypertensive agents on proteinuria and renal function. Arch Intern Med 1995;155(10):1073–1080.

57. Maschio G, Albert D, Janin G, et al. For the Angiotensin-Converting-Enzyme Inhibition in Progressive Renal Insufficiency Study Group. Effect of the angiotensin-converting-enzyme inhibitor benazepril on the progression of chronic renal insufficiency. N Engl J Med 1996;334:939–945.

58. The GISEN Group. Randomised placebo-controlled trial of effect of ramipril on decline in glomerular filtration rate and risk of terminal renal failure in proteinuric, non-diabetic nephropathy. Lancet 1997;349:1857–1863.

59. Giatras I, Lau J, Levey AS. Effect of angiotensin-converting enzyme inhibitors on the progression of nondiabetic renal disease: A meta-analysis of randomized trials. Ann Intern Med 1997;127:337–345.

60. Monane M, Bohn RL, Gurwitz JH, Glynn RJ, Levin R, Avorn J. The effects of initial drug choice and comorbidity on antihypertensive therapy compliance: results from a population-based study in the elderly. Am J Hypertens 1997;10(7 Pt.1):697–704.

61. Israili ZH, Hall WD. Cough and angioneurotic edema associated with angiotensin-converting enzyme inhibitor therapy. A review of the literature and pathophysiology. Ann Intern Med 1992;117:234–242.

62. Hricik DE, Browning PJ, Kopelman R, Goorno WE, Madias NE, Dzau VJ. Captopril-induced functional renal insufficiency in patients with bilateral renal artery stenosis or renal artery stenosis in a solitary kidney. N Engl J Med 1983;308:373–376.

63. Piper JM, Ray WA, Rosa FW. Pregnancy outcome following exposure to angiotensin-converting enzyme inhibitors. Obstet Gynecol 1992;80:429–432.

64. Kaiser G, Ackermann R, Dieterle W, et al. Benazapril and benazeprilat in human plasma and breast milk. Eur J Clin Pharmacol 1989;36(Suppl.):A303.

65. Testa MA, Anderson RB, Nackley JF, Hollenberg NK. Quality of life and antihypertensive therapy in men. A comparison of captopril with enalapril. The Quality-of-Life Study Group. N Eng J Med 1993;328:907–913.

66. Materson BJ, Reda DJ, Williams D. Lessons from combination therapy in Veterans Affairs Studies. Department of Veterans Affairs Cooperative Study Group on antihypertensive agents. Am J Hypertens 1996;9:187S–191S.

67. Rosenthal T, Grossman E, Rathaus M, et al. Treatment of hypertension by enalapril and hydrochlorothiazide separately and together. A multicenter study. Isr J Med Sci 1990;26:2,63–66.

68. Shamiss A, Carroll J, Peleg E. Grossman E, Rosenthal T. The effect of enalapril with and without hydrochlorothiazide on insulin sensitivity and other metabolic abnormalities of hypertensive patients with NIDDM. Am J Hypertens 1995;8:276–281.

69. Messerli FH, Grossman E. Target-organ protection in hypertension and diabetes: The promise of combination therapy. J Cardiovasc Pharmacol 1996;28(Suppl. 4):S45–S48.

70. The Sixth Report of the Joint National Committee on Prevention, Detection, Evaluation, and Treatment of High Blood Pressure. Arch Intern Med 1997;157:2413–2446.

71. Reardon LC, Macpherson DS. Hyperkalemia in outpatients using angiotensin-converting enzyme inhibitors. How much should we worry? Arch Intern Med 1998;158:26–32.

CHAPTER 13

Angiotensin II Receptor Inhibition

Franz H. Messerli
Ehud Grossman
Michael A. Weber
Hans R. Brunner

Pharmacologic blockade of the renin-angiotensin-aldosterone cascade has been found to be a safe and efficacious way to treat hypertension and congestive heart failure. Angiotensin-converting-enzyme (ACE) inhibitors are the most commonly used drugs to achieve this goal and have become a cornerstone in cardiovascular therapy within the past few years.[1-4]

Although, in general, ACE inhibitors are well tolerated, two important adverse effects of ACE inhibitors as a class are cough (common) and angioedema (rare).[5,6] The occurrence of these adverse effects, as well as the quest of achieving a more selective, site-specific blockade of the effects of angiotensin-II (A II), has stimulated the search for other approaches to pharmacologically interrupt the renin-angiotensin aldosterone cascade. Most promising in this respect so far has been the development of the A-II type 1 receptor (AT_1) blockers (ARBs).[7,8]

CHEMISTRY

Several ARB compounds are available; some are still under investigation. ARBs can be chemically classified into biphenyl or nonbiphenyl tetrazoles and nonheterocyclic compounds. Of note, the chemical class does not define whether the ARB binds in a competitive fashion or noncompetitive but apparently surmountable fashion to the AT_1 receptor.

A New Therapeutic Principle

Apart from their effect on angiotensin II, ACE inhibitors have been shown to decrease the metabolism of bradykinin, and thereby, to enhance circulating bradykinin levels which may mediate vasodilation. Additionally, bradykinin levels release nitric oxide as well as increase synthesis of vasoactive prostaglandins. In contrast, ARBs are specifically designed to displace angiotensin II from its type I receptor subtype. Although these drugs may have effects on nitric oxide and bradykinin expression in *in vitro* preparations, there is no evidence as yet of such actions in humans (Table 1).[11]

Receptor Heterogeneity

A II exerts its effects by stimulating the specific receptors on the membrane of various target organ cells.[12,13] At least two principal receptor subtypes can be distinguished by radioligand binding studies and have been labeled as AT_1- and AT_2-receptors.[8,12-16] Although both receptor subtypes appear in different organs in varying proportions, it seems that most, if not all, known cardiovascular effects of A II are mediated by the AT_1 receptor, including vasoconstriction, release of aldosterone from the adrenal cortex, and beta-adrenergic stimulation (Table 2).[8,10,13-16] Most ARBs are selective for the AT_1

TABLE 1. Main Differences between ARBs and ACE Inhibitors.

	ARBs	ACE Inhibitors
Principle mechanism of action	Displacement of A-II from Type 1 Receptor Subtype	Inhibition of ACE
Plasma A-II	↑	↓
Plasma renin activity	↑	↑
Bradykin	—	↑
Postaglandins E_2 and I_2	—	↑
Nitric oxide release	–	↑
Uric acid levels	↓*	–
Effect on AT_1	Yes	Yes
Effect on AT_2, AT_3, AT_4	No	Yes
PAI_1	↑	↓
Cough	uncommon	class-specific

ARB = A-II type 1 receptor blocker
ACE = angiotensin-converting enzyme
↑ = increase
↓ = decrease
– = no change
PAI_1 = plasminogen activator inhibitor
Modified with permission from ref. [10].
*Losartan only

receptor.[14-16] Defining any hemodynamic, humoral, or other functional effects of the AT_2 receptor has not been possible, although some interesting speculations point to issues such as modulation of cell growth in the embryo.[17] During pathologic conditions such as myocardial infarction or left ventricular hypertrophy due to aortic banding and vascular neointimal proliferation, the AT_2 receptor may be re-expressed in the adult in order to facilitate healing or remodeling of damaged tissues. In the microvasculature the AT_1 receptor seems to mediate angiogenesis and vasoconstriction whereas the AT_2 receptor has been shown to inhibit angiogenesis and to promote vasodilation.[18]

The AT_1 receptor (in rats and mice) is composed of two isoforms (AT_{1a} and AT_{1b}).[19-21] The AT_{1a} receptor is predominant in the kidney, liver, vascular smooth muscle, and the heart, whereas the AT_{1b} receptor seems to be predominant in the adrenal tissue. Since the amino acid sequence and the binding properties of the two isoforms are very similar, organ or tissue heterogeneity with regard to receptor isoforms could conceivably account for the differential organ response to A II stimulation and A II blockade.[16] Recently AT_3 and AT_4 receptor subtypes have also been described[20] and remain to be fully characterized pharmacologically (Table 2).

Effect on Systemic Hemodynamics

Experimentally, as well as in clinical studies, ARBs lower arterial pressure by decreasing systemic vascular resistance while maintaining cardiac output and heart rate.[8,14,22-27] The antihypertensive efficacy seems to depend, at least to some extent, on the activity of the renin-angiotensin-aldosterone cascade since it can be abolished by volume expansion or by bilateral nephrectomy.[8,14,25-27] Although heart rate and cardiac output usually remain unchanged with sustained angiotensin receptor blockade, in animals with an activated renin-angiotensin system, a reflexive cardiac acceleration can be observed immediately after dosing.[28-32] Several mechanisms may be responsible for the decrease in systemic vascular resistance caused by ARBs: (1) inhibition of the direct vasoconstrictive effect of A II, (2) decrease in the activity of sympathetic nervous system, (3) decrease in A II-mediated renal tubular sodium reabsorption, (4) decrease in A II-mediated aldosterone release, (5) decrease in the activity of the renin-angiotensin system in the brain, thereby sensitizing baroreceptors, (6) stimulation of the vasodilator prostacyclin through an action at the AT_1 receptor, and (7) decrease in hyperplasia and hypertrophy of vascular (and cardiac) smooth muscle (remodeling, antiproliferative effect). It should be pointed out, however, that only the first of these mechanisms has been clearly documented to be of clinical importance in hypertensive patients.

Uricosuric Effects

Losartan has been shown to exert a uricosuric effect that was dose-dependent in normotensive subjects.[33] Burnier and collaborators showed that this effect was independent of salt

TABLE 2. ANGIOTENSIN II (AT) RECEPTORS.

	AT$_1$		AT$_2$	AT$_3$	AT$_4$
	AT$_{1A}$	AT$_{1B}$			
Location	Lung, liver, vascular smooth muscle, brain, kidney	Adrenals, pituitary glands	Fetal tissue, brain, reproductive tissue	Neuroblastoma cells	Heart, kidney, brain, liver
Selective agonist	None	None	CGP 42112	?	?
Selective antagonist	All compounds listed in Table 1	All compounds listed in Table 1	PD 123319	?	?

? = data unknown
Used with permission from ref. [10].

intake.[34] Similar uricosuric effects were documented in patients with essential hypertension and in hypertensive patients with renal disease.[35,36] The degree of uricosuria does not seem to be dependent on the activity of the renin-angiotensin-aldosterone cascade.[34] The exact mechanism of this uricosuric effect remains unknown, but it seems related to a high anion load in the renal tubules competing with urate reabsorption.[37] The infusion of the active metabolite of losartan (EXP3174) does not increase uric acid excretion nor does the administration of other angiotensin receptor antagonists such as irbesartan.[38,39] This would indicate that the uricosuric properties are specific for losartan and not related to the ARB activity per se. The exact clinical relevance of this uricosuric and hypouricemic effect of losartan remains to be determined. A recent clinical study suggested that the uricosuric effect could be an advantage when losartan is combined with a thiazide diuretic.[40]

Antiatheromatous Effects

In animal experiments, ACE inhibitors have been documented to slow down the progression of, or even decrease, atheromatous lesions,[41] and ARBs have been shown to exert a similar effect in a similar model (Chobanian, personal communication 1998). However, human studies assessing the effects of ACE inhibitors on coronary obstruction and restenosis after transluminal angioplasty have been disappointing.[42] These experimental findings require clarification by a thorough clinical study assessing the effects of A II type-1 receptors on atheromatous lesions in various vascular beds.[43]

Humoral Effects

Plasma immunoreactive A II levels and plasma renin activity have been shown to increase with losartan in a dose-dependent manner,[44-46] suggesting that the negative feedback of A II on renin release from the juxtaglomerular cells is also mediated by the AT_1 receptors. At an equal antihypertensive dose, losartan increased plasma renin activity 1.7-fold and A II twofold, whereas enalapril increased plasma renin activity 2.8-fold and decreased A II by 77%.[46] Concern has been voiced that because of the high plasma A II concentration occurring during A II receptor blockade, abrupt cessation of therapy would cause acute rebound hypertension. However, at least with losartan, no rebound increase in arterial pressure has been observed. Conceivably, the comparatively short half-life of renin and A II may protect the patient from an acute increase in arterial pressure.

Plasma aldosterone concentration in general decreases somewhat with AT_1-receptor blockade, although this decrease has not been very consistent.[35,46-51] Grossman et al.[48] found plasma aldosterone concentrations not to be different from baseline after 12 months of treatment. In the study of Goldberg et al.,[49] 100 mg of losartan decreased aldosterone by 40% after 6 weeks of treatment. Conceivably, alternative pathways leading to aldosterone secretion compensate for losartan's action.

Experimental studies have shown that ARBs also bind to the AT_1 receptors of the sympathetic neurons, thereby decreasing norepinephrine secretion. As a consequence, neither reflexive cardioacceleration nor an increase in plasma norepinephrine is seen with the fall in arterial pressure caused by interruption of the renin-angiotensin-aldosterone cascade.[52-54] Plasma norepinephrine levels in general have a tendency to fall with A II receptor inhibition.[48,49,51] However, at least in one instance an increase in plasma norepinephrine has been seen with a high dose of an ARB.[55]

Metabolic Effects

Because they inhibit angiotensin-stimulated aldosterone release, ACE inhibitors have been shown to partially attenuate the potassium-depleting effect of diuretics.[56] Similarly, ARBs seem to have a modest effect on potassium conservation during concomitant diuretic administration.[40] Also, ACE inhibitors have been shown to be either inert or to have a beneficial effect on some metabolic disturbances associated with essential hypertension.[56,57] Recently losartan was reported to decrease insulin sensitivity as measured by glucose disposal rates in moderately severe hypertensive patients.[58] Since the decrease in glucose disposal rates occurred in parallel with a fall in plasma norepinephrine and blood viscosity suggesting vasodilation and a sympatholytic effect as the common pathophysiologic denominator, ARBs can also be expected to blunt the diuretic-induced increases in insulin resistance. In general, however, most other metabolic values, with the exclusion of uric acid, appear to be unaffected by ARBs.

Clinical Efficacy

Hypertension. ARBs have proven to be efficacious and superior to placebo in large controlled trials.[59-63] The hypotensive effect of the available compounds lasts 24 hours, and therefore they can be used as once daily drugs.[64-80] The antihypertensive effect of ARBs is evident within 2 weeks of starting treatment and maximal at 3 to 6 weeks after treatment initiation. Despite elevated levels of A II, no rebound hypertension was observed after withdrawal of treatment.[67] This class of drugs is also more effective in high renin forms of hypertension.[48] In comparative studies, ARBs were equipotent to angiotensin converting enzyme inhibitors, hydrochlorothiazide, beta-blockers, and calcium antagonists.[47,62,68-73] While all the ARBs are effective antihypertensive agents, irbesartan[74,75] candesartan cilexetil,[76] valsartan,[77] and telmisartan[77a] have demonstrated greater blood pressure reduction than losartan potassium in comparative trials. The ARBs are effective and well tolerated in elderly hypertensive patients.[78,79] In a comparative study valsartan and lisinopril produced comparable reduction in blood pressure in elderly patients, but in contrast to lisinopril, the antihypertensive efficacy of valsartan was unaffected by concomitant administration of nonsteroidal anti-inflammatory drugs.[80] It is not yet known whether responses to ARBs are affected by factors such as ethnicity and gender. Like ACE inhibitors, ARBs have been used alone and in combination with other antihypertensive agents. The most efficacious combination is with diuretics, but combination with calcium antagonists is also recommended.[48,68-71]

Cardiac Effects

Left Ventricular Hypertrophy. Left ventricular hypertrophy (LVH) is a consequence of long-standing hypertension and is considered to be an independent risk factor for cardiovascular morbidity and mortality.[81] Whether reduction of LVH improves morbidity and mortality has to be documented, but indirect evidence suggests that it may be beneficial.[82] Antihypertensive agents are able to regress LVH, but not all agents are equipotent in this regard.[83] A II and aldosterone accelerate myocardial hypertrophy and fibrosis,[84] and therefore blocking the renin-angiotensin-aldosterone system (RAAS) should be a highly effective way to reduce left ventricular mass. Indeed in a recent study Gottdiener et al.[85] showed that diuretics and ACE inhibitors are both equipotent in reducing left ventricular mass (LVM). However, the investigators used captopril twice daily as the ACE inhibitor. Despite not controlling blood pressure throughout a 24-hour period, captopril reduced LVM significantly. A recent meta-analysis by Schmieder et al., reviewing [39] double blind clinical studies done until July 1995, showed clearly that ACE inhibitors reduced LVM more than all other antihypertensive classes.[86]

So far, the results with ARBs are less persuasive. Blockade of the AT_1 receptor is accompanied by an increase in plasma levels of A II and its metabolites. This could be beneficial in stimulating the AT_2 receptors which, if they exist under usual clinical conditions, are unblocked. It appears that activation of the AT_2 receptors inhibits proliferation and might prevent myocardial hypertrophy. Moreover, Mizuno et al.[87] found that cardiac tissue A II, rather than circulating A II, plays an important role in the pathophysiology of left ventricular hypertrophy of spontaneously hypertensive rats. If this is the case in humans, then AT_1 receptor antagonists should be superior to ACE inhibitors in reducing LVM. In various animal models ARBs prevented or regressed left ventricular hypertrophy.[88-92] However, in two small clinical studies no reduction in LVM with the ARB losartan was observed.[93,94] In one study the ARB candesartan cilexetil reduced LVM even at a dose that did not lower blood pressure.[91] In another recent study, blocking the RAAS by the combination of an ACE inhibitor and an ARB reduced blood pressure and LVM more than blocking the system by either drug alone.[88] The results from the large ongoing prospective clinical study LIFE will hopefully clarify this dilemma.[95] In contrast with other ARBs such as valsartan and irbesartan, recently effective reduction in LVM was documented.[96,97]

Cardiac Remodeling. ACE inhibitors have been well documented to be useful in preventing the remodeling of the left chamber that often takes place in the post-myocardial infarction period. It has been hypothesized that these benefits might be mediated by A II, a decrease in aldosterone and/or an increase in bradykinin and to be, at least to some extent, independent of the hemodynamic effects of the ACE inhibitors.[98-101] Experimental data have reported a variable effect of ARBs on left ventricular structure after myocardial infarction in rats.[101,102] Survival after myocardial infarction seems to be similar in rats treated with an ACE inhibitor and those treated with losartan.[103] AT_1 receptor blockade with irbesartan was found to dose-dependently increase survival in post-ischemic congestive heart failure (CHF) rats.[104] Clearly, therefore, clinical studies with ARBs are needed to establish efficacy of this drug class on morbidity and mortality in the post-myocardial infarction patient.

Left Ventricular Function. In the experimental post-infarct model in the Sprague-Dawley rat and in the rapid-pacing sheep model of congestive heart failure, the effects of losartan on left ventricular end-diastolic pressure and volume index, as well as other hemodynamic variables, were virtually identical to the effects of ACE inhibition.[101,105] Thus AT_1 receptor blockade can be expected to have the same favorable therapeutic effect in congestive heart failure as ACE inhibition.

Conceivably, in selected patients with congestive heart failure, ARBs and ACE inhibitors could be combined to achieve a more complete blockade of all effects mediated by circulating and tissue A II. Such a double blockade would interrupt the effects of A II generated from the chymase (non-ACE) pathway,[106] while potentiating the vasodilating effects of bradykinin. These provocative considerations clearly are an incentive for extensive study of these new drug class in patients with congestive heart failure.

Congestive Heart Failure. Congestive heart failure is one of the sequelae of long-standing hypertension. There is good evidence that increased levels of A II and aldosterone with vasoconstriction and sodium retention have adverse effects in CHF. Therefore, blocking the RAAS, whether at the level of A II production (with ACE inhibitor) or at the A II receptor site would be beneficial. Several studies have shown that patients with CHF due to systolic dysfunction, either symptomatic or asymptomatic, with an ejection fraction less than 35%, who received an ACE inhibitor showed a statistically significant reduction in mortality compared with patients who did not receive an ACE inhibitor.[107-109]

In the SAVE study patients with a myocardial infarction and ejection fraction less than 40% in the postinfarction period benefited significantly when an ACE inhibitor was given in addition to routine therapy.[107] Deaths from cardiovascular causes, recurrent myocardial infarction and CHF were reduced. The reduction in total mortality is dependent on pretreatment ejection fraction.[109] A meta-analysis of 16 randomized trials showed that a significant reduction in total mortality was observed only in patients with an ejection fraction of less than 25%.[109]

ARBs induced beneficial hemodynamic effects in several animal models of CHF.[110-112] Valsartan at 10 mg/kg intravenously reduced blood pressure, heart rate, left ventricular pressure, left ventricular end-diastolic pressure and total systemic resistance in dogs with acute heart failure due to coronary artery ligation and in dogs with chronic heart failure due to rapid-ventricular pacing.[111] Similar results were obtained with losartan in rat models of CHF.[110] In clinical studies it has been shown that losartan is beneficial in patients with CHF.[113-117] The acute hemodynamic and neurohormonal response to losartan was evaluated in 66 patients with severe CHF and ejection fraction less than 40%. A dose of 25 mg decreased blood pressure, systemic vascular resistance and pulmonary capillary wedge pressure, associated with moderate reduction in serum aldosterone and plasma noradrenaline.[113] In another study[114] hemodynamic assessment was performed in 134 patients after the first dose and after 12 weeks of losartan treatment. Acutely, losartan at a dose of 50 mg decreased blood pressure and systemic vascular resistance. After 12 weeks of treatment, similar effects were seen on systemic vascular resistance and blood pressure. In addition, capillary wedge pressure fell, cardiac index rose and heart rate decreased. Active treatment was well tolerated and excess cough was not reported. Similar favorable hemodynamic and clinical results have recently been reported in heart failure patients treated with irbesartan versus lisinopril or irbesartan in addition to ACE inhibition therapy.[118-120] A recent 48-week study[115] compared the tolerability and efficacy of a single dose of losartan 50 mg once daily with the ACE inhibitor captopril 50 mg administered three times daily in elderly patients with CHF. Losartan was better tolerated than captopril, and a significant reduction in overall mortality, primarily due to a decrease in sudden death, was observed with losartan compared with captopril. More than 75% of patients in both treatment groups were receiving a diuretic drug or digitalis or both. Thus, it seems that ARBs are as effective as ACE inhibitors and produce less side effects than ACE inhibitors in patients with CHF.

Renal Effects

In a recent meta-analysis including 1594 patients in 10 studies, Giatras et al.[121] showed that ACE inhibitors are more effective than other antihypertensive agents in reducing the development of end-stage nondiabetic renal disease (pooled relative risk was 0.70). Blocking the RAAS by inhibition of the ACE produces a renoprotective effect in diabetic nephropathy and in proteinuric nondiabetic glomerulopathy. Whether this protection is unique to the ACE inhibitors or can be achieved with the ARBs is unknown. In an experimental model of diabetic nephropathy, valsartan prevented the appearance of albuminuria.[122] Because bradykinin may contribute to the efferent arteriolar dilation induced by ACE inhibitors, ARBs could have a smaller effect on glomerular hemodynamics than ACE inhibitors.[123] If so, angiotensin-receptor antagonism would pose less of a threat to glomerular filtration than does ACE inhibition in patients with renal impairment, but it would also be less effective in retarding renal damage in diabetic patients. But in a small group of 11 patients with severe proteinuria unrelated to diabetes, the ARB losartan reduced proteinuria to the same extent as ACE inhibitors suggesting that ARBs have dilatory effects on efferent glomerular arterioles that are similar to ACE inhibitors.[124] Gansevoort and collaborators recently reported a distinct decrease in proteinuria of between 29% and 46% with an ARB in hypertensive patients with renal disease. They also reported that the decrease in proteinuria was similar to that observed for enalapril in the same study.[36,124] Redon[125] pointed out recently that ACE inhibitors or ARBs such as losartan or valsartan have more potential benefits than the other classes of antihypertensive drugs in reducing urinary albumin excretion. Further prospective studies are required before the renoprotective effects of ARBs can be established.

ARBs have been shown to induce natriuresis and kaliuresis in salt-depleted normal volunteers without affecting glomerular filtration rate, and this effect was attenuated by sodium repletion.[34] Similarly, in patients with essential hypertension, ARBs did not affect glomerular filtration rate as assessed by creatinine clearance.[35,126,127] However, in volume-depleted subjects, hypertensive or not, a decrease in creatinine clearance could be observed, which presumably was due to the decrease in arterial tone in the efferent vessel.[128,129] Similar to ACE inhibitor, an increase in creatinine can be observed in susceptible patients.[130] Of note, renal blood flow as measured by effective renal plasma flow was increased by prolonged losartan therapy in hypertensive patients, and since glomerular filtration rate remained unchanged, filtration fraction decreased.[36,124,131]

SAFETY AND ADVERSE EFFECTS

ACE inhibitors are safe and well tolerated with a relatively low rate of adverse events. Monane et al.[132] showed recently that elderly hypertensive patients comply better with ACE inhibitors than with other antihypertensive agents. The overall rate of side effects with ACE inhibitors is about 10% to 20%, with dry, nonproductive cough that may occur in 5-20% as the most frequent and troublesome one.[6] Angioneurotic edema is less common and was reported in 1-2% of the treated patients.[133] First dose hypotension may occur with ACE inhibitors, particularly in patients who are volume depleted.[134] Other side effects include elevation of plasma potassium, particularly in patients with underlying renal insufficiency who are treated with potassium supplements or potassium sparing agents.[135] Deterioration of renal function occurs mainly in patients with renal artery stenoses, either bilateral or in a solitary kidney.[133] Some specific side effects such as taste disturbances, rash, and leukopenia have been reported but are infrequent. Nonspecific side effects such as headache, dizziness, fatigue, diarrhea, and nausea are listed but usually do not cause a problem. ACE inhibitors are contraindicated in pregnancy because they can cause fetal injury and death.[136] The relative incidence of side effects is fairly similar among the various ACE inhibitors. However, in one meticulous study, captopril was superior to enalapril in quality of life measures.[137]

Various studies have examined the safety and tolerability of ARBs.[47,62,63] Pooled analysis of tolerability data from placebo-controlled studies involving 2316 patients treated with valsartan 40 to 160 mg/day showed headache, dizziness and fatigue to be the only adverse events that occurred in more than 1% of patients.[59] A similar profile of adverse effects was observed with irbesartan[61] and with losartan potassium in more than 2900 hypertensive patients.[47] Orthostatic effects and first-dose hypotension appear uncommon, occurring in less than 0.5% of patients treated with ARBs. There are some case reports of patients who developed angioedema during losartan potassium therapy,[138,139] but no cases of angioneurotic edema were observed during controlled trials with valsartan.[59] Unlike the ACE inhibitors, the ARBs do not appear to provoke cough.[140–142] In studies that were designed specifically to assess the incidence and severity of cough in patients with a history of cough during ACE inhibitor therapy, ARBs were less than half as likely as the ACE inhibitor to be associated with cough.[141] In one study[142] hypertensive patients with confirmed propensity for ACE inhibitor induced cough were randomized to 6 weeks' treatment with valsartan 80 mg/day, lisinopril 10 mg/day or hydrochlorothiazide 25 mg/day. The incidences of dry cough were 21.4%, 71.1%, and 19%, respectively. Like ACE inhibitors, ARBs may increase plasma potassium levels particularly in patients with underlying renal insufficiency who are treated with potassium supplements or potassium sparing agents.[59-61] Deterioration of renal function may occur in patients with renal artery stenoses, either bilateral or in a solitary kidney. ARBs are contraindicated in pregnancy because their safety in pregnancy has not been shown.[59-61]

Predictably, hyperkalemia and impairment of renal function can be expected in susceptible patients, particularly in the elderly, in patients with renovascular forms of hypertension, in diabetic patients with hyporeninemic hypoaldoster-onism, and in patients taking potassium-sparing diuretics.

COMPARISON OF VARIOUS ARBs

Most of the compounds differ in terms of pharmacologic half life, potency, protein binding, and metabolization (Table 3). These pharmacological differences notwithstanding, there seems to be some evidence that antihypertensive efficacy varies somewhat among various compounds. In three clinical trials, irbesartan (two trials)[74,75] and candesartan (one trial)[76] achieved superior blood pressure reduction when compared with losartan. Equally, valsartan achieved significantly greater response rates when compared with losartan in another trial.[143] Losartan seems to have a rather shallow dose response curve which is underlined by the fact that it was marketed only in one strength. No other antihypertensive drug has ever been made available in one strength only. Also the JNC VI[144] has indicated that losartan is to be taken either once a day or twice a day, whereas most of the other ARBs are considered to be once a day medications. How clinically important these efficacy differences among ARBs are remains to be determined.

COMBINATION WITH OTHER ANTIHYPERTENSIVE AGENTS

Less than 50% of hypertensive patients will achieve goal blood pressure (< 140/90 mm Hg) with blockers of the RAAS as monotherapy.[48,145,146] Most of these patients will require addition of other antihypertensive agents.[147,148] The combination of hydrochlorothiazide and ACE inhibitors or ARBs should produce an additive hypotensive effect, because the two classes of drugs have a complementary and different pharmacologic mechanism of action. Diuretics stimulate the renin-angiotensin system, and blocking this system is more effective when the system is activated. Several studies have evaluated the efficacy, safety and tolerability of a combination of low dose hydrochlorothiazide and ARB in hypertensive patients. The addition of losartan potassium to hydrochlorothiazide in hypertensive patients whose blood pressure was not adequately controlled by 25 mg hydrochlorothiazide mono-therapy produced a significant decrease in blood pressure already after 1 week of treatment.[40] The antihypertensive response was greater at week 3 than at week 1, with some additional decrease in blood pressure in some groups in later time.

The addition of diuretics to patients whose clinical diastolic blood pressure remained elevated during ARB monotherapy lowered blood pressure further.[48,149-151] Blockers of the renin angiotensin system attenuate the decrease in serum potassium observed with hydrochlorothiazide alone, and may offset the diuretic induced insulin resistance.[152] ARBs may also be successfully combined with calcium antagonists. The combination of ACE inhibitors and calcium antagonists may better protect the kidney in diabetic patients than ACE inhibitors alone, and will reduce the rate of calcium antagonist induced leg edema. ARBs have also been used in combination with calcium antagonists.[71] Corea et al.[71] showed that when added to amlodipine, valsartan, similar to ACE-inhibitors, may reduce peripheral edema. ACE inhibitors were also combined successfully with beta or alpha blockers. However, no such studies with ARBs are available. There is also physiological logic in combining ACE inhibitors with ARBs. ACE inhibitors do not prevent the production of A II by enzymes other than ACE, but increase plasma bradykinins levels by inhibition of their degradation. ARBs block the effects of A II at the receptor site, but they do not increase plasma bradykinins levels. The combination of the two may give maximal blockade of the RAAS with the advantage of elevated levels of bradykinins. It seems, therefore, that in patients who do not experience adverse effects with ACE inhibitors, combination with an ARB may be beneficial. Spinale et al.[112] showed that the combination of benazepril (ACE inhibitor) and valsartan (ARB) may provide unique benefits for left ventricular pump function and neurohormonal systems in the setting of CHF. There is early clinical experience showing that the addition of an ARB to an ACE inhibitor produces a better effect than that achieved by either drug.[153-155] Further studies are required to evaluate the potential benefit of this combination.

TABLE 3. DIFFERENCES BETWEEN VARIOUS ARBs

Pharmacodynamics—Receptors	Irbesartan	Losartan	Valsartan	Candesartan	Telmisartan	Eprosartan
Max AT-1 inhibition	100%	85% (100 mg)	80%	90% (8mg) 1-wk data	96%	100%
Full effect in	3–6 h	6 h	2–6 h	2–4 h	0.5–2 h	1–4 h
24-hr AT-1 inhibition	60% (300mg) 40% (150 mg)	25–40%	30%	50% (8 mg) 1-wk data	40%	?
Affinity AT-1 vs. AT-2	8500 X	1000 X	20000 X	>10000 X	>3000 X	>10000 X
Absorption						
Prodrug	No	Yes	No	Yes	No	No
Bioavailability	60-80%	25–30%	10–35%	15%	42% (40 mg) 58% (160 mg)	13%
Food effect	No	10%↓	40–50%↓	No	No	25%↓
Distribution						
T-max	1.5–2	3–4	2–4	3–4	0.5–1	1–2
Volume of distribution (Vd)	53–93 L	12 L	17 L	5–15 L	500 L	13 L
Protein binding	90%	99.8%	95%	>99%	>99%	98%
Metabolism and Clearance						
Half-life	11–15 h	6–9 h	6 h	9 h	24 h	5–9 h
Renal clearance	<5%	10%	30%	60%	<5%	30%
P450 3A4	No	Yes*	No	No	No	No

ARB = angiotensin receptor blocker
*Losartan is primarily metabolized by P450 2C9.

SUMMARY

Blockers of the renin angiotensin system are safe and effective in lowering blood pressure. There are no prospective studies showing that these classes of drugs reduce morbidity and mortality in hypertensive patients. However, there is compelling evidence that ACE inhibitors are beneficial in subgroups of patients with congestive heart failure, post myocardial infarction, diabetic nephropathy, and nondiabetic renal failure. Use of ACE inhibitors as the first drug of choice in these patients seems to be justified. ARBs are better tolerated than ACE inhibitors in some patients and therefore may become an alternative to ACE inhibitors in this subgroup of hypertensive patients. If ARBs are not preferred as the first choice, they should be substituted for ACE inhibitors when adverse effects develop. Whether to promote ARBs to first-line status in all hypertensive patients is still an open question. Results from ongoing prospective studies of morbidity and mortality in hypertension will answer this key question.

REFERENCES

1. Materson BJ, Preston RA. Angiotensin-converting enzyme inhibitors in hypertension. A dozen years of experience. Arch Intern Med 1994; 154:513–523.

2. Groden DL. Vasodilator therapy for congestive heart failure. Lessons from mortality trials. Arch Intern Med 1993;153:445–454.

3. Cody RJ. Comparing angiotensin-converting enzyme inhibitor trial results in patients with acute myocardial infarction. Arch Intern Med 1994; 154:2029–2036.

4. Hollenberg NK, Raij L. Angiotensin-converting enzyme inhibitors and renal protection. An assessment of implications for therapy. Arch Intern Med 1993; 153:2426–2435.

5. Chu TJ, Chow N. Adverse effects of ACE inhibitors (Letter). Ann Intern Med 1993;118:314.

6. Israili ZH, Hall WD. Cough and angioneurotic edema associated with angiotensin-converting enzyme inhibitor therapy. A review of the literature and pathophysiology. Ann Intern Med 1992;117:234–242.

7. Smith RD, Chiu AT, Wong PC, Herblin WF, Timmermans PBMWM. Pharmacology of nonpeptide angiotensin II receptor antagonists. Annu Rev Pharmacol Toxicol 1992;32:135–165.

8. Timmermans PBMWM, Wong PC, Chiu AT, et al. Angiotensin II receptors and angiotensin II receptor antagonists. Pharmacol Rev 1993;45:205–251.

9. Wexler RR, Greenlee WJ, Irvin JD, Goldberg MR, Prendergast K, Smith RD, Timmermans PB. Nonpeptide angiotensin II receptor antagonists: the next generation in antihypertensive therapy. J Med Chem 1996;39:625–656.

10. Messerli FH, Weber MA, Brunner HR. Angiotensin II receptor inhibition—a new therapeutic principle. Arch Intern Med 1996;156:1957–1965.

11. Siragy HM, Carey RM. The subtype-2(AT2) angiotensin receptor regulates renal cyclic gaunosine 3', 5'-monophosphate and AT1

receptor-mediated prostaglandin E2 production in conscious rats. J Clin Invest 1996; 97:1978–1982.

12. Bumpus FM, Catt KJ, Chiu AT, et al. Nomenclature for angiotensin receptors. A report of the Nomenclature Committee of the Council for High Blood Pressure Research. Hypertension 1991;17:720–721!

13. Timmermans PBMWM, Chiu AT, Herblin WF, Wong PC, Smith RD. Angiotensin II receptor subtypes. Am J Hypertens 1992;5:406–410.

14. Timmermans PBMWM, Benfield P, Chiu AT, Herblin WF, Wong PC, Smith RD. Angiotensin II receptors and functional correlates. Am J Hypertens 1992;5:221S–235S.

15. Bernstein KE, Berk BC. The biology of angiotensin II receptors. Am J Kid Dis 1993;22:745–754.

16. Griendling KK, Alexander RW. The angiotensin (AT1) receptor. Sem Nephrol 1993;13:558–566.

17. Dzau VJ, Mukoyama M, Pratt RE. Molecular biology of angiotensin receptors: target for drug research? J Hypertens Suppl 1994;12:S1–S5.

18. Munzenmaier DH, Greene AS. Opposing actions of angiotensin II on microvascular growth and arterial blood pressure. Hypertension 1996; 27(part 2):760–765.

19. Murphy TJ, Alexander RW, Griendling KK, Runge MS, Bernstein KE. Isolation of a cDNA encoding the vascular type-1 angiotensin II receptor. Nature 1991; 351:233–236.

20. Sasamura H, Hein L, Krieger JE, Pratt RE, Kobilka BK, Dzau VJ. Cloning, characterization, and expression of two angiotensin receptor (AT-1) isoforms from the mouse genome. Biochem Biophys Res Commun 1992;185:253–259.

21. de Gasparo M, Husain A, Alexander W, et al. Proposed update of angiotensin receptor nomenclature. Hypertension 1995;25:924–927.

22. Wong PC, Price WA Jr, Chiu AT, et al. Nonpeptide angiotensin II receptor antagonists: studies with EXP9270 and DuP 753. Hypertension 1990; 15:823–834.

23. Wong PC, Price WA, Chiu AT, et al. Nonpeptide angiotensin II receptor antagonists. VIII. Characterization of functional antagonism displayed by DuP 753, an orally active antihypertensive agent. J Pharmacol Exp Ther 1990;252:719–725.

24. Wong PC, Price WA, Chiu AT, et al. Nonpeptide angiotensin II receptor antagonists. IX. Antihypertensive activity in rats of DuP 753, an orally active antihypertensive agent. J Pharmacol Exp Ther 1990;252:726–732.

25. Wong PC, Price WA Jr, Chiu AT, et al. Hypotensive action of DuP 753, an angiotensin II antagonist, in spontaneously hypertensive rats. Nonpeptide angiotensin II receptor antagonists: X. Hypertension 1990;15:459–468.

26. Bunkenburg B, Schnell C, Baum HP, Cumin F, Wood JM. Prolonged angiotensin II antagonism in spontaneously hypertensive rats. Hemodynamic and biochemical consequences. Hypertension 1991;18:278–288.

27. Inagami T, Murakami T, Higuchi K, Nakajo S. Roles of renal and vascular renin in spontaneous hypertension and switching of the mechanism upon nephrectomy: lack of hypotensive effects of inhibition of renin, converting enzyme, and angiotensin II receptor blocker after bilateral nephrectomy. Am J Hypertens 1991;4: 15S–22S.

28. Brooks DP, Frederickson TA, Weinstock J, Ruffolo RR Jr, Edwards RM, Gellai M. Antihypertensive activity of the non-peptide angiotensin II receptor antagonist, SK&F 108566, in rats and dogs. Arch Pharmacol 1992;345:673–678.

29. Tofovic SP, Pong AS, Jackson EK. Effects of angiotensin subtype 1 and subtype 2 receptor antagonists in normotensive versus hypertensive rats. Hypertension 1991;18;774–782.

30. MacFadyen RJ, Tree M, Lever AF, Reid JL. Effects of the angiotensin II receptor antagonist losartan (DuP 753/MK 954) on arterial blood pressure, heart rate, plasma concentrations of angiotensin II and renin and the pressor response to infused angiotensin II in the salt-deplete dog. Clin Sci 1992; 83:549–556.

31. MacFadyen RJ, Tree M, Lever AF, Reid JL. Haemodynamic and hormonal responses to losartan (DuP 753/MK 954) infusion during cardiac catheterization in conscious salt-deplete dogs. Clin Sci 1993;85:157–163.

32. Criscione L, de Gasparo M, Bühlmayer P, Whitebread S, Ramjoué H-PR, Wood J. Pharmacological profile of valsartan: a potent, orally active, nonpeptide antagonist of the angiotensin II AT1-receptor subtype. Br J Pharmacol 1993,110:761 771.

33. Nakashima M, Uematsu T, Kosuge K, Kanamaru M. Pilot study of the uricosuric effect of DuP-753, a new angiotensin II receptor antagonist, in healthy subjects. Eur J Clin Pharmacol 1992;42:333–335.

34. Burnier M, Rutschmann B, Nussberger J, et al. Salt-dependent renal effects of an angiotensin II antagonist in healthy subjects. Hypertension 1993; 22:339–347.

35. Tsunoda K, Abe K, Hagino T, et al. Hypotensive effect of losartan, a nonpeptide angiotensin II receptor antagonist, in essential hypertension. Am J Hypertens 1993;6:28–32.

36. Gansevoort RT, de Zeeuw D, Shahinfar S, Redfield A, de Jong PE. Effects of the angiotensin II antagonist losartan in hypertensive patients with renal disease. J Hypertens Suppl 1994;12:S37–S42.

37. Burnier MJ, Brunner HR. Angiotensin II receptor antagonists and the kidney. Opinion in Nephrology & Hypertension 1994;3:537–545.

38. Sweet CS, Bradstreet DC, Berman RS, Jallard N, Saenz A, Weidler DJ. Pharmacodynamic activity of intravenous E-3174, an angiotensin II antagonist, in patients with essential hypertension. Am J Hypertens 1994; 7:1035–1040.

39. Ilson B, Boike S, Larouche J, Freed M, Jorkasky D. The angiotensin II receptor antagonist SB 03220 does not increase uric acid excretion in healthy men. J Am Soc Nephrol 1994;5:562–569.

40. Soffer BA, Wright JT Jr, Pratt JH, Wiens B, Goldberg AI, Sweet CS. Effects of losartan on a background of hydrochlorothiazide in patients with hypertension. Hypertension 1995;26:112–117.

41. Chobanian AV. Hypertension, growth factors, and their relevance to atherosclerotic vascular disease. In: Laragh JH, Brenner BM, eds. *Hypertension: Pathophysiology, Diagnosis, and Management.* 2nd ed, Vol. 1. New York, NY: Raven Press, Ltd, 1995:515–521.

42. The Multicenter European Research Trial with Cilazapril after Angioplasty to Prevent Transluminal Coronary Obstruction and Restenosis (MERCATOR) Study Group. Does the new angiotensin converting enzyme inhibitor cilazapril prevent restenosis after percutaneous transluminal coronary angioplasty? Results of the MERCATOR study: a multicenter, randomized, double-blind placebo-controlled trial. Circulation 1992;86:100–110.

43. Pratt RE, Dzau VJ. Pharmacological strategies to prevent restenosis: lessons learned from blockade of the renin-angiotensin system. Circulation 1996; 93:848–852.

44. Munafo A, Christen Y, Nussberger J, et al. Drug concentration response relationships in normal volunteers after oral administration of losartan, an angiotensin II receptor antagonist. Clin Pharmacol Ther 1992;51:513–521.

45. Christen Y, Waeber B, Nussberger J, et al. Oral administration of DuP 753, a specific angiotensin II receptor antagonist, to normal male volunteers. Inhibition of pressor response to exogenous angiotensin I and II. Circulation 1991;83:1333–1342.

46. Goldberg MR, Tanaka W, Barchowsky A, et al. Effects of losartan on blood pressure, plasma renin activity, and angiotensin II in volunteers. Hypertension 1993;21:704–713.

47. Goldberg AI, Dunlay MC, Sweet CS. Safety and tolerability of losartan potassium, an angiotensin II receptor antagonist, compared with hydrochlorothiazide, atenolol, felodipine ER, and angiotensin-converting enzyme inhibitors for the treatment of systemic hypertension. Am J Cardiol 1995;75:793–795.

48. Grossman E, Peleg E, Carroll J, Shamiss A, Rosenthal T. Hemodynamic and humoral effects of the angiotensin II antagonist losartan in essential hypertension. Am J Hypertens 1994;7:1041–1044.

49. Goldberg MR, Bradstreet TE, McWilliams EJ, et al. Biochemical effects of losartan, a nonpeptide angiotensin II receptor antagonist, on the renin-angiotensin-aldosterone system in hypertensive patients. Hypertension 1995;25:37–46.

50. Ohtawa M, Takayama F, Saitoh K, Yoshinaga T, Nakashima M. Pharmacokinetics and biochemical efficacy after single and multiple oral administration of losartan, an orally active nonpeptide angiotensin II receptor antagonist, in humans. Br J Clin Pharmacol 1993;35:290–297.

51. Gottlieb SS, Dickstein K, Fleck E, et al. Hemodynamic and neurohormonal effects of the angiotensin II antagonist losartan in patients with congestive heart failure. Circulation 1993;88: 1602–1609.

52. Doig JK, MacFadyen RJ, Sweet CS, Lees KR, Reid JL. Dose-ranging study of the angiotensin type I receptor antagonist losartan (DuP753/MK954), in salt-deplete normal man. J Cardiovasc Pharmacol 1993;21:732–738.

53. Gavras H, Brunner HR, Turini GA, et al. Antihypertensive effect of the oral angiotensin converting-enzyme inhibitor SQ 14225 in man. N Engl J Med 1978;298:991–995.

54. Mancia G, Parati G, Pomidossi G, et al. Modification of arterial baroreflexes by captopril in essential hypertension. Am J Cardiol 1982;49:1415–1419.

55. van den Meiracker AH, Admiraal PJJ, Janssen JA, et al. Hemodynamic and biochemical effects of the AT1 receptor antagonist irbesartan in hypertension. Hypertension 1995;25:22–29.

56. Weinberger MH. Blood pressure and metabolic responses to hydrochlorothiazide, captopril, and the combination in black and white mild-to-moderate hypertensive patients. J Cardiovasc Pharmacol 1985; 7(Suppl. 1):S52–S55.

57. Weidmann P, Boehlen LM, de Courten M, Ferrari P. Antihypertensive therapy in diabetic patients. J Hum Hypertens 1992;6(Suppl. 2):S23–S36.

58. Moan A, Høieggen A, Nordby G, Eide IK, Kjeldsen SE. Effects of losartan on insulin sensitivity in severe hypertension: connections through sympathetic nervous system activity? J Hum Hypertens 1995;9(Suppl. 5):S45–S50.

59. Markham A, Goa KL. Valsartan. A review of its pharmacology and therapeutic use in essential hypertension. Drugs 1997;54: 299–311.

60. Goa KL, Wagstaff AJ. Losartan potassium: a review of its pharmacology and clinical efficacy in the management of hypertension. Drugs 1996;51: 820–845.

61. Gillis JC, Markham A. Irbesartan: a review of its pharmacodynamic and pharmacokinetic properties and therapeutic use in the management of hypertension. Drugs 1997;54:885–902.

62. Holwerda NJ, Fogari R, Angeli P, et al. Valsartan, a new angiotensin II antagonist for the treatment of essential hypertension: efficacy and safety compared with placebo and enalapril. J Hypertens 1996;14: 1147–1151.

63. Oparil S, Dyke S, Harris F, et al. The efficacy and safety of valsartan compared with placebo in the treatment of patients with essential hypertension. Clin Ther 1996;18:797–810.

64. Neutel J, Weber M, Pool J, et al. Valsartan, a new angiotensin II antagonist: antihypertensive effects over 24 hours. Clin Ther 1997;19:447–458.

65. Byyny RL. Antihypertensive efficacy of the angiotensin II AT1-receptor antagonist losartan: results of a randomized, double-blind, placebo-controlled, parallel-group trial using 24-hour blood pressure monitoring. Ambulatory Blood Pressure Monitoring Study Group. Blood Press Suppl 1996;2:71–77.

66. Heuer HJ, Schondorfer G, Hogemann AM. Twenty-four hour blood pressure profile of different doses of candesartan cilexetil in patients with mild to moderate hypertension. J Hum Hypertens 1997;11 (Suppl. 2):S55–S56.

67. Belcher G, Hubner R, George M, Elmfeldt D, Lunde H. Candesartan cilexetil: safety and tolerability in healthy volunteers and patients with hypertension. J Hum Hypertens 1997;11 (Suppl 2):S85–S89.

68. Hegner G, Faust G, Freytag F, Meilenbrock S, Sullivan J, Bodin F. Valsartan, a new angiotensin II antagonist for the treatment of essential hypertension: efficacy and safety compared to hydrochlorothiazide. Eur J Clin Pharmacol 1997;52:173–177.

69. Dahlof B, Keller SE, Makris L, Goldberg AI, Sweet CS, Lim NY. Efficacy and tolerability of losartan potassium and atenolol in patients with mild to moderate essential hypertension. Am J Hypertens 1995;8:578–583.

70. Lappe JT, Nelson EB, Critchley JAJH, Raskin SJ, Snavely DB, Sweet CS for Losartan vs. Felodipine Investigators. Efficacy and tolerability of losartan potassium (MK-954, DuP 753), compared to felodipine ER in elderly hypertensive patients (abstract). J Hypertens 1994;12(Suppl. 3):80.

71. Corea L, Cardoni O, Fogari R, et al. Valsartan, a new angiotensin II antagonist for the treatment of essential hypertension: a comparative study of the efficacy and safety against amlodipine. Clin Pharmacol Ther 1996;60:341–346.

72. Stumpe KO, Haworth D, Hoglund C, et al. Comparison of the angiotensin II receptor antagonist irbesartan with atenolol for treatment of hypertension. Blood Press 1998;7:31–37.

73. Mimran A, Ruilope L, Kerwin L, et al. A randomised, double-blind comparison of the angiotensin II receptor antagonist, irbesartan, with the full dose range of enalapril for the treatment of mild-to-moderate hypertension. J Hum Hypertens 1998;12:203–208.

74. Kassler-Taub K, Littlejohn TL, Elliot W, et al. Comparative efficacy of two angiotensin II receptor antagonists, irbesartan and losartan, in mild-to-moderate hypertension. Am J Hypertens 1998;11:445–453.

75. Oparil S, Guthrie R, Lewin AJ, et al. An elective titration study of the comparative effectiveness of two angiotensin II receptor blockers, irbesartan and losartan. Irbesortan/Losartan Study Investigators. Clin Therapeut 1998; 20:398–409.

76. Andersson OK, Neldam S. A comparison of antihypertensive effects of candesartan cilexetil and losartan in patients with mild to moderate hypertension. J Hum Hypertens 1997;11 (Suppl. 2):S63–S64.

77. Mallion JM, Siche JP, Lacourciere Y, and the Telmisartan Blood Pressure Monitoring Group. ABPM comparison of the antihypertensive profiles of the selective angiotensin II receptor antagonists telmisartan and losartan in patients with mild-to-moderate hypertension. J Hum Hypertens, in press, 1999.

77a. Hedner T, et al. A comparison of the angiotensin II antagonists valsartan and losartan in the treatment of essential hypertension. Am J Hypertens 1999;12:414–417.

78. Muller P, Flesch G, de Gasparo M, Gasparini M, Howald H. Pharmacokinetics and pharmacodynamic effects of the angiotensin II antagonist valsartan at steady state in healthy, normotensive subjects. Eur J Clin Pharmacol 1997; 52:441–449.

79. Burrell LM, Johnston CI. Angiotensin II receptor antagonists. Potential in elderly patients with cardiovascular disease. Drugs Aging 1997;10:421–434.

80. Bremner AD, Baur M, Oddou-Stock P, Bodin F. Valsartan: long term efficacy and tolerability compared to lisinopril in elderly patients with essential hypertension. Clin Exp Hypertens 1997;19:1263–1285.

81. Levy D, Garrison RJ, Savage DD, et al. Prognostic implications of echocardiographically determined left ventricular mass in the Framingham Heart Study. N Engl J Med 1990;322:1561–1566.

82. Messerli FH, Soria F. Does a reduction in left ventricular hypertrophy reduce cardiovascular morbidity and mortality. Drugs 1992;44(Suppl. 1):141–146.

83. Messerli FH, Oren S, Grossman E. Left ventricular hypertrophy and antihypertensive therapy. Drugs 1988;35(Suppl. 5):27–33.

84. Sun Y, Ramires FJ, Weber KT. Fibrosis of atria and great vessels in response to angiotensin II or aldosterone infusion. Cardiovasc Res 1997;35:138–147.

85. Gottdiener JS, Reda DJ, Massie BM, Materson BJ, Williams DW, Anderson RJ for the VA Cooperative Study Group on Antihypertensive Agents. Effect of single-drug therapy on reduction of left ventricular mass in mild to moderate hypertension: comparison of six antihypertensive agents with placebo. The Department of Veterans Affairs Cooperative Study Group on Anti-hypertensive Agents. Circulation 1997;95:2007–2014.

86. Schmieder RE, Martus P, Kingbell A. Reversal of left ventricular hypertrophy in essential hypertension: a meta-analysis of randomized double-blind studies. JAMA 1996;275:1507–1513.

87. Mizuno K, Tani M, Hashimoto S, et al. Effects of losartan, a nonpeptide angiotensin II receptor antagonist, on cardiac hypertrophy

and the tissue angiotensin II content in spontaneously hypertensive rats. Life Sci 1992; 51:367–374.

88. Nunez E, Hosoya K, Susic D, Frohlich ED. Enalapril and losartan reduced cardiac mass and improved coronary hemodynamics in SHR. Hypertension 1997;29(1 Pt 2):519–524.

89. Ledingham JM, Laverty R. Remodelling of resistance arteries in genetically hypertensive rats by treatment with valsartan, an angiotensin II receptor antagonist. Clin Exp Pharmacol Physiol 1996;23(6–7):576–578.

90. de Simone G, Devereux RB, Camargo MJ, Wallerson DC, Scaley JE, Laragh JH. Reduction of development of left ventricular hypertrophy in salt-loaded Dahl salt-sensitive rats by angiotensin II receptor inhibition. Am J Hypertens 1996;9:216–222.

91. Mitsunami K, Endoh S, Maeda K, Kinoshita M, Okada M, Motomura M. Effects of TCV-116 on hemodynamics and cardiac hypertrophy in patients with essential hypertension [poster]. Satellite symposium to the 15th Scientific Meeting of the ISH; Angiotensin II Receptor Antagonists: can they go beyond ACE inhibitors? March 19, 1994, Melbourne.

92. Bruckschlegel G, Holmer SR, Jandeleit K, et al. Blockade of the renin-angiotensin system in cardiac pressure-overload hypertrophy in rats. Hypertension 1995;25:250–259.

93. Himmelmann A, Svensson A, Bergbrant A, Hansson L. Long–term effects of losartan on blood pressure and left ventricular structure in essential hypertension. J Hum Hypertens 1996;10:729-734.

94. Cheung B. Increased left-ventricular mass after losartan treatment. Lancet 1997;349:1743–1744.

95. Dahlof B, Devereux R, de Faire U, et al. The Losartan Intervention For Endpoint reduction (LIFE) in Hypertension study: rationale, design, and methods. The LIFE Study Group. Am J Hypertens 1997;10:705–713.

96. Kahan T, Malmqvist K, Edner M, Held C, Osbakken M. Rate and extent of left ventricular hypertrophy regression: a comparison of angiotensin II blockade with irbesartan and beta-blockade (abstract). J Am Coll Cardiol 1998;31(Suppl A):212A.

97. Thürmann PA. Angiotensin receptor blockers and left ventricular hypertrophy (abstract). Am Heart J 1998;11(4,Pt 2):252A.

98. Martorana PA, Kettenbach B, Breipohl G, Linz W, Scholkens BA. Reduction of infarct size by local angiotensin-converting enzyme inhibition is abolished by a bradykinin antagonist. Eur J Pharmacol 1990;182:395–396.

99. Bao G, Gohlke P, Qadri F, Unger T. Chronic kinin receptor blockade attenuates the antihypertensive effect of ramipril. Hypertension 1992; 20:74–79.

100. Gohlke P, Bunning P, Unger T. Distribution and metabolism of angiotensin I and II in the blood vessel wall. Hypertension 1992;20:7151–7157.

101. Raya TE, Fonken SJ, Lee RW, et al. Hemodynamic effects of direct angiotensin II blockade compared to converting enzyme inhibition in rat model of heart failure. Am J Hypertens 1991;4(Suppl.):334S–340S.

102. Smits JFM, van Krimpen C, Schoemaker RG, Cleutjens JPM, Daemen MJAP. Angiotensin II receptor blockade after myocardial infarction in rats: effects on hemodynamics, myocardial DNA synthesis, and interstitial collagen content. J Cardiovasc Pharmacol 1992;20:772–778.

103. Milavetz JJ, Raya TE, Johnson CS, Morkin E, Goldman S. Survival after myocardial infarction in rats: captopril versus losartan. J Am Coll Cardiol 1996;27:714–719.

104. Richer-Giudicelli C, Fornes P, Cazaubon C, Nisato D, Giudicelli J–F. Effects of angiotensin II AT1 receptor blockade on survival, systemic and coronary hemodynamics and cardiac remodeling in postischemic heart failure in rats (abstract). Circulation 1997;96(Suppl. I):I–644.

105. Fitzpatrick MA, Rademaker MT, Charles CJ, Yandle TG, Espiner EA, Ikram H. Angiotensin II receptor antagonism in ovine heart failure: acute hemodynamic, hormonal, and renal effects. Am J Physiol 1992; 263:H250–H256.

106. Husain A. The chymase-angiotensin system in humans [editorial]. J Hypertens 1993;11:1155–1159.

107. Pfeffer MA, Braunwald E, Moye LA, et al. for the SAVE Investigators. Effect of captopril on mortality and morbidity in patients with left ventricular dysfunction after myocardial infarction: results of the Survival and Ventricular Enlargement Trials. N Engl J Med 1992;327:669–677.

108. SOLVD Investigators. Effects of enalapril on survival in patients with reduced left ventricular ejection fractions and congestive heart failure. N Engl J Med 1991;325:293–302.

109. Garg R, Yusuf S for the Collaborative Group of ACE Inhibitor Trials. Overview of randomized trials of angiotensin converting enzyme inhibitors on mortality and morbidity in patients with heart failure. JAMA 1995; 273:1450–1456.

110. Liu YH, Yang XP, Sharov VG, et al. Effects of angiotensin-converting enzyme inhibitors and angiotensin II type 1 receptor antagonists in rats with heart failure. Role of kinins and angiotensin II type 2 receptors. J Clin Invest 1997;99:1926–1935.

111. Yamamoto S, Hayashi N, Kometani M, Nakao K. Pharmacological profile of valsartan, a non-peptide angiotensin II type 1 receptor antagonist. 5th communication: hemodynamic effects of valsartan in dog heart failure models. Arzneimittelforschung 1997; 47:630–634.

112. Spinale FG, de Gasparo M, Whitebread S, et al. Modulation of the renin-angiotensin pathway through enzyme inhibition and specific receptor blockade in pacing-induced heart failure: I. Effects on left ventricular performance and neurohormonal systems. Circulation 1997;96:2385–2396.

113. Dickstein K, Gottlieb S, Fleck E, et al. Hemodynamic and neurohumoral effects of the angiotensin II antagonist losartan in patients with heart failure. J Hypertens Suppl 1994;12:S31–S35.

114. Crozier I, Ikram H, Awan N, et al. Losartan in heart failure. Hemodynamic effects and tolerability. Losartan Hemodynamic Study Group. Circulation 1995;191:691–697.

115. Pitt B, Segal R, Martinez FA, et al. Randomised trial of losartan versus captopril in patients over 65 with heart failure (Evaluation of Losartan in the Elderly Study, ELITE). Lancet 1997;349:747–752.

116. Dickstein K, Chang P, Willenheimer R, et al. Comparison of the effects of losartan and enalapril on clinical status and exercise performance in patients with moderate or severe chronic heart failure. J Am Coll Cardiol 1995;26:438–445.

117. Lang RM, Elkayam U, Yellen LG, et al. Comparative effects of losartan and enalapril on exercise capacity and clinical status in

patients with heart failure. The Losartan Pilot Exercise Study Investigators. J Am Coll Cardiol 1997;30:983–991.

118. Havranek EP, Thomas I, Smith WB, et al. Dose-related beneficial long-term hemodynamic and clinical effects of irbesartan in heart failure (abstract). Circulation 1997;96:I–452.

119. Virjay N, Alhaddad IA, Denny DM, et al. Irbesartan compared with lisinopril in patients with mild to moderate heart failure (abstract). J Am Coll Cardiol 1998; 31(Suppl. A):68A.

120. Tonkon M, Awan N, Niazi I, et al. for the Irbesartan Heart Failure Group. Irbesartan combined with conventional therapy, including angiotensin converting enzyme inhibitors in heart failure (abstract). J Am Coll Cardiol 1998;31(Suppl. A):188A.

121. Giatras I, Lau J, Levey AS. Effect of angiotensin-converting enzyme inhibitors on the progression of nondiabetic renal disease: a meta-analysis of randomized trials. Ann Intern Med 1997;127: 337–345.

122. Allen TJ, Cao Z, Youssef S, Hulthen UL, Cooper ME. Role of angiotensin II and bradykinin in experimental diabetic nephropathy. Functional and structural studies. Diabetes 1997;46:1612–1618.

123. Kon V, Fogo A, Ichhikawa I. Bradykinin causes selective efferent arteriolar dilation during angiotensin I converting enzyme inhibition. Kidney Int 1993; 44:545–550.

124. Gansevoort RT, de Zeeuw D, de Jong PE. Is the antiproteinuric effect of ACE inhibition mediated by interference in the renin-angiotensin system? Kidney Int 1994;45:861–867.

125. Redon J. Treatment of patients with essential hypertension and microalbuminuria. Drugs 1997;54:857–866.

126. Hagino T, Abe K, Tsunoda K, Yoshinaga K. Antihypertensive effect of a non-peptide angiotensin II receptor antagonist, MK954, in patients with essential hypertension [Japanese]. Nippon Jinzo Gakkai Shi 1992;34:133–140.

127. Sweet CS, Nelson EB. How well have animal studies with losartan predicted responses in humans? J Hypertens 1993;11:S63–S67.

128. Doig JK, McFadyen R, Sweet CS, Devlin AM, Reid JL. Haemodynamic and renal response to losartan during salt depletion or salt repletion (abstract). J Hypertens 1993; 11(Suppl. 5):S419–S420.

129. Bauer JH, Reams GP, Lau A. Effects of losartan on blood pressure, renin-aldosterone, and renal function in essential hypertension (abstract). J Am Soc Nephrol 1993;4:529.

130. Saine DR, Ahrens ER. Renal impairment associated with losartan (letter). Ann Intern Med 1996;124:775.

131. Shaw W, Snavely D, Shahinfar S. Safety and efficacy of losartan (DuP 753, MK-954) in hypertensive patients with renal impairment (abstract). J Am Soc Nephrol 1994;5:567.

132. Monane M, Bohn RL, Gurwitz JH, Glynn RJ, Levin R, Avorn J. The effects of initial drug choice and comorbidity on antihypertensive therapy compliance: results from a population-based study in the elderly. Am J Hypertens 1997;10(7 Pt 1): 697–704.

133. Hricik DE, Browning PJ, Kopelman R, Goorno WE, Madias NE, Dzau VJ. Captopril-induced functional renal insufficiency in patients with bilateral renal artery stenosis or renal artery stenosis in a solitary kidney. N Engl J Med 1983;308:373–376.

134. Postma CT, Dennesen PJW, de Boo T, Thien T. First dose hypotension after captopril; can it be predicted? A study of 240 patients. J Hum Hypertens 1992;6:205–209.

135. Rimmer JM, Horn JF, Gennari FJ. Hyperkalemia as a complication of drug therapy. Arch Intern Med 1987;147:867–869.

136. Piper JM, Ray WA, Rosa FW. Pregnancy outcome following exposure to angiotensin-converting enzyme inhibitors. Obstet Gynecol 1992;80:429–432.

137. Testa MA, Anderson RB, Nackley JF, Hollenberg NK. Quality of life and antihypertensive therapy in men. A comparison of captopril with enalapril. N Engl J Med 1993;328:907–913.

138. Sharma PK, Yium JJ. Angioedema associated with angiotensin II receptor antagonist losartan. South Med J 1997;90:552-553.

139. Acker CG, Greenberg A. Angioedema induced by the angiotensin II blocker losartan. N Engl J Med 1995;333:1572.

140. Chan P, Tomlinson B, Huang TY, Ko JT, Lin TS, Lee YS. Double-blind comparison of losartan, lisinopril, and metolazone in elderly hypertensive patients with previous angiotensin-converting enzyme inhibitor-induced cough. J Clin Pharmacol 1997;37: 253–257.

141. Lacourciere Y, Brunner H, Irwin R, et al. Effects of modulators of the renin-angiotensin-aldosterone system on cough. Losartan cough study group. J Hypertens 1994;12:1387–1393.

142. Benz J, Oshrain C, Henry D, Avery C, Chiang YT, Gatlin M. Valsartan, a new angiotensin II receptor antagonist: a double-blind study comparing the incidence of cough with lisinopril and hydrochlorothiazide. J Clin Pharmacol 1997;37:101–107.

143. Baruch L. The hemodynamic and hormonal effects of AT1 receptor blockade added to ACE inhibition in heart failure (abstract). Am J Hypertens 1998; 11(4, Pt2):252A.

144. Furberg CD, Psaty BM. JNC VI: timing is everything. Lancet 1997; 350:1413–1146.

145. Materson BJ, Reda DJ, Cushman WC, et al. Single-drug therapy for hypertension in men. A comparison of six antihypertensive agents with placebo. N Engl J Med 1993;328:914–921.

146. MacKay JH, Arcuri KE, Goldberg AI, Snapinn SM, Sweet CS. Losartan and low-dose hydrochlorothiazide in patients with essential hypertension. Arch Intern Med 1996;156:278–285.

147. Schoenberger JA for the Losartan Research Group. Losartan with hydrochlorothiazide in the treatment of hypertension. J Hypertens 1995;13(Suppl. 1):S43–S47.

148. Materson BJ, Reda DJ, Williams D. Lessons from combination therapy in Veterans Affairs Studies. Department of Veterans Affairs Cooperative Study Group on antihypertensive agents. Am J Hypertens 1996;9:187S–191S.

149. Bremner AD, Baur M, Oddou-Stock P, Bodin F. Valsartan: long-term efficacy and tolerability compared to lisinopril in elderly patients with essential hypertension. Clin Exp Hypertens 1997;19:1263–1285.

150. Weber MA, Byyny RL, Pratt JH, et al. Blood pressure effects of the angiotensin II receptor blocker, losartan. Arch Intern Med 1995;155:405–411.

151. Bindschedler M, Degen P, Flesch G, de Gasparo M, Preiswerk G. Pharmacokinetic and pharmacodynamic interaction of single oral doses of valsartan and furosemide. Eur J Clin Pharmacol 1997;52:371–378.

152. Shamiss A, Carroll J, Peleg E, Grossman E, Rosenthal T. The effect of enalapril with and without hydrochlorothiazide on insulin sensitivity and other metabolic abnormalities of hypertensive patients with NIDDM. Am J Hypertens 1995;8:276–281.

153. Hamroff G, Blaufarb I, Mancini D, et al. Angiotensin II-receptor blockade further reduces afterload safely in patients maximally treated with angiotensin-converting enzyme inhibitors for heart failure. J Cardiovasc Pharmacol 1997;30:533–536

154. Azizi M, Guyene TT, Chatellier G, Wargon M, Menard J. Additive effects of losartan and enalapril on blood pressure and plasma active renin. Hypertension 1997;29:634–640.

155. Azizi M, Guyene TT, Chatellier G, Menard J. Pharmacological demonstration of the additive effects of angiotensin-converting enzyme inhibition and angiotensin II antagonism in sodium depleted healthy subjects. Clin Exp Hypertens 1997;19:937–951.

CHAPTER 14

Calcium Antagonists

William H. Frishman
Virmeet Singh

Since their development in 1967, calcium-channel blockers have become increasingly important in the management of various cardiovascular disease. By interfering with the normal transmembrane flux of extracellular calcium ions on which vascular tissue depends for contraction or impulse generation, calcium-channel blockers reduce the contractile activity of the heart and promote coronary and systemic vasodilatation. These effects provide the clinical rationale for the use of calcium antagonists in the management of ischemic heart disease, hypertrophic cardiomyopathy, and certain arrhythmias. Because systemic vasodilatation can be expected to reduce elevated arterial blood pressure, interest has focused on the use of calcium-channel blockers in the medical management of systemic hypertension.[1]

Most of the early calcium-channel blockers used in hypertension were relatively short-acting, requiring repeated daily dosing to maintain adequate blood pressure control. However, the use of novel controlled-release drug delivery systems with the shorter-acting calcium-channel blockers and long-acting agents have allowed for once- and twice-daily dosing of these drugs, which has improved patient compliance while reducing the incidence of some adverse reactions.

RATIONALE FOR USE OF CALCIUM-CHANNEL BLOCKERS IN HYPERTENSION

The beneficial effects of the calcium antagonists in hypertension relate to their ability to induce systemic arterial vasodilatation. In isolated human blood vessels, the dihydropyridines, like nifedipine, have been demonstrated to produce concentration-dependent relaxation of noradrenaline and adrenaline-induced constriction of arteries and veins. In clinical use, the partial venodilator effects of nifedipine are usually overcome by the sympathetic reflex activity elicited by the drug, leaving arterial dilatation as the predominant vascular effect. The potent beta-adrenergic stimulating responses elicited by nifedipine also result in increases in heart rate and myocardial contractility.

Studies of the cardiac effects of verapamil have found the drug to produce little change in heart rate or cardiac output. Like nifedipine, the principal hypotensive action of verapamil is mediated by peripheral vasodilation with reduction in peripheral vascular resistance. However, with verapamil, the reflex sympathetic stimulation noted with nifedipine and other vasodilators is blunted due to the drug's concomitant negative inotropic and negative chronotropic effects. Administration of diltiazem and mibefradil also produces little change in heart rate or cardiac output. The comparative hemodynamic and electrophysiological effects of the various calcium blockers are shown in Table 1; the other pharmacologic properties are compared in Tables 2 to 4.

The most important characteristic of all calcium-channel blockers is their ability to effectively inhibit the inward flow of charge-bearing calcium ions when the calcium ion channels become permeable. Previously, the term "slow channel" was used, but it is now recognized that the calcium ion current develops faster than previously thought, and that there are at least two types of calcium channels, the L and T. The conventional calcium channel, which has been known to exist for a long time, is called the L-channel and is blocked by all the calcium-channel antagonists; the T-type channel appears at more negative potentials than the L-type, and probably plays an important role in the initial depolarization of sinus and AV nodal tissue.[2] Specific blockers for the T-type channel are not yet available, but they could be expected to inhibit the sinus and AV nodes profoundly.

Despite the widespread clinical use of calcium-channel blockers for the treatment of hypertension, there are only few long-term studies (Syst Eur, Syst China, HOT) evaluating cardiovascular and cerebrovascular morbidity and mortality outcomes with these treatments in the general population. In 1995 there were two published reports suggesting an increased risk of myocardial infarction and mortality in hypertensive patients receiving short-acting calcium channel blockers (verapamil, diltiazem, nifedipine) as treatment compared with patients receiving other antihypertensive therapies, which included diuretics and beta blockers.[3] These reports were case control studies which have built within their experimental design significant methodologic flaws. A great debate appeared in the medical literature regarding the safety of calcium channel blockers as a class for treating hypertension.[4,5] Based on the available evidence, the FDA has advised physicians not to use the short-acting calcium channel blockers to treat hypertension, but placed no restrictions on the first-line supplementary use of sustained-release calcium channel blocker formulations or longer-acting formulations available for this indication. The investigators of the Systolic Hypertension in Europe (Syst Eur)[6] trial and Syst-China Collaborative group trial[6a] recently concluded that among elderly patients with isolated systolic hypertension, antihypertensive drug treatment starting with nitrendipine

TABLE 1. PHARMACOLOGIC EFFECTS OF THE CALCIUM-CHANNEL BLOCKERS.

Agent	Heart Rate Acute	Heart Rate Chronic	Conduction SA	Conduction AV	Myocardial Contractility	Peripheral Vasodilator	Cardiac Output	Coronary Blood Flow	Myocardial O$_2$ Demand
Diltiazem	↓	↓	↓	↓	↓	↑	↔	↑	↓
Diltiazem SR	↓	↓	↓	↓	↓	↑	↔	↑	↓
Diltiazem CD	↓↔	↔	↓	↓	↓	↑	↑	↑	↓
Dilacor XR^R	↓↔	↔	↓	↓	↓↔	↑	↑↔	↑	↓
Tiazac^R	↓↔	↔	↓	↓	↓↔	↑	↑↔	↑	↓
Verapamil	↓	↓	↓	↓	↓	↑	↔	↑	↓
Verapamil SR	↓	↓	↓	↓	↓	↑	↔	↑	↓
Verelan^R	↓	↓	↓	↓	↓	↑	↑↔	↑	↓
Verapamil Coer	↓	↓	↓	↓	↓	↑	↑↔	↑	↓
Nifedipine	↑↑	↑↔	↔	↑↔	↓	↑↑	↑↔	↑	↓
Nifedipine GITS	↑↔	↔	↓	↓	↓	↑↑	↑↔	↑	↓
Adalat CC^R	↑↔	↔	↓	↓	↓	↑↑	↑↔	↑	↓

Nicardipine	↑↔	↑↔	↔	↑↔	↔	←	←	↑↔	→
Nicardipine SR	↑↔	↑↔	↔	↑↔	↔	←	↑↔	←	→
Nicardipine IV	←		↔	↑↔	↔	←	↑↔	←	↓↑↔
Amlodipine	↑↔	↔	↔	↓	→	←	↔	↑↔	→
Isradipine	↑↔	↑↔	↓↑↔	↑↔	↔	←	↑↔	←	→
Dynacirc CR^R	↑↔	↑↔	↓↑↔	↑↔	↔	←	↑↔	←	→
Felodipine ER	↑↔	↑↔	↔	↑↔	↔	←	↑↔	←	→
Nisoldipine ER	↑↔	↑↔	↔	↑↔	↔	←	↑↔	←	→

SA = sinoatrial; AV = atrioventricular; ↑ = increase; ↓ = decrease; ↔ = no change; V = variable; GITS = gastrointestinal therapeutic system; IV = intravenous; SR, CD, XR, ER = extended release

TABLE 2. CLINICAL CHARACTERISTICS OF CALCIUM CHANNEL BLOCKERS.[2]

Agent	Dosage Oral	Dosage IV	Onset of Action Oral	Onset of Action IV	Therapeutic PC	Site of Metabolism	Active Metabolites	Excretion (%)
Diltiazem	30–90mg q6–8h	75–150µg/kg 10–20mg	<30 min	<10 min	50–200ng/ml	Deacetylation N-deacetylation O-demethylation Major hepatic first-pass effect	Yes	60 (fecal) 2–4 (unchanged in urine)
Diltiazem SR	60–120mg q12h		30–60 min		50–200ng/ml		Yes	
Diltiazem CD	180–360mg q24h		30–60 min		50–200ng/ml		Yes	
Dilacor XR[R]	180–540mg q24h		30–60		40–200ng/ml		Yes	
Tiazac[R]	120–360mg q24h		1–2 h		40–200 ng/ml		Yes	
Verapamil	80–120mg q6–12h	150µg/kg 10–20mg	<30 min	<5 min	>100ng/ml	N-dealkylation O-demethylation Major hepatic first-pass effect	Yes	15 (fecal) 70 (renal) 3–4 (unchanged in urine)
Verapamil SR	240–480mg q12 or 24h		<30 min		>50ng/ml		Yes	15 (fecal) 70 (renal)

Drug	Dose		Onset	Peak	Therapeutic level	Metabolism		Excretion
Verelan[R]	120–480mg q24h				>50 ng/ml	Yes	Yes	16 (fecal) / 70 (renal)
Verapamil Coer 24	180–240mg q24h	4h				Yes	16 (fecal)	70 (renal) / 3–4 (unchanged in urine)
Nifedipine	10–40mg q6-8h	5–15µg/kg	<20 min	3 min SL	25–100ng/ml	A hydroxycarbolic acid and a lactone with no known activity. Major hepatic first-pass effect	No	20–40 (fecal) / 50–80 (renal) / <0.1 (unchanged in urine)
Nifedipine GITS	30–120mg q24h		2 h				No	
Adalat CC[R]	30–90mg		1–2h				No	
Nicardipine	10–20mg TID	1.15mg/h	<20 min	<5 min	28–50ng/ml	Major hepatic first-pass effect	No	35 (fecal) / 60 (renal) / <1 (unchanged in urine)
Nicardipine SR	30–60mg BID			20	28–50 ng/ml			35 (fecal) / 60 (renal) / <1 (unchanged in urine)
Nicardipine IV	4–5mg/h min			20	10–100ng/ml	Hepatic	No	
Amlodipine	5–10mg q24h		90–120 min		6–10ng/ml	Oxidation Extensive but slow	No	20–25 (fecal) / 60 (renal)

TABLE 2. CONTINUED.

			in vitro		hepatic metabolism		
Isradipine	2.5–10mg q12h		120 min	nd	Hepatic de-esterification and aromatization	No	10 (unchanged in urine)
Dynacirc CR^R	5–10mg q24h	1–2h				No	30 (fecal) 70 (renal) 0 (unchanged in urine)
Felodipine ER	5–20mg q24h		2–5h	2–20nmol/L	Hepatic microsomal P-450 system oxidation Major hepatic first-pass effect	No	10 (fecal) 60–70 (renal) <0.5 (unchanged in urine & feces)
Nisoldipine ER	20–40mg q24h				Hepatic hydroxylation	Yes	80 (renal), <1 unchanged in urine

IV = intravenous; PC = plasma concentrations; BID = twice daily; TID = thrice daily; SL = sublingual; nd = no data

Adapted from ref. [2] Frishman WH, Sonnenblick EH: Calcium channel blockers. In, Schlant RC, Alexander RW (eds): *Hurst's The Heart*, 8th ed. New York: McGraw Hill 1994: 1291-1308.

TABLE 3. PHARMACOKINETICS OF THE CALCIUM-CHANNEL BLOCKERS AND SUSTAINED-RELEASE PREPARATIONS.[2]

Agent	Trade	Absorption (%)	Bioavailability (%)*	Protein Binding (%)	Volume of Distribution (L/kg)	$T_{1/2}$ β (hrs)	Clearance (ml/min/kg)	Time to Peak Plasma Concentration (hrs)
Diltiazem	Cardizem^R	>90	35–60	78	5.0	4.1–5.6	15	2–3
Diltiazem SR	Cardizem SR^R	>90	35–60	78	5.0	5–7	15	6–11
Diltiazem CD	Cardizem CD^R	>95	40	70–80	5.0	5–8	15	10–14
Diltiazem XR	Dilacor XR^R	>95	40	70–80	5.0	5–10	15	4–6
Diltiazem ER	Tiazac^R	>90	40	70–80	3–4.5	6–11		
Verapamil	Calan^R, Isoptin^R	>90	10–20	90	4.3	6±4 IV 8±6 po	13±7	1–2
Verapamil SR	Calan SR^R, Isoptin SR^R	>90	10–20	90	4.3	4.5–12	13±7	1–2
Verapamil SR	Verelan^R	>90	20–35	90	162–380	12		7–9
Verapamil Coer 24	Covera HS^R	>90	20–30	90		6–12		1
Nifedipine	Procardia^R	>90	65	90	1.32	≈5	500–600	0.5
Nifedipine GITS	Procardia XL^R	>90	85	>95	1.32	3.8–16.9	500–600	6 to plateau

continued

Table 3. CONTINUED.

Nifedipine ER	Adalat CC^R	>90	85	>90	7	2.5–5		0.5–2.0 min
Nicardipine	Cardene^R	>90	≈30	>90	0.66	≈2 IV 1–2po*	14	
Nicardipine SR	Cardene SR^R	>90	35	>95		8.6	0.6	1–4
Nicardipine IV	Cardene IV^R							
Amlodipine	Norvasc^R	>90	60–65	>95	21	35–45	7	6–12
Isradipine	Dynacirc^R	90–95	17	97	2.9	8.8	10	1.5
Isradipine GITS	Dynacirc CR^R	>90	15–24	95		(biphasic: early 2h; late 8h)		1.5
Felodipine	Plendil^R	>95	15–25	>99	10	15.1±2.6	12	2.5–5
Nisoldipine	Sular^R	87	5	>99	7–12	6–12		

* = extraction ratio; IV = intravenous; po = oral
Adapted from ref. [2] Frishman WH, Sonnenblick EH. Calcium channel blockers. In, Schlant RC, Alexander RW (eds): *Hurst's The Heart*, 8th ed. New York: McGraw Hill 1994:1291–1308.

TABLE: 4. ADVERSE EFFECTS OF CALCIUM-CHANNEL BLOCKERS.

Agent	Overall (%)	Headache	Dizziness	GI	Flushing	Paresthesia	↓SA/AV Conduction	CHF	Hypotension	Pedal Edema	Worsening of Angina	Palpitations
Diltiazem	~5	+	+	+	+	–	3+	+	+	+	–	+
Diltiazem SR	~5	+	+	+	+	–	3+	+	+	+	–	+
Diltiazem CD	~5	+	+	+	+	–	+	+	+	+	–	+
Diltiazem XRR	~5	+	+	+	–	+	+	–	+	+	–	+
Diltiazem ER	~5	+	+	+	–	+	+	–	+	+	–	+
Verapamil	8	+	+	3+	–	–	3+	2+	+	+	–	+
Verapamil SR	~8	+	+	3+	–	–	3+	2+	+	+	–	+
Verapamil CR	~8	+	+	3+	–	–	3+	2+	+	+	–	+
Verapamil Coer24	~8	+	+	3+	–	–	3+	2+	+	+	–	+
Nifedipine	~20	3+	3+	+	3+	+	–	+	+	2+	+	++
Nifedipine GITS	~10	+	+	+	+	+	–	+	+	+	–	+
Nifedipine ER	~15	+	+	+	+	+	–	+	+	+	–	+

continued

TABLE 4. CONTINUED.

Nicardipine	~20	3+	3+	+	3+	+	−	−	+	+	2+	+	++
Nicardipine SR	~20	+	+	+	+	+	−	+	+	−	+	−	+
Nicardipine IV		+	+	−	+	−	−	−	+	+	−	+	+
Amlodipine	~15	2+	+	+	+	+	−	−	+	−	2+	−	+
Isradipine	~15	2+	2+	+	+	+	−	−	+	−	2+	−	+
Isradipine GITS	~15	2+	+	+	+	+	−	−	+	−	2+	−	+
Felodipine ER	~20	2+	2+	+	2+	+	−	−	+	−	2+	−	+
Nisoldipine ER	~15	2+	+	+	+	−	−	−	+	−	2+	−	+

GI = gastrointestinal; SA = sinoatrial node; AV = atrioventricular node; CHF = congestive heart failure; − = no report; + = rare; 2+ = occasional; 3+ = frequent. Adapted from ref. [1] with permission.

reduces the rate of cardiovascular complications and both fatal and non-fatal stroke. A large number of studies are now in progress comparing calcium channel blockers to other antihypertensive treatments, which will help to resolve this safety issue with this treatment modality once and for all. The recent Joint National Committee for the Prevention, Detection, Evaluation and Treatment of High Blood Pressure-VI (JNC-VI) report also advises against the use of short-acting calcium antagonists for the treatment of hypertension in patients with co-existent coronary artery disease.[7] In older patients with isolated systolic hypertension, diuretics are the preferred class of antihypertensive medications, but long-acting dihydropyridine calcium antagonists are considered appropriate alternatives in these patients.[7]

Another observation that has recently surfaced regards the effect of grapefruit juice ingestion on the pharmacokinetics and hemodynamics of several calcium channel blockers. Studies have demonstrated that grapefruit juice can increase the bioavailability of orally-administered felodipine, nisoldipine, nifedipine, and to a lesser extent other dihydropyridine derivatives.[8] This has been shown to be secondary to the downregulation of intestinal CYP3A4 protein expression by these drugs with increased drug absorption.

CLINICAL USE OF CALCIUM-CHANNEL BLOCKERS IN SYSTEMIC HYPERTENSION

Verapamil

Verapamil, a phenylalkylamine calcium-channel blocker, is a well established treatment for angina, cardiac arrhythmias, hypertrophic cardiomyopathy, and in sustained-release delivery systems, for systemic hypertension. Verapamil's antihypertensive efficacy results from the drug's ability to reduce systemic vascular resistance. Sustained-release verapamil formulations, including a new delayed- and sustained-release formulation, have been proven as effective in lowering blood pressure over 24 hours when used once daily as have the immediate-release verapamil formulations which require more frequent daily dosing.[9]

Studies in hypertensive patients have shown verapamil can lower mean arterial blood pressure at rest and after exercise. This is not associated with a change in cardiac output because of the counterbalancing negative chronotropic and inotropic effects of verapamil. Verapamil is not recommended in patients with heart failure or conduction abnormalities of the heart, as it may not induce sufficient vasodilation to overcome its negative inotropic and chronotropic effects.

Verapamil has minimal to no effect on renal function, plasma lipids and glucose homeostasis, and a variable effect on hepatic blood flow and portal pressure. It has been shown to inhibit platelet aggregation induced by collagen, epinephrine and adenosine diphosphate.

Verapamil has been shown to be as effective as other first-line antihypertensive treatments, including beta blockers, diuretics, angiotensin converting enzyme (ACE) inhibitors, and other calcium-channel blockers. Verapamil has additionally shown efficacy when used as a second- and third-line agent in refractory patients. Verapamil has been used in patients with pulmonary hypertension, concomitant systemic hypertension and angina pectoris, renovascular hypertension, hypertension in pregnancy, and as an IV formulation in hypertensive crisis. In oral forms, it may reduce the risk of recurrent cardiac events in survivors of an acute myocardial infarction.

Diltiazem

Diltiazem, a benzothiazepine calcium-channel blocker, has been shown to be effective in the treatment of patients with angina pectoris, supraventricular tachycardia including atrial fibrillation/flutter, and in sustained-release delivery systems for mild to moderate systemic hypertension.[10] Diltiazem lowers blood pressure as a result of peripheral vasodilatation, which is unaccompanied by reflex tachycardia probably secondary to suppression of the sinoatrial node. Diltiazem may improve left ventricular performance by enhancing myocardial relaxation and diastolic function coupled with afterload reduction, despite a mild negative inotropic effect. The drug has been shown to reduce coronary artery spasm and improve patency of stenotic lesions during exertion with increased perfusion of myocardium at risk of ischemia.

Diltiazem may improve renal function in patients with hypertensive nephropathy and has not been shown to reduce renal blood flow or alter glomerular filtration rate. No long-term effect is known to occur on serum electrolyte levels, fluid retention, and glucose or lipid homeostasis.

Diltiazem's success as a antihypertensive agent is comparable to other medications including hydrochlorothiazide, ß-blockers, ACE inhibitors and other calcium-channel blockers. In stable angina pectoris, it has shown equivalence to propranolol, nifedipine, and verapamil. Diltiazem's efficacy in unstable angina has been comparable to that of intravenous nitroglycerin and oral propranolol. Beneficial cardioprotective effects (in protecting against recurrent cardiac events) have been observed in patients who had survived a non-Q-wave myocardial infarction.

Diltiazem should be used with caution in patients with atrioventricular conduction delays and is contraindicated in patients with sick sinus syndrome, second or third degree atrioventricular block, hypotension, acute myocardial infarction, and pulmonary congestion. Intravenous diltiazem is effective in unstable angina pectoris, controlling paroxysmal supraventricular tachycardia and atrial fibrillation/flutter, and as an intracoronary parenteral treatment to prevent vasospasm during coronary angioplasty.

Nifedipine

Two sustained-release formulations of nifedipine have been shown to be effective in the treatment of mild-to-moderate hypertension.[11] The nifedipine gastrointestinal therapeutic system (GITS) has been shown to reduce blood pressure by approximately 20%, and patients are usually spared the post-dose tachycardia seen with short-acting conventional nifedipine formulations.

Nifedipine mainly acts as a peripheral arterial vasodilator with a small, direct negative inotropic effect in vitro and after intracoronary administration to humans. This is usually not observed after oral administration. Despite nifedipine's action to enhance SA and AV nodal conduction, it is similar to diltiazem and verapamil in its antianginal effects. Nifedipine improves coronary blood flow, especially to areas supplied by stenotic arteries, improves exercise tolerance in patients with effort angina, and relieve coronary vasospasm in variant (Prinzmetal's) angina.

Although there is conflicting evidence of nifedipine's effect on the serum lipid profile, it does appear to reduce the progression of new atherosclerotic plaques in patients with mild-to-moderate coronary artery disease, however, with no favorable effect on mortality. Nifedipine does not appear to affect glucose tolerance, but has significant diuretic, natriuretic, kaliuretic, and uricosuric actions.

Studies indicate that the sustained-release formulations of nifedipine (GITS and Adalat CC®) are at least as effective as hydrochlorothiazide, with mean blood pressure reductions ranging from 8% to 22%, and an overall antihypertensive response rate of 60% to 80% in patients with hypertension. There is, however, little change in blood pressure in normotensive subjects. Nifedipine GITS is also approved for patients with angina pectoris. Efficacy has additionally been observed with Raynaud's phenomenon, hypertension in pregnancy, and pre- and post-operative management of pheochromocytoma.

Nifedipine is well tolerated, with side effects being mild and transient, usually related to the drug's vasodilatory actions. These include headache, flushing, dizziness, pedal edema. Sustained-release nifedipine is generally better tolerated than immediate-release nifedipine because of a slower absorption, a more gradual onset of action, and lower peak plasma concentrations.

Nicardipine

Nicardipine, a dihydropyridine calcium-channel blocker, is effective in the treatment of angina and in conventional and sustained-release delivery systems for systemic hypertension.[12] It produces a dose-related decrease in mean arterial blood pressure and increase in heart rate, with its greatest effects observed at rest rather than during exercise. It has also been observed that patients taking both nicardipine and beta-adrenergic blockers have lower blood pressure and systemic vascular resistance than being on beta blockers alone. In addition, nicardipine will normalize heart rate, cardiac output, and ventricular relaxation which are decreased after beta blocker therapy. Nicardipine appears to reduce coronary vascular resistance to a greater extent than systemic vascular resistance, and is known to increase coronary blood flow in patients with coronary artery disease. Nicardipine may also improve ventricular function in patients with coronary artery disease, reducing left ventricular lactate production by improving myocardial perfusion and aerobic metabolism in chronically ischemic areas. Other effects of nicardipine include an increase in renal blood flow, glomerular filtration rate, plasma renin activity and a modest natriuretic effect. There may also be a potent dose-related cerebral vasodilating effect.

Studies have indicated that nicardipine is at least as effective as hydrochlorothiazide, propranolol, and verapamil in patients with mild to moderate hypertension. In addition, nicardipine is comparable in effectiveness to nifedipine, verapamil, diltiazem, propranolol, and atenolol in patients with angina pectoris. An intravenous formulation of nicardipine is being marketed for the parenteral treatment of systemic hypertension; it is the first calcium antagonist to be approved for this use.[13]

Isradipine

Isradipine, a dihydropyridine calcium-channel blocker in both immediate-release and sustained-release formulations, is used for the treatment of systemic hypertension. Clinical studies have demonstrated its efficacy as a monotherapy or in combination with beta blockers, diuretics or ACE inhibitors for long-term management of patients with mild to moderate hypertension.[14]

Isradipine offers the advantage of having little myocardial depressant activity, a selective action on the coronary, cerebral and skeletal vasculatures, and a potent vasodilatory action. Compared with nifedipine, isradipine has a lesser negative inotropic effect and rarely causes reflex tachycardia. This drug has a sustained diuretic and natriuretic effect, and plasma renin activity has been shown to either increase or remain unchanged. Isradipine appears to have anti-atherogenic potential and does not adversely affect the serum lipid profile, however, no mortality benefit has been observed.[15]

In long-term trials, isradipine has been found to normalize systolic and diastolic blood pressure in up to 85% of patients with mild to moderate hypertension. Its efficacy is comparable to that of nifedipine, hydrochlorothiazide, propranolol, atenolol, prazosin, and diltiazem. In comparative trials with nifedipine and isosorbide dinitrate, it was similar in improving the subjective and objective symptoms of patients with chronic stable angina.

Isradipine's major side effects of headache, flushing, ankle edema, dizziness, and palpitations/tachycardia are generally mild, dose related, and transient, with improvement after the initial weeks of therapy. Isradipine is known to elevate peak plasma propranolol concentration, but does not alter steady state digoxin levels.

Amlodipine

Amlodipine is a long-acting dihydropyridine calcium-channel blocker, is approved for use in patients with either systemic hypertension or angina pectoris. Clinical trials have demonstrated its efficacy in the long-term management of these conditions. In comparative studies, amlodipine was at least as effective as atenolol, verapamil, hydrochlorothiazide, or captopril in patients with hypertension, and as effective as diltiazem or nadolol in patients with angina pectoris.[16]

Amlodipine is similar to other dihydropyridine calcium-channel blockers, demonstrating coronary and peripheral vasodilating activity. It has a gradual onset of antihypertensive effect, with a sustained action allowing once-daily dosing. Amlodipine increases renal blood flow and glomerular filtration rate, and reduces renovascular resistance without significantly affecting plasma renin activity, aldosterone, and catecholamine levels. The drug appears to have no long-term effect on sodium homeostasis. Amlodipine does not have a significant cardiodepressant effect, and has been used safely in patients with mild congestive heart failure as an adjunctive therapy to ACE inhibitors, digoxin, and diuretics.[1]

In addition, amlodipine is thought to have antiatherosclerotic, antithrombotic, and antihypertrophic actions. Unlike verapamil, diltiazem, and nifedipine, amlodipine does not undergo extensive hepatic first-pass metabolism, although it is extensively and slowly metabolized by the liver. Its rate of elimination is significantly reduced in the elderly and in patients with hepatic cirrhosis. No significant pharmacokinetic changes are found in patients with renal impairment.[17]

Amlodipine is generally well tolerated with the most common adverse effects being peripheral edema and flushing. Unlike other dihydropyridine calcium-channel blockers, it usually does not cause reflex tachycardia. Despite the observation that nifedipine can increase plasma digoxin concentration, neither this interaction nor any other significant drug interactions have been found with amlodipine.

Felodipine

Felodipine, a dihydropyridine calcium-channel blocker, was initially studied in a conventional tablet formulation; however, more recent experience has been with an extended-release (ER) formulation which has permitted once-daily dosing.[18a] In patients with mild to moderate essential hypertension, felodipine ER is at least as effective as other calcium-channel blockers, beta blockers, diuretics, and ACE inhibitors, and has been shown to be effective in combination with controlled-release metoprolol and enalapril.

Felodipine is a selective arterial dilator of vascular smooth muscle, without the negative inotropic effects of nifedipine and amlodipine seen at doses producing equivalent vasodilation. This drug may initially increase heart rate, stroke volume, and cardiac output with a subsequent return to baseline. However, a sustained increase in stroke volume and cardiac output may be experienced in patients with heart failure during long-term therapy.

Hypertensive patients may experience an acute neurohumoral response to felodipine, which disappears after one week of therapy. These responses include increases in plasma renin activity, plasma levels of angiotensin II, catecholamine, and atrial natriuretic factor, as well as diuresis, natriuresis, and kaluresis. Felodipine appears to have no effect on glomerular filtration rate and creatinine clearance, although renal vascular resistance is decreased and renal blood flow may be marginally increased. There appear to be no significant effects on blood levels of lipids and glucose.

When ingested, felodipine ER forms a gel on contact with gastrointestinal fluid which is gradually dissolved to release the drug at a slow, constant rate without the pronounced plasma drug peak seen with conventional formulations. Both increasing patient age and hepatic cirrhosis have been associated with a decreased plasma clearance of conventional felodipine tablets. No pharmacokinetic changes being observed in patients with renal failure.

Trials have indicated that the addition of felodipine ER, 5 to 20 mg once daily, in patients with severe hypertension inadequately controlled by a beta blocker and/or diuretic can produce additional reductions in blood pressure. As with other calcium-channel blockers, reductions in left ventricular hypertrophy with felodipine have been noted. Similar to other calcium-channel blockers, felodipine is suitable for hypertensive patients with diabetes, renal dysfunction, Raynaud's phenomenon, asthma, or gout. It has been used as an adjunctive therapy in patients with congestive heart failure who are receiving ACE inhibitors, digoxin, and diuretics.

Felodipine's adverse effect profile, which is improved due to the lower plasma peak in the ER formulation, is similar to other dihydropyridines, and includes peripheral edema, headache, flushing and dizziness. Drugs that induce (antiepileptics) and inhibit (cimetidine, erythromycin) the hepatic cytochrome P450 system, may affect plasma felodipine concentrations. In patients with congestive heart failure, conventional formulation felodipine is associated with increased plasma drug concentrations, while the ER formulation has no significant effect on plasma drug levels in heart failure patients. In addition, conventional felodipine decreases the absorption of orally-administered theophylline.

Nisoldipine

Nisoldipine, a new dihydropyridine calcium-channel blocker similar in structure to nifedipine, is available only in a sustained-release formulation for once daily dosing. It has been used in clinical trials for the treatment of patients with systemic hypertension and angina pectoris, and in a limited experience in the treatment of patients with congestive heart failure. It acts predominantly by inhibiting the entry of calcium ions into excitable tissue, resulting in peripheral and coronary vasodilation. Nisoldipine-induced peripheral vasodilation is estimated to be 5 to 10 times that of nifedipine, but less potent in its effects on cardiac conduction tissue. Oral doses of the drug produce dose-dependent decreases in both resting and exercise blood pressure values.

Many human studies using intravenous nisoldipine have shown increases in heart rate. The effect on heart rate after oral dosing is more variable. One study showed no effect on heart rate at rest or during peak exercise, whereas another study showed increased heart rate at rest and during exercise.[19] Nisoldipine is a potent coronary vasodilator, shown to decrease coronary vascular resistance and increase coronary blood flow in humans.

The most optimal dosing regimen has not been established in clinical trials. The drug appears to have a favorable side effect profile.

CONTROLLED-RELEASE DRUG DELIVERY SYSTEMS AMONG CALCIUM-CHANNEL BLOCKERS

Controlled-release drug delivery systems allow once and twice daily dosing of shorter-acting antihypertensive agents, which can enhance patient compliance and reduce the side effects seen with the basic formulations (Table 5). The goal, although not always realized, is to attain zero-order drug kinetics with a constant rate of drug release with time. This is inevitably affected by the pattern of gastrointestinal motility in the fed and fasted states; gastrointestinal transmit time from the stomach to the ileocecal valve; splanchnic blood flow; increasing pH from the stomach to the colon; declining liquid media for dissolution from the stomach to the colon; and differing areas of gastrointestinal absorption throughout the gastrointestinal tract. The most common oral controlled-release formulations include a polymeric coated reservoir or homogenous drug–polymer matrix system based on diffusional principles; an encapsulation or matrix formulation dissolutional system via bioerosion or degradation; and osmotic pump systems.[20]

The Nifedipine GITS introduced in 1989, consists of a semipermeable membrane surrounding a bilayer core composed of an active drug layer of nifedipine suspension and a pharmacologically-inert and osmotically-active layer. Water absorption throughout the gastrointestinal tract swells the pill allowing zero-order drug release via a laser-drilled hole over 24 hours. Food increases the peak concentration of the GITS tablet by about 28% and decreases the time-to-maximum concentration. When compared with long-acting propranolol, nifedipine GITS was found to be more effective in lowering systolic and diastolic blood pressure.[11]

Nifedipine CC (Adalat CC) consists of an external coat and an internal core, both containing nifedipine. The coat is a slow-release formulation for release in the upper gastrointestinal tract, and the core is a fast-release formulation for immediate release in the colon. Nifedipine CC should be taken on an empty stomach since C_{max} is increased by 60% with food intake.

There are three controlled-release delivery systems currently available in the United States for verapamil: the Calan SR/Isoptin SR formulations, Verelan, and Verapamil-Coer. In the Calan/Isoptin formulations, the effect of immediate-release verapamil is prolonged via the drug's incorporation into a matrix of the natural polysaccharide sodium alginate. Once in contact with gastrointestinal fluid, the pill swells and verapamil diffuses through a gel-like matrix, with total release over approximately seven hours. Gastrointestinal absorption and bioavailability are decreased when taken with food, with peak plasma levels 2.1 times greater and the area under the curve 1.76 times greater than in the fasting state. When compared with immediate-release verapamil, verapamil SR causes an equivalent dose-dependent reduction in blood pressure, but a more favorable side effect profile. Verelan, approved in 1990, is a formulation designed to release verapamil without respect to the fasting or fed states. This spheroidal oral drug absorption system (SODAS) consists of multiple 1 mm drug spheres stored in a rate-controlling polymer all within

TABLE 5. DELAYED RELEASE DRUG DELIVERY SYSTEMS OF LONG-ACTING CALCIUM-CHANNEL BLOCKERS.

Agent	System
Nifedipine GITS Isradipine GITS	A semipermeable membrane surrounds an osmotically active drug core. The core has 2 layers—an "active" layer containing drug and pharmacologically inert but osmotically active "push" layer. After ingestion, the tablet overcoating is quickly dissipated in the gastrointestinal tract, allowing water to enter the tablet through the semi-permeable membrane. The push layer swells and exerts pressure against the active drug layer releasing isradipine through laser-drilled table orifice.
Verapamil (Calan SR[R]/ Isoptin SR[R])	Diffusional System—verapamil is incorporated into a matrix of the natural polysaccharide sodium alginate which sells in contact with GI fluid. Verapamil diffuses out over 7 hours.
Verelan[R]	Dissolutional System—the spheroidal oral drug absorption system (SODAS) consists of multiple 1mm spheres surrounded by rate-controlling polymers all stored in a hard gelatin capsule. A fraction of the beads are released immediately with the rest distributed within the GI tract. Dissolution is independent of pH and food.
Verapamil Coer	Delayed-release osmotor pump system—two-stage drug delivery with an outer membrane, an underlying subcoat, a drug reservoir, and a "push layer"—the outer member and subcoat delay water absorption and drug release for 4–5 hours after dosing. When enough moisture has been absorbed, the push layer expands and forces the drug through pores in outer membrane.
Felodipine ER	Diffusional System—upon contact with GI fluid, felodipine diffuses over 12 hours, first from an outer hydrophilic gel layer and then from an outer reservoir, permitting once daily dosing.
Diltiazem Cardizem SR[R]	Dissolutional System—diltiazem beads contain a variably thick pharmaceutical coating which dissolves over 3–12 hours in the GI tract. Twice daily dosing required.
Cardizem CD[R]	Diffusional System—in a water dependent process, 2 populations of SR beads, thin and thick coated, release diltiazem over the first 12 hours and then the second 12 hours, respectively, for once daily dosing.
Dilacor XR[R]	Dissolutional System— tablet swelling causes release of 3 or 4 60 mg diltiazem tablets beyond an outer hard gelatin coating over 24 hours for once daily dosing. The outer slow-hydrating coat ensures drug release at a constant rate.
Tiazac[R]	Diltiazem hydrochloride in extended release beads at doses of 120, 180, 240, 300 and 360 mg.
Nicardipine SR	Dissolutional System—a two component capsule contains an immediate-release powder and a slow-release spherical granule, the former containing 25% and the latter

TABLE 5. CONTINUED.

Agent	System
	75% of the total nicardipine dose. The granule's polymer of methacrylic acid ensures insolubility at pH <5.0, and the limited spheroidal surface area available for dissolution creates a sustained release effect once past the duodenum.
Nisoldipine SR Adalat CC[R]	Dissolutional System—Consists of an external coat and an internal core, both of which contain the drug. The coating is formulated for slow release in the upper gastrointestinal tract, where absorption is rapid, while the core is formulated for immediate release in the colon where absorption is slower, and permitting once a day dosing.

a hard gelatin capsule. Wide distribution and dissolution within the gastrointestinal tract occurs independent of pH and food, with a proportion of the beads being released immediately. In vitro dissolution is prolonged to 7.3 hours compared with the traditional SR verapamil tablet of 5.0 hours.[21,22] Verapamil-Coer utilizes a two-stage delivery system with an outer delay coat and an inner osmotic push-pull system similar to nifedipine and isradipine GITS. The formulation is administered once daily, at bedtime, and will cause a delay in the release of verapamil for 4–6 hours and then deliver the drug in a sustained-release fashion for 10–12 hours. Blood pressure is reduced to the greatest extent during the day time when blood pressure is generally the highest (especially in the morning), and to a lesser but significant extent during the nighttime when blood pressure is generally the lowest, as part of the circadian rhythm.[23] The Verapamil-Coer is also approved for once daily use in angina pectoris.[23a] A clinical morbidity and mortality trial is now taking place in hypertensive patients comparing once daily use of Verapamil-Coer, administered at bedtime, to atenolol and hydrochlorothiazide, administered in the morning.

An extended-release formulation of the dihydropyridine calcium-channel blocker felodipine is available in the United States. This is a tablet consisting of a felodipine reservoir embedded in a hydrophilic gel-forming substance surrounded by an outer felodipine primary layer, activated upon contact with gastrointestinal fluid. Felodipine is released by diffusion at a controlled rate over 12 hours, with time-to-maximum concentration of a 10 mg dose being 3 hours for the extended-release formulation and 1 hour for the immediate-release formulation.

Nicardipine SR is a sustained-release hard gelatin capsule containing 30, 45, or 60 mg of nicardipine hydrochloride. Each capsule is composed of a powder component and a spherical granule. Both parts contain inactive ingredients (i.e., starch), but the former also contains 25% active nicardipine and the latter 75% active drug. This system permits twice daily dosing of nicardipine for hypertension instead of thrice daily dosing as with the immediate-release preparation of the drug.[21]

Sustained-release nisoldipine is similar to nifedipine CC (Adalat CC), consisting of an external coat and an internal core, both of which contain the drug. The coating is formulated for slow release in the upper gastrointestinal tract, where absorption is rapid, while the core is formulated for immediate-release in the colon, where absorption is slow, permitting once a day dosing.

Isradipine GITS is similar to nifedipine GITS, and consists of a semipermeable membrane surrounding an osmotically active drug core. The core has 2 layers, and "active" layer containing drug and a pharmacologically inert, but osmotically active, "push" layer. After ingestion, the tablet overcoat is quickly dissipated in the gastrointestinal tract, allowing water to enter the tablet through the semipermeable membrane. The push layer swells and exerts pressure against the active drug layer, releasing isradipine through laser-drilled tablet orifice.

Four delayed-release formulations of diltiazem are now available: an SR formulation requiring twice daily dosing and three once daily formulations (CD, XR, and Tiazac). Diltiazem SR is a multiparticulate formulation consisting of beads with a pharmaceutical coating of variable thickness which dissolves over 3–12 hours in the gastrointestinal tract. Cardizem CD contains SR beads of thin and thick copolymer coats. Thin beads release 40% of the diltiazem dose in the first 12 hours, with the rest dispensed over the ensuing 12 hours in a water-dependent diffusional process. The number of beads determines the strength of the capsule. With Dilacor XR, the sustained release is accomplished via a three layer, 60 mg tablet composed of a core of diltiazem HCl and hydrophilic and hydrophobic material lying between two inactive external layers containing the same hydrophilic and hydrophobic material and an additional non-soluble excipient. Slow hydration of the outer layers controls the core hydration, with regulation of diltiazem's release being determined by the surface area-volume dimensions, matrix porosity and tablet swelling. Available dosages are 180 and 240 mg tablets, containing either 3 or 4 short-acting diltiazem 60 mg tablets respectively. Studies thus far demonstrate that this new once daily sustained-release formulation of diltiazem effectively lowers systolic and diastolic blood pressure in patients with mild-to-moderate essential hypertension.[24,25] It appears to be safe and well tolerated with adverse experiences being generally mild in nature; its incidence of side effects is similar to that of placebo. Tiazac, the most recently approved sustained-release formulation of diltiazem hydrochloride, uses a system of extended release beads.

CONCLUSION

Each calcium-channel antagonist exerts its effects through inhibition of slow-channel-mediated calcium ion transport. However, many of the drugs appear to accomplish this by different mechanisms, with differing effects on various target organs that can be of clinical relevance in individual patients.[26]

TABLE 6. SOME ONGOING CLINICAL TRIALS COMPARING CALCIUM-CHANNEL BLOCKERS WITH OTHER ANTIHYPERTENSIVE MEDICATIONS.

Trial	Participants	Sample Size	Drugs Compared	Primary Outcome	Length of Study (year completed)
NORDIL	Mild-moderate Htn aged 50–69 with primary HTN	12,000	Diltizem vs diuretics or ß blockers	Fatal acute MI, fatal stroke, sudden death, other fatal and nonfatal	5 years (1999)
INSIGHT	HTN higher-risk* patients; aged 55–80	6,600	Long-acting nifedipine vs diuretics	Total CV disease	3 years (1999)
CONVINCE	Mild-moderate HTN higher-risk patients aged >55	15,000	Controlled onset ER verapamil vs diuretics or ß blockers	Prevention of fatal and nonfatal MI and stroke, death	4–6 years (2000–2002)
ALLHAT	HTTN, higher-risk patients, aged ?55	40,000	CCB vs diuretics vs ACE inhibitors vs ß blockers	Mortality and MI	6 years (2002)

NORDIL = Nordic Diltiazem Trial; INSIGHT = International Nifedipine Study Intervention as a Goal in Hypertension Treatment; HOT = Hypertensional Optimal Treatment/International Study; CONVINCE = Controlled Onset Verapamil Investigation of Cardiovascular Endpoints; ALLHAT = Antihypertensive and Lipid Lowering to Prevent Heart Attack Trial
Adapted from ref. [1] with permission.

Results from ongoing morbidity and mortality trials in patients with systemic hypertension and congestive heart failure will impact how calcium channel antagonists will be used as antihypertensive treatments in the future (Table 6).

REFERENCES

1. Frishman WH. Calcium-channel blockers. In, Frishman WH, Sonnenblick EH (eds): *Cardiovascular Pharmacotherapeutics*. New York: McGraw-Hill 1997:101–130.

2. Frishman WH, Sonnenblick EH. Beta-adrenergic blocking drugs and calcium channel blockers. In, Alexander RW, Schlant RC, Fuster V, et al. (eds.). *Hurst's The Heart*, 9th ed. New York: McGraw-Hill 1997:1583–1618.

3. Pahor M, Guralnik JM, Corti C, et al. Long-term survival and use of antihypertensive medications in older persons. JAGS 1995;43: 1191–1197.

4. Stelfox HT, Chua G, O'Rourke K, Detsky AS: Conflict of interest in the debate over calcium channel antagonists. N Engl J Med. 1998;338:101–106.

5. Psaty BM, Heckbert SR, Koepsell TD, et al. The risk of myocardial infarction associated with antihypertensive drug therapies. JAMA 1995;274:620–625.

6. Staessen JA, Fagard R, Thijs L, et al. Randomized double-blind comparison of placebo vs active treatment for older patients with isolated systolic hypertension: The Systolic Hypertension in Europe (SYST-EUR) Trial Investigators. Lancet 1997;350(9080): 757-764.

6a. Liu L, Gong L, Wang JG for the SYST-China Investigators: Stroke incidence in the placebo-controlled Chinese Trial on isolated systolic hypertension in the elderly (abstract). J Am Coll Card 1998;31/2 (Suppl A):129A.

7. The Sixth Report of the Joint National Committee on the Prevention, Detection, Evaluation and Treatment of High Blood Pressure. Arch Intern Med 1997;157:2413–2446.

8. Lundahl J, Regardh CG, Edgar S, Johson G. Effect of grapefruit juice ingestion—pharmacokinetics and hemodynamics of intravenous and orally administered felodipine in healthy men. Eur J Clin Pharmacol 1997;52:139–145.

9. McTavish D, Sorkin EM: Verapamil. An updated review of its pharmacodynamic and pharmacokinetic properties and therapeutic uses in hypertension. Drugs 1989;38(1):19-76.

10. Buckley MT, Grant SM, Goa KL, McTavish D, Sorkin EM. Diltiazem: A reappraisal of its pharmacologic properties and therapeutic use. Drugs 1990;39(5):757–806.

11. Murdoch D, Brogden RN. Sustained-release nifedipine formulations. An appraisal of their current uses and prospective roles in the treatment of hypertension, ischaemic heart disease and peripheral vascular disorders. Drugs 1991;41(5):737–79.

12. Sorkin EM, Clissold DP. Nicardipine. A review of its pharmacodynamic and pharmacokinetic properties and therapeutic efficacy in the treatment of angina pectoris, hypertension and related cardiovascular disorders. Drugs 1987;33:296–345.

13. IV Nicardipine Group: Efficacy and safety of intravenous nicardipine in the control of postoperative hypertension. Chest, 1991;99:393–98.

14. Fitton A, Benfield P. Isradipine. A review of its pharmacodynamic and pharmacokinetic properties and therapeutic use in cardiovascular disease. Drugs 1990;40(1):31–74.

15. Borhani NO, Mercuri M, Borhani PA, et al. Final outcome results of the Multicenter Isradipine Diuretic Atherosclerosis Study (MIDAS). A randomized controlled trial. JAMA 1996;276(10): 784–791.

16. Murdoch D, Heel RC. Amlodipine. A review of its pharmacodynamic and pharmacokinetic properties, and therapeutic use in cardiovascular disease. Drugs 1991;41(3):478–505.

17. Frishman WH, Hershman D. Amlodipine. In, Messerli FH (ed): *Cardiovascular Drug Therapy*, 2nd ed. Philadelphia: W.B. Saunders Co., 1996:1024–1040.

18. Todd PA, Faulds D. Felodipine. A review of the pharmacology and therapeutic use of the extended-release formulation in cardiovascular disorders. Drugs 1992;44(2):251–77.

18a. HOT Study Group Steering Committee. Effects of intensive blood pressure lowering and acetylsalicylic acid in patients with hypertension: Principal results of the Hypertension Optimal Treatment (HOT) randomised trial. Lancet 1998;351:1755–1762.

19. Mitchell J, Frishman W, Heiman M. Nisoldipine: a new dihydropyridine calcium channel blocker. J Clin Pharmacol 1993;33:46-52.

20. Prisant ML, Bottini B, DiPiro JT, Carr AA. Novel drug-delivery systems for hypertension. Am J Med 1992;93 (Suppl. 2A):45S–55S.

21. Gradman AH, Frishman WH, Kaihlanen PM, Wong SC, Friday K. Comparison of sustained release formulations of nicardipine and verapamil for mild to moderate systemic hypertension. Am J Cardiol 1992;70:1571–1575.

22. Frishman WH, Lazar EJ. Sustained-release verapamil formulations for treating hypertension. J Clin Pharmacol 1992;32:455–462.

23. White WB, Anders RJ, MacIntyre JM, Black HR, Sica DA, and the Verapamil Study Group: Nocturnal dosing of a novel delivery system of verapamil for systemic hypertension. Am J Cardiol 1995;76: 375–380.

23a. White WB, Black HR, Weber MA, et al. Comparison of effects of controlled-onset extended release verapamil at bedtime and nifedipine gastrointestinal therapeutic system on arising on early morning blood pressure, heart rate, and heart rate-blood pressure product. Am J Card 1998;81:424–431.

24. Graney WF. Clinical experience with a once-daily extended-release formulation of diltiazem in the treatment of hypertension. Am J Med 1992;93(Suppl. 2A):56S–64S.

25. Frishman WH. A new extended-release formulation of diltiazem HCl for the treatment of mild to moderate hypertension. J Clin Pharmacol 1993;33:612–622.

26. Frishman WH. Calcium channel blockers. In, Frishman WH, Sonnenblick EH (eds): *Cardiovascular Pharmacotherapeutics: Companion Handbook*. New York: McGraw-Hill, 1998:73–106.

CHAPTER 15

Rational Antihypertensive Therapy: Overview

Franz H. Messerli

Hypertension is, by definition, primarily a hemodynamic disorder, and arterial pressure can be considered the product of cardiac output and vascular resistance. Thus, the relationship among arterial pressure, vascular resistance, and cardiac output can be expressed in a simple mathematical formula (Figure 1). It follows that any increase in arterial pressure has to occur by an increase in cardiac output, an increase in vascular resistance, or both. A variety of studies from all over the world have documented that the hemodynamic pattern leading to arterial hypertension is heterogeneous, depending on demographic factors as well as on a myriad of pressor/antipressor mechanisms.[1-3] Several recent studies have clearly documented that the hemodynamic pattern in essential hypertension is age dependent (Figures 2 and 3).[4]

THE YOUNG PATIENT

Since the pioneering observation by Widimsky et al.,[5] several other authors have documented that, in young patients, borderline or early established essential hypertension is characterized hemodynamically by an increase in cardiac output, mostly owing to an increase in heart rate.[5-9] Systemic vascular resistance usually remains within normal limits. The term inappropriately normal has been used to characterize this phenomenon because in normotensive subjects one would expect resistance to be low in the presence of an elevated cardiac output. Some few young hypertensive patients exhibit increased sensitivity to beta-adrenergic stimulation (hyperbeta-adrenergic state)[10] but more common is a decreased response to vagal inhibition (hypovagotonic state).[11] In parallel with the elevated cardiac output, renal blood flow is often slightly increased and intravascular volume is normal to mildly contracted, with a shift of total blood volume from the capacitance vessels (veins) to the cardiopulmonary circulation. The increase in cardiopulmonary

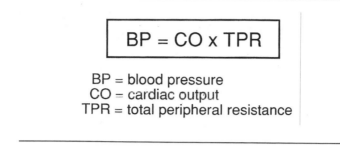

$$BP = CO \times TPR$$

BP = blood pressure
CO = cardiac output
TPR = total peripheral resistance

Figure 1. *Blood pressure, cardiac output, and total peripheral resistance are related by a mathematical formula.*

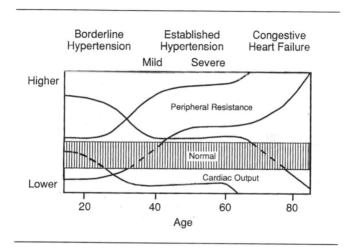

Figure 2. *Cardiac output is elevated in young patients with juvenile hypertension, whereas total peripheral resistance is normal, but , as the patient grows older and hypertension becomes more severe, cardiac output reverts to normal and total peripheral resistance becomes elevated. A high peripheral resistance is the hemodynamic hallmark of established essential hypertension. With a progressive increase in afterload, cardiac output starts falling, congestive heart failure ensues, and resistance becomes even higher. Reproduced with permission from Messerli FH. Individualization of antihypertensive therapy: An approach based on hemodynamics and age. J Clin Pharmacol 1981;21:517–528.*

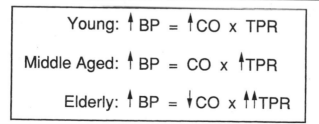

Figure 3. *The mathematical formula establishing the relationship among blood pressure, cardiac output, and total peripheral resistance changes dramatically with age. In young patients, the hemodynamic cause of elevated pressure is an increase in cardiac output. In elderly patients, the elevation of arterial pressure is caused by very high peripheral resistance in the presence of low cardiac output because of latent or overt congestive heart failure.*

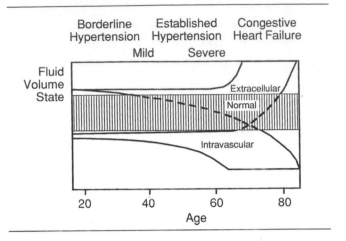

Figure 4. *Intravascular blood volume progressively contracts with age and severity of hypertension, reaching its lowest levels between ages 60 and 80 years. Once congestive heart failure develops, however, fluid volume retention may manifest itself clinically as edema. Intravascular volume remains contracted and extracellular fluid volume is expanded in patients with congestive heart failure.*

volume closely correlates with the elevated cardiac output. Freis[12] used the descriptive term *cardiogenic hypertension* to characterize the main hemodynamic abnormality in these young patients.

THE MIDDLE-AGED PATIENT

As a young patient with hypertension ages, a physiologic inversion takes place; that is, cardiac output reverts to normal and systemic vascular resistance becomes elevated (see Figure 2). In fact, elevated vascular resistance must be considered the hemodynamic hallmark of established essential hypertension. The left ventricle attempts to compensate for the increase in afterload, relative wall thickness increases in an attempt to bring wall stress back to normal, and progressive left ventricular hypertrophy (LVH) of the concentric type (wall thickening at the expense of chamber volume) develops. At the same time, intravascular volume becomes more and more contracted (Figure 4).[4,13] Renal blood flow tends to fall rapidly as hypertensive cardiovascular disease becomes more severe because of progressive nephrosclerosis.[14,15] Because, at least initially, the glomerular filtration rate remains well preserved, an increase in filtration fraction is commonly observed.

THE ELDERLY PATIENT

Elderly hypertensive patients are characterized by a low cardiac output and a very high systemic vascular resistance. In a careful matching study,[16] we documented that cardiac output was about 25% lower in elderly hypertensive patients than in younger patients with the same arterial pressure.

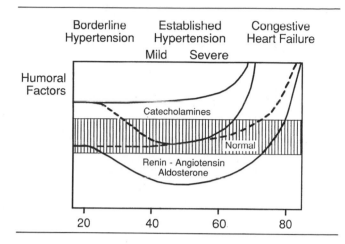

Figure 5. *The activity of the renin-angiotensin system declines through-out age and is at its lowest levels in elderly persons. In patients with con-gestive heart failure, reactivation of the renin-angiotensin system occurs, which maintains arterial pressure in the presence of falling cardiac out-put. In contrast, plasma catecholamines increase progressively throughout life. An additional increase in catecholamines is often seen in persons with congestive heart failure. Reproduced with permission from Messerli FH. Clinical determinants and consequences of left ventricular hypertro-phy. Am J Med 1983;75:51–63.*

These cross-sectional data were corroborated and expanded in an elegant long-term, follow-up study by Lund-Johansen (see Chapter 2) reporting an increase in resistance and a fall in cardiac output with age. Intravascular volume becomes even more contracted in elderly patients, making them sen-sitive to further volume depletion (see Figure 4).[16] Target organ damage, such as distinct LVH, hypertensive cardiopa-thy, nephrosclerosis, and cerebral vascular damage is often encountered. More than two thirds of elderly patients with mild hypertension have LVH by echocardiographic criteria (Figure 5).[17] Ultimately, the left ventricle can no longer com-pensate for the ever-increasing afterload and congestive heart failure, with its characteristic neuroendocrine features, ensues (Figure 6).

NEUROHUMORAL BACKGROUND OF HEMODYNAMIC CHANGES

Although the exact etiology of so-called essential hyperten-sion remains as elusive as ever, a variety of hypothetical mechanisms have been proposed to explain the pathogene-sis of the elevation in arterial pressure. Increased activity of the sympathetic nervous system has been documented in most patients with borderline or early essential hypertension (Figure 7).[18] This increased sympathetic activity is predomi-nantly confined to the beta-adrenergic system, whereas the alpha-adrenergic system remains less affected. It is, there-fore, not surprising that in the hemodynamics of early hypertension a predominantly beta-adrenergic pattern is

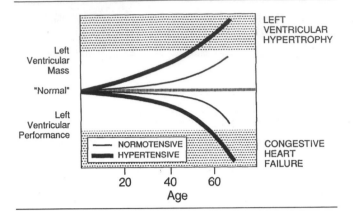

Figure 6. *Left ventricular mass increases with age in normotensive subjects and left ventricular pump function declines somewhat. Both of these changes are greatly accelerated in hypertensive patients. Thus, instead of developing left ventricular hypertrophy (LVH) late in life or not at all, a patient with hypertension may already fulfill echocardiographic criteria of LVH at age 40. A similar pattern can be observed for left ventricular pump function.*

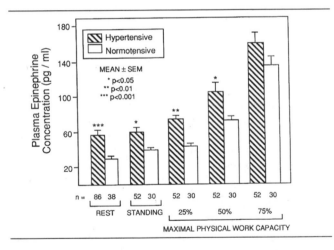

Figure 7. *Plasma epinephrine levels are slightly more elevated in hypertensive subjects than in normotensive control subjects. This is true at rest as well as during physical exercise and it may reflect excessive sympathetic activity in essential hypertension. Modified from Kiowski W, Bühler FR, Bolli P, et al. Hypertonie und adrenerge Kreislaufregulation Einflüsse von Alter und Blutdruck. In: Bergener M, Grobecker H, eds. Hypertonie in Alter: Norvariante oder Krankheit? Stuttgart: Schattauer, 1984: 51–64.*

observed with an elevated cardiac output, heart rate, etc. Because beta-receptors produce vasodilation, systemic vascular resistance (which depends both on alpha-receptors and beta-receptors) remains unchanged.

The chronic, excessive bombardment of beta-receptors with catecholamines ultimately leads to down-regulation or desensitization of these receptors.[19–22] In the heart, such down-regulation would lead to a fall in cardiac output and heart rate. Indeed, heart rate response to exercise and other stimuli

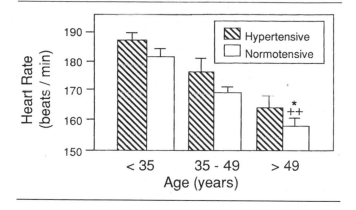

Figure 8. *The greatest increase in heart rate with exercise is seen in young patients. The increase declines progressively with age in both hypertensive and normotensive subjects. Modified from Kiowski W, Bühler FR, Bolli P, et al. Hypertonie und adrenerge Kreislaufregulation Einflüsse von Alter und Blutdruck. In: Bergener M, Grobecker H, eds. Hypertonie in Alter: Norvariante oder Krankheit? Stuttgart: Schattauer, 1984: 51–64.*

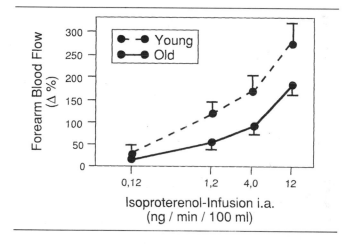

Figure 9. *Isoproterenol stimulates beta-receptors and, therefore, produces vasodilation. As can be seen, this vasodilation is much less pronounced in elderly than in young patients. Modified from Kiowski W, Bühler FR, Bolli P, et al. Hypertonie und adrenerge Kreislaufregulation Einflüsse von Alter und Blutdruck. In: Bergener M, Grobecker H, eds. Hypertonie in Alter: Norvariante oder Krankheit? Stuttgart: Schattauer, 1984: 51–64.*

has been documented to decrease with age (Figure 8).[18] In vascular smooth muscle, down-regulation of beta-receptors leads to a loss of vasodilatory properties (Figure 9)[18] and, in turn, to predominantly alpha-receptor effects. As a consequence of this imbalance, vasoconstriction and thus an increase in systemic vascular resistance take place.

Vasoconstriction becomes progressively stronger, and the increase in intravascular pressure may elicit so-called myogenic reactivity.[22] The increased wall stress results in a massive flux of extracellular calcium into the distended smooth muscle cell, which further intensifies vascular smooth muscle tone.

As a result of the increased wall stress, smooth-muscle hypertrophy takes place more gradually, and the vascular wall thickens. Vascular hypertrophy is a compensatory mechanism that brings wall stress back to normal. However, such remodeling of the resistance vessel with an increase in the wall-to-lumen ratio has been documented to further shift to the left of the dose-response curve of smooth muscle contraction and to make it steeper. Thus, for any given pressor stimulus, the hypertrophied vessel responds with a greater increase in arterial pressure than does a nonhypertrophied vessel (Folkow hypothesis).[23,24] Folkow et al.[23,24] suggested that vascular hypertrophy not only accelerates hypertension but, as a hereditary process, even precedes its development and is the primary event responsible for pressure elevation

Thus, at least three different mechanisms contribute to the increase in arterial pressure in the resistance vessels: (1) neurohumoral factors (noradrenaline, downregulation of $beta_2$ receptors, angiotensin II, or a relative imbalance between pressor and depressor mechanisms); (2) myogenic reactivity; and (3) structural adaptation (increased wall-to-lumen ratio).

IMPLICATIONS FOR ANTIHYPERTENSIVE THERAPY

Clearly, it is neither feasible nor practical before initiation of therapy to identify the predominant mechanism of pressure elevation in every patient with essential hypertension. However, a few simple clinical guidelines allow the practicing physician to define, as least to some extent, the underlying hemodynamic and neurohumoral patterns.

A young patient with mild essential hypertension as well as elevated cardiac output, increased heart rate, and other symptoms and signs of sympathetic activity is an ideal candidate for *beta-blockade* or antioadrenergic therapy. Both of these drug classes have been shown to bring the hemodynamic pattern in such patients back to normal. Thus, symptoms and signs of increased sympathetic activity diminish in parallel with a fall in arterial pressure.

In a patient with early established essential hypertension, in whom an imbalance between alpha- and beta-adrenergic activity is suspected and in whom there is an increase in systemic vascular resistance, an alpha-blocker may be a good choice. Alpha$_1$-blockers lower arterial pressure by reversing the functional component of increased systemic vascular resistance. Thus, they may be particularly useful in patients in whom no distinct structural adaptations have taken place. Alpha-blockers have the additional advantage of exerting beneficial effects on lipoproteins. Because many patients with uncomplicated hypertension have abnormally elevated cholesterol and triglyceride levels, alpha-blockers may lower the burden of total cardiovascular risk more than one would expect from their blood pressure lowering effects.

The *angiotensin-converting enzyme (ACE) inhibitors* and the *angiotensin receptor blockers (ARBs)* are certainly the drugs of choice in all situations characterized by enhanced activity of the renin-angiotensin-aldosterone cascade. This comprises some patients with early hypertension but also some with late essential hypertension and particularly congestive heart failure. Concomitant disorders, such as LVH, glucose intolerance, or early hypertensive renal disease with microproteinuria, may further favor selection of an ACE inhibitor. Because ACE inhibitors are metabolically inert and may even improve insulin resistance, they are good agents for patients with essential hypertension who have increased insulin resistance.

Calcium antagonists are the agents of choice when enhanced myogenic reactivity in the resistance vessels is suspected. Like ACE inhibitors, calcium antagonists are metabolically inert and have been shown to reduce LVH and to have some renal protective effects. Clearly, the presence of concomitant disorders such as impaired left ventricular filling, coronary artery disease, or peripheral vascular disease further favors the use of calcium antagonists. Some of the third-generation calcium antagonists can even be used in combination with ACE inhibitors (or possibly with ARBs) in patients with congestive heart failure.

REFERENCES

1. Laragh JH. Vasoconstriction—volume analysis for understanding and treating hypertension: The use of renin and aldosterone profiles. In: Laragh JH, ed. Hypertension manual. New York: Yorke Medical Books, 1973: 823.

2. Messerli FH, Laragh JH. Hypertension. In: Messerli FH, ed. Cardiovascular drug therapy. Philadelphia: W.B. Saunders, 1990: 20–22.

3. Messerli FH, Schmieder RE, Nunez BD. Heterogeneous pathophysiology of essential hypertension: Implications for therapy. Am Heart J 1986;112:886–893.

4. Messerli FH. Individualization of antihypertensive therapy: An approach based on hemodynamics and age. J Clin Pharmacol 1981;21:517–528.

5. Widimsky J, Fejfarova MH, Fejfar Z. Changes in cardiac output in hypertensive disease. Cardiologica 1957;31:381–389.

6. Frohlich ED, Kozul VJ, Tarazi RC, et al. Physiological comparison of labile and essential hypertension. Circ Res 1970;27(Suppl. I):155–169.

7. Julius S, Pascual AV, Sannerstedt R, et al. Relationship between cardiac output and peripheral resistance in borderline hypertension. Circulation 1971;43:382–390.

8. Sannerstedt R, Julius S. Systemic haemodynamics in borderline arterial hypertension: Responses to static exercise before and under the influence of propranolol. Cardiovasc Res 1972;6:398–403.

9. Messerli FH, De Carvalho JGR, Christie B, et al. Systemic and regional hemodynamics on low, normal and high cardiac output borderline hypertension. Circulation 1978;58:441–448.

10. Frohlich ED, Tarazi RC, Dustan HP. Hyperdynamic beta-adrenergic circulatory state: Increased beta-receptor responsiveness. Arch Intern Med 1969;123:1–7.

11. Julius S, Esler M. Autonomic nervous cardiovascular regulation in borderline hypertension. Am J Cardiol 1975;36:685–696.

12. Freis ED. Hemodynamics of hypertension. Physiol Rev 1960;40:27–55.

13. Frohlich ED, Tarazi RC, Dustan HP. Re-examination of the hemodynamics of hypertension. Am J Med Sci 1969;257:9–23.

14. Reubi FC, Weidmann P, Hodler J, et al. Changes in renal function in essential hypertension: Am J Med 1978;64:556–563.

15. Messerli FH, Frohlich ED, Dreslinski GR, et al. Serum uric acid in essential hypertension: An indicator of renal vascular involvement. Ann Intern Med 1980;93:817–821.

16. Messerli FH, Sundgaard-Rüse K, Ventura H, Glade L, et al. Essential hypertension in the elderly: Haemodynamics, intravascular volume, plasma renin activity, and circulating catecholamine levels. Lancet 1983;2:983–986.

17. Messerli FH. Clinical determinants and consequences of left ventricular hypertrophy. Proceedings of a Symposium: Left Ventricular Hypertrophy in Essential Hypertension—Mechanisms and Therapy. Am J Med 1983;75(3A):51–56.

18. Kiowski W, Bühler FR, Bolli P, et al. Hypertonie und adrenerge Kreislaufregulation Einflüsse von Alter und Blutdruck. In: Bergener M, Grobecker H, eds. Hypertonie in Alter: Norvariante oder Krankheit? Stuttgart: Schattauer, 1984: 51–64.

19. Lakatta EG. Alterations in the cardiovascular system that occur in advanced age. Fed Proc 1979;38:163–167.

20. van Brummelen P, Bühler FR, Kiowski W, et al. Age-related decrease in cardiac and peripheral vascular responsiveness to isoprenaline: Studies in normal subjects. Clin Sci 1981;60:571–577.

21. Pan HY, Hoffman BB, Pershe RA, et al. Decline in beta adrenergic receptor-mediated vascular relaxation with aging in man. J Pharmacol Exp Ther 1986;239:802–807.

22. Lakatta EG, Gerstenblith G, Angell CS, et al. Diminished inotropic response of aged myocardium to catecholamines. Circ Res 1975;36:262–269.

23. Folkow B, Grimby G, Thulesius O. Adaptive structural changes of the vascular wall in hypertension and their relation to the control of peripheral resistance. Acta Physiol Scand 1958;44:255–272.

24. Folkow B. Physiological aspects of primary hypertension. Physiol Rev 1982;62:347–504.

CHAPTER 16

Nonpharmacological Blood Pressure Reduction

Gregory Y.H. Lip
D. Gareth Beevers

The nonpharmacological approach to the reduction of blood pressure is relevant to all grades of hypertension and is also relevant to a great many people who would usually be considered to have normal blood pressures. The prudent diet recommended by practically all members of the medical community has potential benefits in the prevention of coronary heart disease and strokes as well as the control of hypertension.

There is now reliable evidence that the onset of hypertension can be delayed by the use of an appropriate alteration in dietary habits.[1] Furthermore, even among patients whose hypertension is severe enough to require drug therapy, there is evidence that these therapies can be potentiated by appropriate nonpharmacologic maneuvers and, occasionally, these drugs can be discontinued.[2,3]

The current approach to blood pressure control, referred to by the late Geoffrey Rose as the "high risk" strategy, is essentially a "late" strategy and requires continuous efforts to detect, diagnose, and treat new hypertensive individuals, which can be costly and labor-intensive, although opportunistic screening in primary care by practice nurses may help the problem. However, this approach only deals with part of the blood pressure problem and ignores the large proportion of the population with blood pressures above optimal, but who are not frankly hypertensive. The complementary strategy, "population-wide approach," with its emphasis on primary prevention, aims to lower average blood pressure in populations, stem the rise in blood pressure with age, and reduce the prevalence of high-normal and high blood pressure. Nonpharmacological measures, such as diet and lifestyle changes, may be one method of achieving this aim. For example, a 2 mm Hg reduction in population average blood pressure (perhaps by population salt restriction) could result in a 5% reduction in ischaemic heart disease and an 11% reduction in stroke mortality, a benefit which is about the same as the effective treatment of all hypertensives with diastolic pressures above 105 mm Hg.

It is interesting to note that although most recommendations on modifications on dietary habits are not particularly controversial, the medical community has been slow to respond to the increasing reliable literature on this topic. It can be argued that a dietitian or nutritionist should have an integral role in both the primary and secondary health team and has the potential substantially to influence the health of the population.

Nonpharmacological measures may be particularly useful in view of the increasing cost of antihypertensive drugs as well as their side effects. The purpose of this chapter is to examine nonpharmacologic approaches to blood pressure reduction in the light of their clinical usefulness and feasibility.

SALT

The "salt hypothesis" might have been regarded as controversial until about ten years ago. Recent analyses, including the INTERSALT project, which compared 52 populations, and a major meta-analysis of the epidemiology by Law and colleagues now mean that, despite individual "negative" studies, there can be little doubt that high salt intake is important in the pathogenesis of hypertension.[4-6] The subsequent reanalysis of the INTERSALT data file confirmed that, in urban societies, high salt intake is closely related to the rise in blood pressure that occurs with advancing age. In the INTERSALT reanalysis,[7] it was found that in a within-population analysis, where individual 24-hour urinary sodium excretion rose by 100 mmol (for example 70 vs. 170 mmol) this was associated with rise in blood pressure, on average by 3/0 to 6/3 mm Hg. In the cross-population analysis from 52 INTERMAP centers, a rise in median 24-hour sodium excretion by 100 mmol was associated with an increase in blood pressure by 10–11/6 mm Hg. This difference in blood pressure would be expected to translate into an increase of mortality of 34% from stroke and 21% from ischaemic heart disease.[8] In primitive communities where salt intake is low, blood pressure does not rise with age and, correspondingly, hypertension is rare. For example, rural populations with low salt diet consumption (for example, in Kenya) have low blood pressures, but following migration to the cities where salt intake increased, blood pressure increased.[9] Hypertension and its complications are virtually unheard of in societies which consume little salt. The meta-analysis of the published salt restriction studies also shows that substantial reductions in blood pressure can be achieved by relatively modest reductions in salt intake. In Western societies, daily salt intake varies between 150 mmol and 200 mmol of sodium per day. A reduction to around 100 mmol can bring about clinically useful reductions in blood pressure. This can be achieved simply by not adding salt to the food at the table, avoiding notoriously salty foods such as hamburgers, and restricting the amount of salt used in cooking. Many people believe that if the salt content in a meal is reduced, the flavor of the food can be better appreciated. The high salt intake in Western communities dates from the days when sodium chloride was necessary as an additive to food to prevent it from rotting during winter months. Since the invention of the refrigerator, embalming food in sodium chloride is no longer necessary. Sadly, however, the food industry has fought a rear-guard action attempting to rubbish the salt hypothesis and persuade the poor and unhealthy to continue to consume large quantities of salt.

Carefully controlled, randomized trials have shown that there is a dose-dependent relationship between dietary salt intake and blood pressure.[10] To avoid the confounding effects of patient awareness, it is necessary to conduct studies using placebo versus active slow-sodium tablets. When patients were studied while adhering to a low-sodium diet and taking placebo slow-sodium tablets, their blood pressures were low; whereas, when, in a double-blind manner, they switched to active slow-sodium tablets and salt intake rose again, blood pressures also rose (Figure 1).[11]

It is probably spurious to subdivide populations into those considered to be salt sensitive and those who are salt resistant. Clearly, salt sensitivity is distributed in a manner similar to that of blood pressure itself. There is evidence, however, that patients who are most salt sensitive are those who have low plasma renin levels. When they are deprived of salt, their low renin levels rise only modestly and, as a result, there is a lessor pressor effect related to a rise in plasma angiotensin II levels. These data suggest strongly that patients with low renin and, in particular, older patients and patients of African origin are more salt sensitive than white patients or younger patients.[12]

There is also some evidence to suggest that persons with higher pressures are more salt sensitive that are those with only modestly raised or normal blood pressure.[12,13] This relationship between the height of the blood pressure and salt responsiveness may also be related to plasma renin

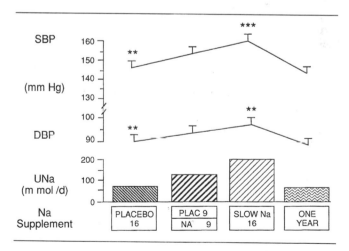

Figure 1. *Randomized, controlled trial of different levels of salt intake in hypertension. Patients were all salt restricted to 50 mmol/day and were then given 9 to 16 slow-sodium (slow-Na) tablets for four weeks each. Data at one year demonstrate that participants were able to maintain a low sodium intake on a long-term basis. Modified from MacGregor GA, Markandu ND, Sagnella GA, et al. Double-blind study of three sodium intake and long-term effects of sodium restriction in essential hypertension. Lancet 1989;2:1244–1247, with permission.*

levels as, in general, hypertensives have lower renin levels than normotensives.

The meta-analysis by Law and coworkers suggested that many of the so-called negative studies of salt restriction and blood pressure are negative only because they did not go on for long enough.[6] It is probable that salt restriction does not exert its full effect on blood pressure until after four or even eight weeks and many studies, therefore, lack the power to detect any change.

At a population level, there is some evidence that salt restriction can reduce the rise in blood pressure that occurs with advancing age and also, in borderline hypertensives, delay the onset of hypertension.[1,14] Epidemiologic evidence and surveillance data, largely from Japan and Portugal, two countries where average salt consumption is high, strongly suggest that a reduction of salt intake in the whole population can lead to a fall in the prevalence of hypertension and a reduction in the incidence of stroke.[15] This can occur with no great cost to the community or any significant increase in other medical conditions.

There is convincing evidence that salt restriction, like diuretic therapy, has useful additive effects when used in conjunction with the angiotensin-converting enzyme (ACE) inhibitors and beta-adrenergic receptor blockers.[16] However, salt restriction, unlike diuretic therapy, has few side effects.

The degree of salt restriction advocated by the medical community is eminently feasible. A great many healthy persons are already consuming relatively small amounts of salt in their diets. These people are frequently of higher social class and have a low mortality from cardiovascular disease.

POTASSIUM

The dietary intake and physiologic metabolism of sodium and potassium are closely related. Some evidence suggests that a relatively high potassium intake, achieved with increased consumption of fruit and vegetables, may have some independent protective effect against cardiovascular disease.[17] Epidemiological data have suggested an inverse relationship between potassium intake and blood pressure. In North America, the striking differences in blood pressure between black and white people may be related to a lower intake of potassium among black people than among whites, and this, in turn may explain the increased susceptibility to stroke among blacks.[18] In the INTERSALT study,[19] potassium excretion was negatively and significantly related to blood pressure, especially in the elderly. Overall, an average difference of 10 mmol in potassium corresponded to a reduction in mean BP by 0.7 mm Hg. Similarly, in a large prospective study of nutritional factors and development of hypertension among American men, a low potassium intake was a predictor for the development of hypertension with a relative risk of 1.54 for subjects in the lowest quintile of potassium intake.[20] A higher potassium intake by 10 mmol/day has also been associated with 40% lower stroke mortality in a study of 859 elderly people.[14]

Many authors have questioned whether potassium is more important than sodium in the pathogenesis of hypertension and in the nonpharmacologic approach to blood pressure reduction. In practical terms, these two monovalent cations should be considered together; a low-salt diet can best be achieved by an increase in potassium intake. Randomized, controlled trials of potassium supplementation, in general, show that this maneuver can lead to a fall in blood pressure, which may, in part, be related to an increased natriuresis itself induced by potassium loading.[21] No one, however, advocates the use of potassium chloride tablets in the management of hypertension; the potassium loading studies strongly suggest that an increase in dietary potassium intake to around 80 mmol/day to 100 mmol/day can lead to clinically useful reductions in blood pressure, and this can be achieved without difficulty by adopting a prudent diet.

As with the data on sodium and blood pressure, it appears that the effects are related to the cation (sodium or potassium), rather than to the anion, which might be chloride, bicarbonate, or citrate. In practical terms, the human diet is largely comprised of sodium chloride and potassium chloride in varying quantities, and there is little evidence that chloride itself is a major determinant of blood pressure.

ALCOHOL

It was not until the late 1970s that the medical community became aware of the importance of alcohol intake in the pathogenesis of hypertension.[22] In the INTERSALT study, a highly significant correlation between blood pressure and heavy drinking (above 300 ml of alcohol/week) was found.[4] Analysis from the same study showed that differences in systolic blood pressure between alcohol drinkers and nondrinkers existed at all levels of intake above 50 ml/week.[23]

There remains some controversy whether small quantities of alcohol are protective, but this is unimportant compared with the unanimity that high alcohol intake can cause high blood pressure and strokes.[24,25] A great many reliable studies, some of which were placebo controlled (inasmuch as a placebo for alcohol is feasible), show that a moderation of alcohol intake can lead to clinically useful reductions in blood pressure (Figure 2).[26–28] No convincing evidence exists that total abstinence is necessarily beneficial and, indeed, there is some evidence that small quantities of alcohol may have independent beneficial effects on coronary heart disease, possibly mediated by effects on plasma lipid levels.[29] There is, therefore, nothing to suggest that clinicians should advocate total abstinence. The general recommendation is that the maximum alcohol intake for men is 21 units (roughly equivalent to 10.5 pints of beer) per week and in women 14 units (equivalent to 7 pints of beer) per week.

Intake above this carries some hazard to health; in the management of hypertension, moderation of alcohol intake can be regarded as beneficial while in no way interfering with a pleasant life style.

Study 1

Blood pressure mmHg

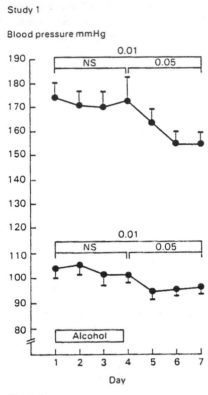

Study 2

Blood pressure mmHg

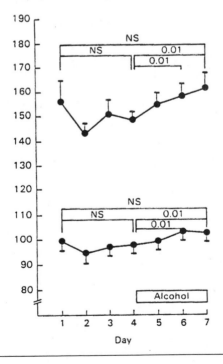

Figure 2. *Effect of cessation of alcohol consumption in the form of beer in hypertensive patients. Modified from Potter JF, Beevers DG. Pressor effect of alcohol in hypertension. Lancet 1984;1:119–122, with permission.*

OBESITY

There is reliable evidence that obesity is closely related to high blood pressure even after adjustment for the error induced by the measurement of blood pressure in obese arms.[30] The exact mechanisms whereby obesity can cause an increase in blood pressure remains uncertain. Like hypertensives and non-insulin-dependent diabetics, obese persons display some evidence of insulin resistance, and this might be a final common pathway toward an elevation of blood pressure.[31] Obesity is also characterized by an increased accumulation of fat tissue, increased metabolic demands and enhanced cardiac output. The high afterload (caused by increased peripheral vascular resistance) gives an additional burden to the left ventricle, leading to left ventricular hypertrophy. Increased sympathetic nervous activity is another mechanism involved in the relationship between obesity and hypertension.

Many studies show that a reduction in body weight is associated with a reduction in blood pressure at a rate of about 1 mm Hg/kg of body weight (Figure 3).[32-34] The effect of weight reduction is independent of salt restriction, but a greater fall in blood pressure is achieved if both measures are implemented. We know of one negative study in which, amazingly, body weight fell, but there was a small rise in blood pressure.[35] This particular study should, however, be seen in the context of a great many other studies, which have shown that reduction of obesity causes a fall in blood pressure.[36] For example, the meta-analysis by Staessen et al.[36] of all studies from 1954 to 1985 concluded that a 1 kg fall in body weight was followed by a mean blood pressure reduction of 1.6/1.3 mm Hg: the reduction of blood pressure was

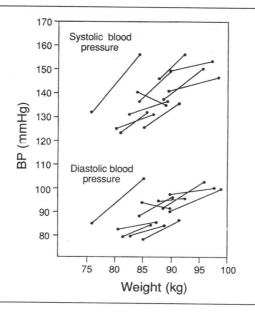

Figure 3. Overview of studies of weight reduction and blood pressure reduction. Each line represents one published study. Modified from Beevers DG, MacGregor GA. Hypertension in practice. London: Dunitz, 1987, with permission.

particularly more prominent when the initial blood pressure was higher, and was independent of the degree of obesity.

Again, it is impossible to look at obesity in isolation. In the process of restricting calorie intake and achieving a more desirable body weight, an individual will inevitably reduce his or her salt intake, increase potassium, and at the same time reduce the consumption of animal fats. One of the major problems faced by people with obesity is that restricting weight is extremely difficult. Patients frequently become disheartened when, after enormous efforts, they find they have reduced their weight by around 5 kg but are still considered obese. Some evidence suggests that dietitians are better able to achieve a reduction in obesity when compared with clinicians giving advice alone.[37]

CIGARETTE SMOKING

The relationship between cigarette smoking and blood pressure is complex. It is important to note that cigarette smoking is an independent risk factor for premature cardiac or stroke death, which exerts its effect in synergism with the effects of high blood pressure and high plasma cholesterol levels.[38,39] It comes as a surprise to many clinicians to learn that, in general, cigarette smokers have lower blood pressures than do nonsmokers and that people who have stopped smoking may sustain a small rise in blood pressure and body mass index.[40] However, the benefits of restricting smoking greatly outweigh any small adverse effect on blood pressure. Furthermore, the benefits of smoking cessation are considerably greater than any benefits from drug treatment of mild hypertension in low-risk individuals. This inverse relationship between cigarette smoking and blood pressure is seen at all levels except in the accelerated or malignant phase of hypertension (characterized by retinal hemorrhages, cotton wool spots with or without papilledema).[41] Although there is an association between malignant hypertension and cigarette smoking, the mechanism is unknown. Atheromatous renal artery stenosis is also more common in smokers.

It is the duty of the clinician to assist the patient in all ways to restrict or totally abandon cigarette smoking. This advice must be seen as relevant to the whole health of the patient and also, by virtue of passive smoking, the health of his or her family. While blood pressure will not be affected particularly, there can be a major impact in coronary heart disease, chest diseases, strokes, peptic ulcer disease, and many other medical conditions.

STRESS

It is commonly held that a high level of environmental or personal stress may be related to raised blood pressure. In fact, the epidemiologic data in favor of this hypothesis are not particularly reliable.[42] Various well-conducted, randomized, controlled trials of stress management in the reduction of blood pressure have provided conflicting results.[43,44] There is, however, no reason to believe that reduction of stress does any harm even though there is no convincing evidence that it has any beneficial effect on blood pressure. It is likely that a high level of environmental stress does not so much cause hypertension but rather a false elevation of blood pressure particularly at a time when it has been measured in a clinical environment. The clinician should, therefore, make efforts to avoid the inappropriate use of antihypertensive drugs in patients who, when attending a clinic, are clearly very anxious. A clue to this diagnosis may be the detection of an inappropriately fast pulse rate in relation to the blood pressure. Frequently, clinicians will observe that mild hypertensives who have a high level of stress will "settle down" if the blood pressure is measured on repeated occasions in a quiet and relaxing environment. Alternatively, ambulatory blood pressure measurement may be employed, which would be particularly useful in cases of "white-coat hypertension."[45] Thus, stress management may well exert this effect by reducing the incidence of false elevations of blood pressure rather than any effect on the pathogenesis of hypertension. This area remains controversial although stress management could be regarded as beneficial to the well being of the individual.

CALCIUM

The relationship between calcium and blood pressure is complex. In general, hypertensives have slightly higher levels of serum total calcium than do normotensives, although they may have slightly lower levels of serum ionized calcium.[46,47] Some evidence suggests that the dietary intake of calcium is lower in hypertensives than in normotensives, and this has led to studies of dietary calcium supplementation.[48] In general, these studies have provided conflicting results, and a recent and useful meta-analysis of the world literature on calcium loading and blood pressure strongly suggests that calcium loading has no effect on blood pressure at all.[49] A high-calcium diet is achieved by increased intake of dairy products, which also causes an increase in dietary intake of fat. Such an increase in dietary fat intake must be regarded as potentially harmful and, for this reason, calcium supplementation by dietary means cannot be recommended in the management of hypertension.

EXERCISE

It was initially difficult to be certain whether increasing physical exercise had beneficial effects on blood pressure. During active exertion, there is a sharp rise in systolic blood pressure, while during the ensuing rest period blood pressures fall to low levels. Epidemiologic studies comparing persons who exercise regularly with those who do not tend to be confounded by the tendency of many regular exercisers simultaneously to adopt more healthy diets and to avoid obesity. Recent reliable short-term studies of different levels of physical exercise in volunteers do, however, strongly suggest that regular exercise several times per week does independently lower blood pressure (Figure 4).[50] It remains

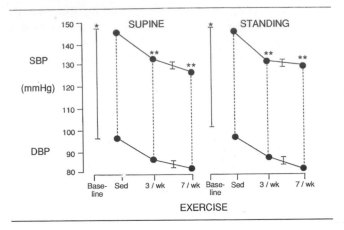

Figure 4. *Effect of three levels of exercise (sedentary and exercising three or seven times per week) in mild hypertensive patients. Modified from Nelson L, Jennings GL, Esler MD, Korner PI. Effect of changing levels of physical activity on blood pressure and haemodynamics in essential hypertension. Lancet 1986;2:473–476, with permission.*

uncertain whether this is due to a fall in cardiac output, a fall in peripheral resistance, or both. In a recent meta-analysis by Fagard,[51] dynamic physical training resulted in a mean net-weighted reduction of blood pressure by 5.3/4.8 mm Hg. Hypertensive patients tended to have a greater response, with a fall in mean blood pressure by 13/8 mm Hg, when compared to normotensive subjects who had a fall in mean blood pressure by 3/2 mm Hg.

Common sense dictates that obese, middle-aged coronary-prone patients should not be advised suddenly to take up vigorous or exhausting sports. Instead, a program of graded, supervised increases in physical activity should be encouraged. Among fit, young, mild hypertensives, it should be emphasized that regular exercise along with other measures outlined in this chapter can sometimes mean that drug therapy can be avoided, postponed, or, occasionally discontinued.

OTHER NONPHARMACOLOGICAL MANEUVERS

Various papers have been published over the years on the intake of magnesium and selenium, together with the suggestions that high levels of lead and cadmium might be harmful. Many of these studies are invalidated by failure to take into account the important confounding variables and, at the present state of knowledge, they cannot be regarded as having an important role in the management of hypertension.

ANIMAL FAT INTAKE

As with cigarette smoking, serum cholesterol levels have an independent effect on coronary heart disease. The whole topic of dietary fats and coronary heart is huge and beyond the scope of this chapter, particularly with publication of large well-conducted randomized trials such as the 4S and WOSCOPS Study demonstrating that lipid lowering significantly reduces cardiovascular events. In hypertension, per se, outcome trials such as ALLHAT and ASCOT are investigating the role of lipid lowering in hypertensives. The prudent life style recommended by almost all clinicians does, along with a restriction of obesity, salt intake, and moderation of alcohol intake, include reduction of the saturated fat component of the diet. This can be achieved by eating less animal fat in the form of full cream milk and full fat cheese and avoiding fried foods. There is no reliable evidence that this reduces blood pressure in either the short or long term. It should be remembered, however, that many hypertensive patients have very high serum cholesterol levels up to 10 mmol/1 and would be found, on detailed investigation, to have familial hypercholesterolemia. In these patients, there is little controversy that restricting the fat content in the diet and reducing serum cholesterol levels by use of cholesterol-lowering drugs is beneficial. Rigorous restriction of fat intake in an attempt to reduce cholesterol when this is only moderately elevated has yet to be shown to be beneficial, although epidemiologic evidence in favor of the cholesterol hypothesis is very convincing.[38] Despite these negative results, there is evidence that the adoption of a vegetarian diet itself does cause a worthwhile reduction in blood pressure in mild hypertensives, although it is uncertain what component of the vegetarian diet is responsible.[52]

THE PREVENTION OF HYPERTENSION

Studies designed to prove that any particular dietary maneuver is beneficial in the prevention of hypertension are extremely difficult to achieve. One study in newborn infants suggested that salt restriction at a modest level can cause a smaller rise in blood pressure with age,[14] and one reliable study of the use of a package of nonpharmacologic regimes in borderline or hypertension-prone persons suggested that these maneuvers delayed the onset of clinical hypertension in adults.[1]

NONPHARMACOLOGICAL MANEUVERS AND THE DISCONTINUATION OF ANTIHYPERTENSIVE DRUGS

There are now at least two reliable studies to suggest that some patients may safely discontinue their antihypertensive medication if, at the same time, they make strenuous efforts to control their diets with alcohol restriction, salt restriction, and an increased potassium intake in the form of fruit and vegetables, a low-fat diet, and smoking cessation.[2,3] At one time it was taught that antihypertensive treatment once initiated was for life, but this may not be so among mild hypertensives whose blood pressures are easily controlled with one drug. In these cases, cessation of therapy can frequently be achieved as long as there are appropriate alterations in dietary habits and careful follow-up.

TABLE 1. DIETARY AND LIFE STYLE MODIFICATIONS AS NON-PHARMACOLOGICAL APPROACHES TO BLOOD PRESSURE REDUCTION AND CORONARY RISK REDUCTION.

	Blood Pressure Reduction	Coronary Risk Reduction
Weight control	+++	++
Alcohol reduction	+++	+
Salt restriction	++	?
Moderate exercise	++	++
High potassium intake	+	?
Calcium supplements	−	−
Vegetarian like diets	+	+
Dietary fish oils	+	+++
Stopping smoking	−	+++
Relaxation techniques	−	?

− denotes no effect
? denotes equivocal effect
+, ++, +++ denote weak, moderate or strong positive effect respectively
Modified from Lydakis C, Lip GYH, Beevers M, Beevers DG, Diet, Lifestyle and Blood Pressure. Coronary Health Care 1997;J:130–37.

CONCLUSIONS

The recommendations made in this chapter on salt consumption, potassium intake, alcohol use, calcium intake, the fat content of the diet, and cigarette smoking can all be seen in the context of the adoption of a healthy life style and avoidance of excessive quantities of any particular food. These maneuvers should also be seen in relation to the importance of avoiding obesity. The effects of dietary and lifestyle modifications as nonpharmacological approaches to blood pressure reduction and coronary risk reduction are summarized in Table 1.

The striking differences in disease between the social classes are clearly of environmental origin. In general, in urban societies, people with high social class tend to be thinner and to have a healthier diet than people of low social class. The dietary maneuvers suggested, therefore, are those that are achievable. The only problem is that the high social class diet (low-fat, low-salt, high-potassium) is relatively expensive. Poorer people, who often live in suboptimal conditions, may find it easier to rely on the frying pan and a high consumption of "junk food." In this context, the medical and nursing professions have the duty to attempt to influence individuals as well as legislators in the avoidance of unhealthy foods. The striking reduction of coronary heart disease and stroke in the United States is an example of what can be achieved, and other countries should take note.

REFERENCES

1. Stamler R, Stamler J, Gosh FC, Civinelli J, et al. Primary prevention of hypertension by nutritional hygienic means. Final report of a randomized controlled trial. JAMA 1989;262:1801–1807.

2. Langford HG, Blaufax MD, Oberman A, et al. Dietary therapy slows the return of hypertension after stopping prolonged medication. JAMA 1985;253:657–664.

3. Stamler R, Stamler J, Grimm R, et al. Nutritional therapy for high BP. Final report of a four year randomized controlled trial. The Hypertension Control Programme. JAMA 1987:257;1989–1991.

4. INTERSALT Cooperative Research Group. INTERSALT: An international study of electrolyte excretion and blood pressure. Results for 24 hour urinary sodium and potassium excretion. Br Med J 1989; 297: 319–328.

5. Law MR, Frost CD, Wald NJ. By how much does dietary salt reduction lower blood pressure. I —Analysis of observational data among populations. Br Med J 1991;302:811–815.

6. Law MR, Frost CD, Wald NJ. By how much does dietary salt reduction lower blood pressure? III—Analysis of data from trials of salt reduction. Br Med J 1991;302:819–824.

7. Elliott P, Stamler J, Nichols R, Dyer A, Stamler A, Kesteloot H, Marmot M. For the INTERSALT Cooperative Research Group. INTERSALT revisited: further analysis of 24-hour sodium excretion and blood pressure within and across populations. Br Med J 1996;312:1249–1253.

8. MacMahon S, Peto R, Cutler J, Collins R, Sorlie P, Neaton J et al. Blood pressure, stroke, and coronary heart disease. Part 1: Prolonged differences in blood pressure: Prospective observational studies corrected for the regression dilution bias. Lancet 1990;335:765–774.

9. Poulter NK, Khaw KT, Hopwood BE, Mugambi M, Peart WS, Rose G, Sever PS. The Kenyan Luo migration study: observations on the initiation of the rise in blood pressure. Br Med J 1990;300:967–972.

10. MacGregor GA, Markandu ND, Sagnella GA, et al. Double-blind study of three sodium intakes and long-term effects of sodium restriction in essential hypertension. Lancet 1989; 2:1244–1247.

11. MacGregor GA, Markandu ND, Best FE, et al. Double-blind–randomised cross-over trial of moderate sodium restriction in essential hypertension. Lancet 1982;1:351–355.

12. Grobbee DE, Hofman A. Does sodium restriction lower blood pressure? Br Med J 1986;293:27–29.

13. MacGregor GA. Sodium is more important than calcium in essential hypertension. Hypertension 1985;7:628–637.

14. Hofman A, Hazebrock A, Valkenburg HA. A randomized trial of sodium intake on blood pressure in newborn infants. JAMA 1983;250:370–373.

15. Perry IJ. What has caused the widespread decline in stroke mortality? J Irish Coll Physicians Surg 1990;19:257–259.

16. Singer DRJ, Markandu ND, Sugdon AL, Miller MA, MacGregor GA. Sodium restriction in hypertensive patients treated with a converting enzyme inhibitor and thiazide. Hypertension 1991;17:798–803.

17. Khaw K-T, Barrett-Connor E. Dietary potassium and stroke associated mortality. A 12 year prospective population study. N Engl J Med 1987; 316: 235–240.

18. Langford HG. Dietary potassium and hypertension: Epidemiologic data. Ann Intern Med 1983;98:770–772.

19. Elliott P, Dyer A, Stamler R. On behalf of the INTERSALT Cooperative Research Group. The INTERSALT study: Results for 24-hour sodium and potassium, by age and sex. J Hum Hypertens 1989;3:323–330.

20. Acherio A, Rimm EB, Giovannucci EL, Colditz GA, Bosner B, Willett WC, Sacks F, Stampfer MI. A prospective study of nutritional factors and hypertension among US men. Circulation 1992;86: 1475–1484.

21. Cappuccio FP, MacGregor GA. Does potassium supplementation lower blood pressure? A meta-analysis of published trials. J Hypertens 1991;9:465–473.

22. Klatsky AL, Friedman GD, Sigelaub AB, Gerard MJ. Alcohol consumption and blood pressure: Kaiser Permanente multiphasic health examination data. N Engl J Med 1977;296:1194–1200.

23. Marmot MG, Elliott P, Shipley MJ, Dyer AR, Ueshima H, Beevers DG, Stamler R, Kesteloot H, Rose __, Stamler J. Alcohol and blood pressure: The INTERSALT study. Br Med J 1994;308:1263–1267.

24. Maheswaran R, Gill JJ, Davies P, Beevers DG. High blood pressure due to alcohol. A rapidly reversible effect. Hypertension 1991; 17:787–792.

25. Gill JS, Zezulka AV, Shipley MJ, et al. Stroke and alcohol consumption. New Eng J Med 1986;315:1041–1046.

26. Potter JF, Beevers DG. Pressor effect of alcohol in hypertension. Lancet 1984;1:119–122.

27. Puddey I, Beilin LJ, Vandongen R. Regular alcohol use raises blood pressure in treated hypertensive subjects. Lancet 1987; 1: 647–651.

28. Veshimalt, Ogihara T, Baba S, et al. The effect of reduced alcohol consumption on blood pressure: A randomised controlled single-blind study. J Hum Hypertens 1987;1:113–119.

29. Moore RD, Pearson TA. Moderate alcohol consumption and coronary artery disease. A review. Medicine 1986;65:242–267.

30. Kannel WB, Brand N, Skinner JJ, Dawber TR, McNamara PM. The relation of obesity to blood pressure and the development of hypertension. Ann Intern Med 1967;67:48–59.

31. Reaven GM. Role of insulin resistance in human disease: Banting lecture. Diabetes 1988;37:1595–1607.

32. Fletcher AP. The effect of weight reduction upon the blood pressure of obese hypertensive women. Q J Med 1954;23:331–345.

33. Fagenberg B, Anderson OK, Isaksson B, Bjorntorp P. Blood pressure control during weight reduction in obese hypertensive men: Separate effects of sodium and energy restriction. Br Med J 1984;288:11–14.

34. MacMahon SW, MacDonald FJ, Bernstein L, Andrews G, Blacket RB. Comparison of weight reduction with metoprolol in treatment of hypertension in young overweight patients. Lancet 1985;i: 1233–1236.

35. Haynes RB, Harper AC, Costley SR, et al. Failure of weight reduction to reduce mildly elevated blood pressure: A randomized trial. J Hypertens 1984;2:535–539.

36. Staessen J, Fagard R, Amery A. The relationship between body weight and blood pressure. J Hum Hypertens 1988;2:207–217.

37. Ramsay LE, Ramsay MH, Hettiarachchi J, Davies DL, Winchester J. Weight reduction in a blood pressure clinic. Br Med J 1978; 2:244–245.

38. Stamler J, Wentworth D, Neaton JD. Is relationship between serum cholesterol and risk of premature death from coronary heart disease continuous or graded? JAMA 1986;256:2823–2828.

39. Shinton RA, Beevers DG. Meta-analysis of relationship between cigarette smoking and stroke. Br Med J 1989;298:798–794.

40. Green SB. Smoking and blood pressure change—a seven year follow up. J Chron Dis 1977;30:401–413.

41. Bloxham CA, Beevers DG, Walker JM. Malignant hypertension and cigarette smoking. Br Med J 1979;i:581–583.

42. Gill JS, Beevers DG. The relationship of hypertension and its treatment with stress and well-being. Stress Med 1985;1:279–286.

43. Patel C, Marmot MG, Terry DG, et al. Trial of relaxation in reducing coronary risk: Four year follow-up. Br Med J 1985;290: 1103–1106.

44. Van Montfrancs GA, Kavenmaker JM, Wielling W, Dunning AJ. Relaxation therapy and continuous ambulatory blood pressure in mild hypertension: A controlled study. Br Med J 1990;300:1368–1372.

45. Pickering TG, James GD, Boddie C, Harshfield GA, Blank S, Laragh JH. How common is white coat hypertension? JAMA 1988; 259:225–228.

46. Sangal AK, Beevers DG. Serum calcium and blood pressure. Lancet 1982;ii:493.

47. Buckley BM, Smith SC, Beevers M, et al. Lack of evidence of low ionized calcium levels in system hypertension. Am J Cardiol 1987; 59:878–880.

48. Harlan WR, Hull AL, Schmonder RL, Landis RJ, Thompson FE, Larkin FA. Blood pressure and nutrition in adults: The National Health and Nutrition Examination Survey. Am J Epidemiol 1984; 120:17–28.

49. Cappuccio FP, Siani A, Strazzullo P. Oral calcium supplementation and blood pressure: An overview of randomized controlled trials. J Hypertens 1989;7:941–946.

50. Nelson L, Jennings GL, Esler MD, Korner PI. Effect of changing levels of physical activity on blood pressure and haemodynamics in essential hypertension. Lancet 1986;2:473–476.

51. Fagard R. The role of exercise in blood pressure control: supportive evidence. J Hypertens 1995;13:1223–1227.

52. Margetts BM, Beiling LJ, Vangougon R, Armstrong BK. Vegetarian diet in mild hypertension: A randomized controlled trial. Br Med J 1986;293:1468–1471.

CHAPTER 17

Established Hypertension: Initial Therapy

Norman M. Kaplan

For the purposes of this chapter, sustained or established hypertension is defined as the presence of blood pressures above 140/90 mm Hg on most readings taken during the hours when patients are awake and ambulating. Such patients presumably will not have suffered overt target organ damage (as was covered in Part II). Before these patients begin therapy, the persistence of usually elevated pressures, preferably taken out of the doctor's office, will separate them from those with "early" hypertension (as was covered in Chapter 15).

LIFE-STYLE MODIFICATIONS

Once they have been identified, all patients with sustained or established hypertension should be treated in order to lower their pressures to levels that are less likely to induce target organ damage. However, some patients may be adequately managed, at least temporarily, by nondrug therapies,[1] now better referred to as life-style modifications (Table 1). All of the measures that are appropriate to the patient's needs should be enthusiastically offered and vigorously pursued because each has the potential to effectively lower the blood pressure by about 5 mm Hg in most hypertensives who follow them. Although not all modifications will work on all patients, none should be onerous or harmful and, because most will also improve the other cardiovascular risk factors so often present in hypertensive patients, their use should be encouraged in every patient with established hypertension.

There is consensus in the medical community that smoking cessation and weight reduction are useful. Questions continue to be raised about the value of most of the other life-style modifications.

Moderate Sodium Restriction

Hypertensive patients vary in their pressure sensitivity to varying amounts of dietary sodium intake, but the majority

TABLE 1. LIFE-STYLE MODIFICATIONS FOR HYPERTENSION.

Stop smoking for overall cardiovascular health.

Lose weight, particularly for upper body obesity.

Reduce sodium intake to no more than 100 mmol/d
(2.4 g sodium or 6 g sodium chloride).

Moderate alcohol intake (no more than two usual portions per day
for men, one portion for women).

Exercise (isotonic) regularly.

Maintain adequate potassium, calcium, and magnesium intake.

---

will have a 5 mm Hg to 10 mm Hg fall in systolic pressure after 4 to 6 weeks on a diet with 50–100 mmol/day less sodium than the usual intake of 150 mmol/day to 170 mmol/day.[2]

Such moderate sodium restriction is not difficult to accomplish, particularly with the increasing presence of labels on processed foods that make it possible to identify and avoid high-sodium choices, such as tomato juice, that have a deceptively nonsalty taste.

No major deprivations beyond avoidance of some processed meats, cheeses, and pickled condiments are needed. Such moderate sodium restriction can be followed by all persons who are able to select their foods, either at home or in restaurants.

Moderate Alcohol Intake

Too much alcohol (i.e., more than three usual portions of beer, wine, or whiskey per day) often raises the blood pressure and may lead to serious alcohol abuse. Too little alcohol (i.e., none at all) increases the risk of developing coronary disease. The right amount of alcohol (i.e., one half to two usual portions each day) will not raise the blood pressure and will reduce coronary risks.[3] Therefore, hypertensive patients who have no other reason to avoid alcohol (for example, reformed alcohol abusers) need not be asked to abstain but rather should be encouraged to drink in moderation.

Regular Isotonic Exercise

Most controlled studies document a 5 mm Hg to 10 mm Hg fall in diastolic pressures after six weeks of regular isotonic exercise, three to four periods a week for 30 min to 45 min at 70% of maximal capacity. The antihypertensive effect of exercise likely involves down-regulation of sympathetic nervous system activity and may also involve up-regulation of insulin sensitivity.[4]

Increased Potassium Intake

A number of reports confirm the value of increased potassium intake as a preventative measure but, more obviously, as a therapeutic maneuver.[4] Although formulated potassium supplements may be too expensive, inexpensive salt substitutes containing potassium chloride can be used. The best way to increase potassium intake is to substitute natural foods—almost all of which are high in potassium and low in sodium—for processed foods, most of which are higher in sodium and lower in potassium.

Evidence of the effectiveness of other life-style modifications is inadequate to recommend their routine use, although some patients may benefit from them. These include relaxation and increased consumption of calcium, magnesium, fish oils, or garlic.

Drug Therapy

As detailed in previous chapters, five major classes of antihypertensive drugs are suitable for initial monotherapy and, if necessary, subsequent additive therapy.[1] The sixth class of currently available antihypertensive drugs—the centrally acting alpha-agonists—may also be used, as may reserpine, but their propensity to induce both bothersome side effects and reactive sodium retention has led to their being relegated by most authorities to less than favored status.

Initial Monotherapy and Subsequent Titration

Most patients with established hypertension should be started with only one drug at a low dose.[5] Of course, some patients need immediate and drastic reduction of dangerously high pressure in the face of impending cardiovascular catastrophes. However, the number of such hypertensive urgencies is small compared with the overwhelming majority of patients who are at little, if any, immediate risk but who need an effective and well-tolerated lifelong regimen in order to reduce the long-term consequences of hypertension.

Even with fairly high pressure levels (i.e., 180/110 mm Hg), some patients may respond markedly well to low doses of any drug. There is little reason to overdose the minority who are so sensitive because the less sensitive majority will also be better served by a slow, gradual descent of pressure rather than by a precipitous crash. Most side effects are related to pressure changes that are either too fast or too great in response to "usual" doses of antihypertensive drugs. The risk for such inadvertent overdosing is particularly high for fragile elderly patients,[6] as will be described in Chapter 21.

Rather than providing the full reduction in pressure that is the eventual goal of therapy with the first dose, the safer and more comfortable course is for the physician to slowly titrate the pressure downward, taking three to six months to achieve this goal. This usually means starting at the lower range of doses with only one drug. For some drugs, even a low dose may prove to be markedly effective. An excellent demonstration of the full effectiveness of what most would assume to be a low dose is that of Carlsen and coworkers,[7] who administered varying doses of the thiazide diuretic, bendrofluazide, to groups of hypertensive patients (Table 2). Note the full effectiveness of the lowest dose, equivalent to 12.5 mg of hydrochlorothiazide, which invoked none of the significant metabolic disturbances seen with the higher doses.

In truth, most drugs are likely being started at doses that are too high. Instead of 12.5 mg of hydrochlorothiazide, 6.25 mg may be enough if used in combination with another agent.

TABLE 2. EFFECTS OF VARYING DOSES OF DIURETIC ON BLOOD PRESSURE, BLOOD CHEMISTRIES, AND LIPIDS.

Change from Week 0 to Week 10	0	1.25	2.5	0.0	10.0
Blood pressure (mm Hg)	-3/3	-13/10	-14/11	-13/10	-17/11
Potassium (mmol/l)	+0.09	-0.16	-0.20	-0.33	-0.45
Glucose (μmol/l)	-0.08	-0.19	0.14	0.04	0.27
Cholesterol (mmol/l)	-0.06	-0.03	0.00	0.12	0.25

From Carlsen J, Kober L, Torp-Pedersen C, Johansen P. Relation between dose of bendrofluazide, antihypertensive effect, and adverse biochemical effects. Br Med J 1990;300:975–978.

TABLE 3. PREVALENCE OF OTHER CORONARY RISK FACTORS IN PATIENTS WITH HYPERTENSION.

Risk Factor	Percentage
Cigarette smoking	35
Hypercholesterolemia	40
Low high-density lipoprotein	25
Left ventricular hypertrophy	30+
Upper body obesity	40
Glucose intolerance	30
Hyperinsulinemia	50
Physical inactivity	50

Instead of 100 mg of metoprolol, 25 mg may be enough. The need for "starting low and going slow" is becoming obvious, particularly in the elderly. Recall that only 12.5 mg of chlorthalidone was adequate to markedly reduce the pressure in almost half of the participants of the Systolic Hypertension in the Elderly Program.[8] Even if such low doses are not fully effective for most patients, they will be more than enough for some and will begin gradual downward titration of the pressure, the appropriate way to treat established hypertension.

Management of Other Coronary Risk Factors

While the pressure is being reduced, attention must be directed toward the multiple other coronary risk factors found more frequently among hypertensive patients than among nonhypertensive subjects (Table 3). Although the prevalence of smoking is shown to be no higher in hypertensives than in normotensives, this estimate is probably too low because almost all measurements of blood pressure in those who smoke are made some hours after the last cigarette was smoked. As has now been amply demonstrated by ambulatory monitoring, the pressure rises with each cigarette smoked but returns to a lower level within 15 min to 30 min.[4] Therefore, the contribution of smoking to hypertension has been inadvertently underestimated.

To minimize these risk factors, the life-style modifications shown in Table 1 may be particularly helpful. When drugs are needed, their potential adverse or beneficial influences on concomitant risk factors should be considered (Table 4). The negative effects shown for diuretics and beta-blockers may largely reflect their use in relatively high doses. Certainly data such as are shown in Table 2 suggest that less mischief will be seen when drugs are administered in lower doses.

Individualized Therapy

Beyond the potential effects various drugs may have on concomitant coronary risk factors, they are know to impact favorably or adversely on other diseases commonly found in hypertensive patients (Table 5). The partial listing of comorbid conditions obtained from a questionnaire administered to more than 2,000 hypertensives indicates the likelihood that most patients with hypertension will also have one or more additional problems. Some of these problems simply accompany aging; others are precipitated or accentuated by hypertension.

Whatever the reason for their presence, coexisting conditions should be identified and antihypertensive drugs chosen

TABLE 4. THE EFFECTS OF DIFFERENT ANTIHYPERTENSIVE AGENTS ON CORONARY RISK FACTORS.

	Diuretics	Beta-Blockers	Alpha-Blockers	Calcium Antagonists	ACE Inhibitors
Blood pressure	+	+	+	+	+
Cholesterol	−		+		
HDL cholesterol		−			
Left ventricular hypertrophy	+/−	+	+	+	+
Glucose intolerance	−	−	+		+
Hyperinsulinemia	−	−	+		+
Physical activity		−	+		+

ACE = angiotensin-converting enzyme
HDL = high-density lipoprotein
+ = positive effect
− = negative effect

TABLE 5. COMORBID CONDITIONS AMONG 2,706 HYPERTENSIVE PATIENTS.

Comorbid Condition	Percentage
Diabetes	18.1
Arthritis	36.1
Back problems	4.4
Chronic lung disease	7.4
Angina	8.0
Myocardial infarction	2.2
Congestive heart failure	5.9
None	37.3

that will not make them worse but, instead, will prove beneficial for both the hypertension and the other conditions (Table 6). This partial listing of the more common concomitant conditions provides a basic formula for selecting antihypertensive drugs for individual patients. Some choices are obvious and well accepted; for example, a diuretic or, more likely, an angiotensin-converting enzyme (ACE) inhibitor is preferable to other drugs for a hypertensive patient with congestive heart failure. Others are less well documented but nonetheless reasonable. For example, an alpha-blocker should be selected for a hypertensive patient with dyslipidemia. Still others seem rational but remain unproven, such as the choice of an ACE inhibitor for a diabetic patient to prevent diabetic nephropathy.

The Overall Plan

By using the format shown in Table 6, one should be able to select a drug for every hypertensive that, at least on paper, can be expected to be effective both for the hypertension and for any other disorder that accompanies the hypertension. In clinical practice, however, as many as a third or more of patients do not have the expected antihypertensive effect or experience bothersome side effects from whatever drug is chosen. Therefore, the substitution of a second agent from another category will be needed in a sizable number of patients despite the clinician's most educated guess regarding initial monotherapy (Figure 1). For many other patients, a less-than-adequate response will be provided by moderate doses of the initial drug. In this instance, two choices are possible: increase the dose of the initial drug or add a second drug from another class. The latter alternative will probably be more effective than the former, particularly if the goal is avoidance of dose-dependent side effects.

TABLE 6. RELATIVE PREFERENCES OF ANTIHYPERTENSIVE DRUGS.

Coexisting Condition	Diuretics	Beta-Blockers	Alpha-Blockers	Calcium Antagonists	ACE Inhibitors
Older age	++	+/-	+	+	+
Black race	++	+/-	+	+	+/-
Coronary disease	+/-	++	+	++	+
Congestive failure	++	+	+	-	++
Cerebrovascular disease	+	+	+/-	++	+
Renal insufficiency	++	+/-	+	++	++
Diabetes	-	-	++	+	++
Dyslipidemia	-	-	++	+	+
Asthma or COPD	+	-	+	+	+

++ Preferred
+ Suitable alternative
+/- Usually not preferred
- Usually contraindicated
ACE = angiotensin-converting enzyme
COPD = chronic obstructive pulmonary disease

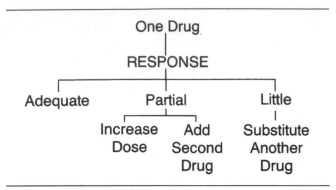

Figure 1. *Individualized approach to the therapy of hypertension. The choice of initial therapy is based on multiple clinical features. From Kaplan NM. Clinical hypertension, 6th ed. Baltimore: Williams & Wilkins, 1994:248–253.*

CONCLUSION

The general guidelines shown in Figure 1 and Table 6 should aid in the management of most patients with established hypertension. The final consideration is to decide on the goal of therapy. For most patients, that seems to be achievement of blood pressure of 130 mm Hg to 140 mm Hg systolic and 80 mm Hg to 85 mm Hg diastolic. Although the existence of a paradoxical increase in coronary risk at lower pressures (i.e., a J curve)[9] remains controversial, most patients seem to derive little benefit from lower pressures than these for maximal long-term protection from cardiovascular complications. Until prospective data document or discount the presence of such a J curve, prudence dictates that a gentle, gradual reduction of pressure to around 135/85 mm Hg is the safest goal for most patients with established hypertension.

REFERENCES

1. The Sixth Report of the Joint National Committe on Prevention, Detection, Evaluation, and Treatment of High Blood Pressure. Arch Intern Med 1997;147:2413–2446.

2. Cutler, JA, Follman O, Allender PS. Randomized trials of sodium reduction. Am J Clin Nutr. 1997;65(Suppl.):6435–6515.

3. Thun, MJ, Peto R, Lopez AD et al. Alcohol consumption and mortality among middle-aged and elderly U.S. adults. N Engl J Med 1997;337:1705–1714.

4. Kaplan, NM. Chapter 6: Therapy of primary hypertension: Nondrugs. In *Clinical Hypertension*, 7th ed. Baltimore: Williams & Wilkins, 1998.

5. Kaplan, NM. The appropriate goals of antihypertensive therapy: Neither too much nor too little. Ann Intern Med 1992;116:686–690.

6. Beard K, Bulpitt C, Mascie-Taylor H, O'Malley K, Sever P, Webb S. Management of elderly patients with sustained hypertension. Br Med J 1992;304:412–416.

7. Carlsen JE, Kober L, Torp-Pedersen C, Johansen P. Relation between dose of bendrofluazide, antihypertensive effect, and adverse biochemical effects. Br Med J 1990;300:975–978.

8. SHEP Cooperative Research Group. Prevention of stroke by antihypertensive drug treatment in older persons with isolated systolic hypertension. Final results of the Systolic Hypertension in the Elderly Program (SHEP). JAMA 1991;265:3255–3264.

9. Fletcher AE, Bulpitt CJ. How far should blood pressure be lowered? N Engl J Med 1992;326:251–254.

CHAPTER 18

Combination Therapy in the Management of Hypertension

Murray Epstein
Franz H. Messerli

The principle of polypharmacy has gained almost universal acceptance for those patients with certain conditions, such as angina, who do not respond to a single agent. Moreover, the treatment of hypertension often includes the use of combination therapy (addition of a drug with a complementary mechanism of action to another) in order to enhance the blood pressure lowering effect of a single agent. Until recently, the concept of using fixed dose combination therapy to treat hypertension has been slow to gain widespread current acceptance.[1] The recent introduction and approval by the Food and Drug Administration (FDA) of several fixed-dose ACE inhibitor/calcium antagonist combinations has increased awareness of this concept and increased the usage of fixed-dose combinations for the management of hypertension.[2]

In the following sections, we will consider the rationale for combining two different antihypertensive agents. Tables 1 and 2 summarize the potential advantages of fixed-dose antihypertensive combination medications.

ENHANCED ANTIHYPERTENSIVE EFFICACY

The rationale for prescribing fixed dose combinations of antihypertensive agents relates in part to the concept that antihypertensive efficacy may be enhanced when two classes of agents are combined. First, there is increasing awareness of heterogeneity in responsiveness to treatment.[3] Crossover studies demonstrate that patients who respond to one class of drug do not necessarily respond to a different class.[4,5] Consequently, good blood pressure control could be achieved in a larger proportion of patients by use of low doses of two drugs that act on different physiological systems.

* Portions of this chapter were adapted with permission from Epstein, M, Bakris G. Newer approaches to antihypertensive therapy: use of fixed dose combination therapy. *Arch Intern Med* 1996;156:1969–1978.

TABLE 1. POTENTIAL ADVANTAGES OF FIXED-DOSE ANTIHYPERTENSIVE COMBINATION MEDICATIONS.

1. Simplicity of use and convenience for patient and physician
2. Simple titration process (of the combination per se)
3. Improved compliance, with possibly enhanced efficacy
4. Potentiation of antihypertensive effects
   A. Additive or synergistic effect
   B. Permitting of full blood pressure lowering effect in patients tending to have less than full response to one component
5. Reduction in side effects by allowing lowering of dosage of one or both components, e.g. less thiazide-induced hypokalemia when using ACE-inhibitor/thiazide combination.
6. Offsetting of undesirable side effects, e.g., obviation of calcium antagonist-induced edema by addition of ACE inhibitor.
7. Cost of fixed-dose combinations is usually less than the cost of the constituents prescribed separately.

Adapted with permission from Epstein M, Oster JR. Hypertension. *Practical Management*. Miami: Battersea, 1988:128.

TABLE 2. COMBINATION THERAPY IN HYPERTENSION: SYNERGISTIC EFFECT ON TOLERABILITY.

Drug A	Drug B	Drug B Improves
DHP-Ca-antagonist	Beta blocker	Palpitations
DHP-Ca-antagonist	ACE inhibitor	Peripheral edema
Diuretic	ACE inhibitor	Hypokalemia, insulin resistance
Antiadrenergic	Diuretic	Edema, pseudoresistance
Diuretic	Alpha blocker	Dyslipidemia

DHP-Ca-antagonists = dihydropyridine calcium antagonist

Second, combination therapy serves to countervail the counterregulatory mechanisms that are triggered whenever pharmacologic intervention is initiated. It is well established that when an antihypertensive drug is administered to attenuate or countervail the effects of one of the pathophysiologic mechanisms mediating hypertension, counterregulatory mechanisms are evoked that act to limit the efficacy of the pharmacologic intervention.[1,2,6,7] For example, when sodium depletion is induced by diuretics, there is a stimulation of the sympathetic nervous system,[8] a stimulation of the renin-angiotensin-aldosterone system[9] and possibly a release of vasopressin. All three of these mechanisms will serve to restore blood pressure to its pretreatment level.

Arterial vasodilators, such as hydralazine or minoxidil, also stimulate both the sympathetic nervous and renin-angiotensin systems.[6,7,10] In addition, these agents induce profound sodium avidity by the kidney and hence, volume expansion. Moreover, short-acting dihydropyridine (nifedipine-like) calcium antagonists increase sympathetic neuronal tone much like other vasodilators.[11-13] Longer acting calcium antagonists also increase sympathetic tone albeit not to the same extent as the short-acting agents.[11,12] Conversely, long-acting nondihydropyridine calcium antagonists, such as verapamil or diltiazem do not increase sympathetic neuronal tone.[12,14] Combination therapy, by adding a second drug, which acts to attenuate or countervail these counter-regulatory mechanisms, enhances the antihypertensive effects of the first agent.

ENHANCED TOLERABILITY AND REDUCTION OR LIMITATION OF SIDE EFFECTS BY LOW-DOSE COMBINATION THERAPY FOR HYPERTENSION

For initial therapy of most hypertension, full doses of multiple drugs in combination are not routinely prescribed because of inability to titrate each of the constituents and to separate individual side effects while unnecessarily exposing patients to superfluous therapy. However, if low doses of two antihypertensive agents with different modes of action are combined, this may benefit hypertensive patients by minimizing the dose-dependent adverse effects since smaller doses of drugs are used to achieve control.

The concept has been nicely demonstrated by Fagan[15] (Figure 1). With a low dose of drug A, only a partial therapeutic effect is obtained and adverse effects (A′) are minimal. If the dose is raised to B, the greater effect will be accompanied by more adverse effects (B′). However, if a low dose of another drug is added, with its minimal side effects, the extra benefit will be obtained without more adverse effects, which will remain at A′.

This notion has recently been validated by multifactorial trials that have documented that low doses of bisoprolol fumarate (an ultra cardioselective beta-blocker) and hydrochlorothiazide (HCTZ) in combination decreased systolic

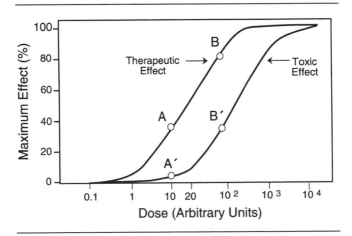

Figure 1. Linear dose-response curves showing theoretical therapeutic and toxic effects. The horizontal axis is a logarithmic scale with arbitrary dose units. The vertical axis is a linear scale showing percentage of maximal possible response. (Reproduced with permission from Fagan TC. Arch Intern Med 1994; 154:1430–1431. Copyright 1994, American Medical Association).

and diastolic blood pressures with few adverse effects.[16] This demonstration that efficacy was achieved with no more side effects than placebo eventuated the United States FDA to approve this low-dose combination as first-line therapy.[17]

Another relevant concept for consideration of fixed combination therapy is enhanced tolerability. In brief, this notion suggests that one drug of a fixed combination can antagonize some of the adverse effects of the second drug.[1,18] Ideally, the side effect profile of the components of a combination should be mutually counteractive, or at least nonadditive, and never additive (Tables 1 and 2). Good examples of potential counteractive effects include the attenuation of thiazide-induced urinary losses of potassium and magnesium by potassium-sparing diuretics and the reduction of hydralazine-induced tachycardia with reserpine. Others include the mitigation by beta-blockers or captopril of diuretic-induced hypokalemia, prevention of propranolol-induced reduction in cardiac output with hydralazine, and prevention of peripheral edema with dihydropyridine calcium antagonists by ACE inhibitors. It must be emphasized that some adverse effects can be exacerbated by inappropriate combination therapy (Table 3).

IMPROVED COMPLIANCE

An important consideration in evaluating a role for fixed dose combination therapy is the issue of compliance. As detailed elsewhere, despite the availability of many newer antihypertensive agents, hypertensive patients continue to remain at higher risk of premature death than the general population.[13,20] This persistence of morbidity and mortality may be accounted for by the frequent failure to achieve adequate blood-pressure reduction. For instance, the Nutrition and Health Examination Survey in the United States found that nearly 80% of treated hypertensive patients failed to attain a target blood pressure of <140 mm Hg systolic and 90

TABLE 3. ADVERSE DRUG REACTIONS AS A RESULT OF COMBINATION THERAPY.

Drug A	Drug B	Drug B Potentially Aggravates
Diuretic	Vasodilators	Hypokalemia
HRL-Ca antagonist	Beta blocker	Atrioventricular block, bradycardia
Alpha-blocker	Diuretic	First dose hypotension
ACE-inhibitors	Diuretic	Decrease in GFR
ACE-inhibitors	Potassium sparing diuretic	Hyperkalemia
Diuretic	Beta blockers	Hyperglycemia
Hydralazine	DHP-Ca Antagonist	Palpitation, myocardial ischemia

HRL = heart rate lowering
DHP = dihydropyridine
GFR = glomerular filtration rate

mm Hg diastolic.[21,22] The extent of the problem is revealed by a recent European survey indicating that the experience in Europe is similar.[23] Although there are several initiatives that may serve to bridge this gap,[24] a pivotal approach is the use of agents with more acceptable side-effect profiles, thereby enhancing patients' compliance. One such initiative is the use of the newer fixed-dose combination agents.

In addition to an enhanced tolerability profile, the treatment regimen can be simplified by using fixed-dose combinations in order to reduce the number of tablets the patient is required to take. Fewer tablets should lessen the likelihood for the patient to confuse medications and prevent treatment failure that might result from missed doses.[1,2]

COST OF DRUGS

Another substantive consideration that impacts directly on the success of therapeutic interventions is the cost of drugs. The cost of medications is one of the major reasons for poor adherence to antihypertensive medication which results in less than optimal blood pressure control for many patients. An interesting attribute of fixed-dose combinations is the reduced cost in many instances. The cost of fixed-dose combinations is often less than the cost of the constituents prescribed separately in part because of the requirements of government health reimbursement systems. In the United States, the cost of all four fixed combinations of ACE inhibitors and calcium antagonists is less than the cost of the two component drugs purchased separately.[25]

ENHANCEMENT OF FAVORABLE EFFECTS ON TARGET ORGANS

Several lines of evidence suggest that combinations of different agents, especially calcium antagonists used in combination with ACE-inhibitors, may have additive effects not only on blood pressure but also on preservation of target organs such as the heart and kidney and the vascular tree (Table 4). It has been proposed that these two classes may act in a complementary or synergistic fashion to either favor regression of left ventricular hypertrophy,[26-29] or to retard the progression of renal disease in patients with chronic renal insufficiency.[30,30a]

FIXED-DOSE VS. FREE-COMBINATION ANTIHYPERTENSIVE THERAPY

The value of fixed-dose as opposed to free-combination antihypertensive therapy is still debated.[1] What are the potential advantages of fixed-dose combinations? They are certainly very convenient for both patients and physician. Fixed-dose combinations are expected to improve compliance by minimizing the number of pills to be taken every day. The doses contained in the fixed-dose combination tend, if anything, to be lower than those used habitually in free prescriptions.

TABLE 4. POSSIBLE SYNERGISM RESULTING FROM A
COMBINATION OF A CALCIUM ANTAGONIST AND AN
ACE INHIBITOR.

	DHP-Calcium Antagonist	HRL Calcium Antagonist	ACE Inhibitor
Kidneys			
↑ Renal blood flow	Yes	Yes	Yes
↑ Efferent vasodilation	Little	Yes	Yes
↑ Afferent vasodilation	Yes	Yes	Yes
↓ Microproteinuria	Little	Yes	Yes
"Renoprotection"	Unknown	Possible	Yes
Vascular Tree			
↓ Endothelin mediated vasoconstriction	Yes	Yes	No
↓ Endothelin release	No	No	Yes
↓ Nitric oxide release	No	No	Yes
↑ Arterial compliance	Yes	Yes	Yes
↓ Vascular hypertrophy	Yes	Yes	Yes
↓ Atherogenesis*	Yes	Yes	Yes
Heart			
↓ Left ventricular hypertrophy	Yes	Yes	Yes
↑ Left ventricular filling	Yes	Yes	No
↑ Contractility, unloading	Some	No	Yes
↑ Coronary flow	Yes	Yes	Some

ACE = Angiotensin converting enzyme, DHP = Dihydropyridine,
HRL = Heart rate lowering, ↑ = increase, ↓ = decrease
*Experimental data only
Used with permission from Messerli FH, Michalewicz L: Am J Hypertens
1997;10:148S.

SPECIFIC COMBINATIONS

The availability of five main groups of antihypertensive agents provides ten possible combinations of two drugs. Several of these recently approved combinations include: fixed dose combinations of calcium antagonists with ACE-inhibitors, ACE-inhibitors with diuretics, and dihydropyridine calcium antagonists in combination with β-adrenoreceptor blockers. Table 5 lists combination drugs that are currently available for treating hypertension.

ACE Inhibitor/Diuretic Combinations

ACE inhibitors are known to reduce arterial pressure by reducing angiotensin II production. Hence, while they are effective antihypertensive agents in all subjects, their antihypertensive efficacy is enhanced when the renin-angiotensin system is activated. This is clearly shown in a recently reported, double-blind placebo controlled, parallel-group trial by the Canadian Working Group. These investigators added a diuretic to enalapril and showed a superior antihypertensive efficacy with a combination over enalapril alone.[31] Since diuretics increase the activity of the renin-angiotensin system and are vasodilators in their own right, it is logical to combine these two groups of drugs to potentiate reductions in arterial pressure.

TABLE 5. COMBINATION DRUGS FOR HYPERTENSION.

Drug	Trade Name
Beta adrenergic blockers and diuretics	
Atenolol, 50 or 100 mg/chlorthalidone, 25 mg	Tenoretic
Bisoprolol fumarate, 2.5, 5, or 10 mg/hydrochlorothiazide, 6.25 mg	Ziac*
Metoprolol tartrate, 50 or 100 mg hydrochlorothiazide, 25 or 50 mg	Lopressor HCT
Nadolol, 40 or 80 mg/bendroflumethiazide, 5 mg	Corzide
Propranolol hydrochloride, 40 or 80 mg/ hydrochlorothiazide, 25 mg	Inderide
Propranolol hydrochloride (extended release), 80, 120, or 160 mg/hydrochlorothiazide, 50 mg	Inderide LA
Timolol maleate, 10 mg/hydrochlorothiazide, 25 mg	Timolide
ACE inhibitors and diuretics	
Benazepril hydrochloride, 5, 10, 20 mg/ hydrochlorothiazide, 6.25, 12.5, or 25 mg	Lotensin HCT
Captopril, 25 or 50 mg/hydrochlorothiazide, 15 or 25 mg	Capozide*
Enalapril maleate, 5 or 10 mg/hydrochlorothiazide, 12.5 or 25 mg	Vaseretic
Lisinopril, 10 or 20 mg/hydrochlorothiazide, 12.5 or 25 mg	Prinzide, Zestoretic
Angiotensin II receptor antagonists and diuretics	
Losartan potassium, 50 mg/hydrochlorothiazide, 12.5 mg	Hyzaar
Valsortan, 80 and 160 mg/hydrochlorothiazide, 12.5 mg	
Calcium antagonists and ACE inhibitors	
Amlodipine besylate, 2.5 or 5 mg/benazepril hydrochloride, 10 or 20 mg	Lotrel
Diltiazem hydrochloride, 180 mg/enalapril maleate, 5 mg	Teczem
Verapamil hydrochloride (extended release), 180/2, 240/1, 240/2, or 240/4 mg/ trandolapril, 1, 2, or 4 mg	Tarka
Felodipine, 5 mg/enalapril maleate, 5 mg	Lexxel
Diuretic combinations	
Triamterene, 37.5, 50, or 75 mg/hydrochlorothiazide, 25 or 50 mg	Dyazide, Maxide
Spironolactone, 25 or 50 mg/hydrochlorothiazide, 25 or 50 mg	Aldactazide
Amiloride hydrochloride, 5 mg/hydrochlorothiazide, 50 mg	Moduretic
Other combinations	
Guanethidine monosulfate, 10 mg/hydrochlorothiazide, 25 mg	Esimil
Hydralazine hydrochloride, 25, 50, or 100 mg/hydrochlorothiazide, 25 or 50 mg	Apresazide
Methyldopa, 250 or 500 mg/hydrochlorothiazide, 15, 25, 30, or 50 mg	Aldoril
Reserpine, 0.125 mg/hydrochlorothiazide, 25 to 50 mg	Hydropres
Reserpine, 0.10 mg/hydralazine hydrochloride, 25 mg/hydrochlorothiazide, 15 mg	Ser-Ap-Es
Clonidine hydrochloride, 0.1, 0.2, or 0.3 mg/ chlorthalidone, 15 mg	Combipres
Methyldopa, 250 mg/chlorothiazide, 150 or 250 mg	Aldochlor
Reserpine, 0.125 or 0.25 mg/chlorthalidone, 25 or 50 mg	Demi-Regroton
Reserpine, 0.125 or 0.25 mg. chlorothiazide, 250 or 500 mg	Diupres
Prazosin hydrochloride, 1, 2, or 5 mg/ polythiazide, 0.5 mg	Minizide

*Approved for initial therapy

While several studies have demonstrated that addition of thiazide diuretics to ACE inhibitors increased blood pressure reductions, several recent studies have also examined fixed-dose combinations.[32-34] ACE inhibitor monotherapy is least effective in low-renin states and/or in salt-sensitive patients, such as black subjects and the elderly.[35] When combined with a diuretic, however, the two drug classes appear to work synergistically to lower blood pressure in patients with high, normal or low renin levels, with response rates of 80% and above.[36,37] The response rates are generally higher than those achieved with a beta-blocker/diuretic combination.[38]

Diuretic-induced hypokalemia is usually abolished by the addition of an ACE inhibitor. The neutral or beneficial effects of ACE inhibitors on serum lipids, glucose intolerance, and hyperinsulinemia might be expected to attenuate the adverse metabolic effects of diuretic monotherapy. However, clinical trials of ACE inhibitor/hydrochlorothiazide combinations have produced controversial results,[39,40] showing a deterioration in some metabolic parameters with these combinations.

Of note, there is evidence that ACE inhibitor/diuretic combinations may prevent the hypertensive vascular trophic effects and coronary artery vasoconstriction that are amplified by diuretic-induced increases in angiotensin II.[41,42] An ACE inhibitor plus a low-dose diuretic is therefore a particularly good combination for hypertensive patients with congestive heart failure, left ventricular hypertrophy, or diabetic nephropathy.[43] It is also very effective in patients with severe hypertension,[37] in the elderly and in African-American patients in whom monotherapy with ACE inhibition has been unsuccessful.[44]

Angiotensin Receptor Blocker (ARB)/ Diuretic Combinations

Similar synergistic effects as exist between ACE inhibitors and diuretics can be expected to occur with the combination of ARBs and diuretics. Several factorial design studies have documented that this combination is additive. ARBs in monotherapy have been found to be less effective in patients characterized by low renin states and/or salt sensitivity such as the African American and the elderly. However, when combined with a diuretic, the two drug classes have been shown to synergistically lower arterial pressure with high normal and low renin plasma activity, achieving response rates of 80% and above. At the present time two fixed ARBs/diuretics combinations are available in the US, i.e., losartan and hydrochlorothiazide (Hyzaar) and valsartan and hydrochlorothiazide (Diovan HCT).

Beta-Blocker/Diuretic Combinations

While beta-blockers are known to reduce arterial pressure, the precise mechanisms are not fully established. However, beta-blockers are known to enhance renal sodium retention and promote peripheral vasoconstriction.[45] Consequently, the addition of a diuretic would not only act to counteract these renal and peripheral vascular effects but may, if used at lower doses, not worsen cardiac risk factors such as cholesterol or insulin resistance. Many fixed dose combinations of beta-blocker with diuretics have been available for clinical use for over 20 years.[46-49] However, based on our current level of knowledge regarding dosing of these two agents and worsening of cardiac risk factors, the fixed dose combination that seems the most appropriate is a low dose/fixed dose combination of the beta-blocker in fixed dose combination with 6.25 mg of a thiazide diuretic. In theory this combination reduces the risk of beta-blocker-induced congestive heart failure and has a possible cardioprotective effect.[43] The attenuation of diuretic-induced hypokalemia by beta-blockade has also been suggested, although this effect has proven somewhat unreliable. Indeed, fixed-dose combinations of a beta-blocker/thiazide/potassium-sparing agent have been considered necessary by some.[50]

In spite of these benefits, the utility of beta-blocker/diuretic combinations is limited, especially with long-term use, by the tendency of both drug classes to raise serum triglycerides, glucose and uric acid, and to cause sexual dysfunction. Furthermore, the negative effect of beta-blockers on peripheral vascular resistance combined with diuretic-related volume depletion may compromise perfusion in susceptible patients. Interestingly enough, no study has shown that the addition of a beta-blocker to the diuretic enhances the benefits of the diuretic per se. Thus, potentially all beneficial effects on morbidity and mortality with beta-blocker/diuretic combinations may be due to diuretics alone.

A recent double-blind placebo controlled trial in 218 hypertensive subjects compared the blood pressure lowering efficacy of the fixed dose combination of bisoprolol with low dose hydrochlorothiazide with either amlodipine or enalapril.[51] There was no significant difference in the blood pressure-lowering response between the fixed dose combination and amlodipine. However, both treatments were better than enalapril.[51] This observation was corroborated by another multicenter randomized, double-blind, placebo controlled trial wherein the fixed dose combination of a beta-blocker with low dose hydrochlorothiazide was shown to have greater antihypertensive efficacy than either of its components.[52] Moreover, a lower side effect profile was noted with the combination.[52] In concert these studies support the notion that even antihypertensive agents known to have adverse side effects individually may, when combined at lower doses, provide lower side effect profiles and greater antihypertensive efficacy.

Beta-Blocker/Calcium Antagonist Combinations

Hemodynamically, beta-blockers combine well with calcium antagonists of the dihydropyridine class, since the former limit cardiovascular performance and decrease cardiac output, while the latter vasodilate and increase cardiac output. Furthermore, beta-blockade can prevent the tachycardia and sympathetic nervous system activation that occurs with dihydropyridines.[43,53] The antihypertensive effects of the two drug classes are additive, and the combination is well tolerated. In a study comparing atenolol/nifedipine SR with either agent, close, vasodilatory adverse effects normally attributable to calcium antagonists, such as ankle edema, flushing and tachycardia, were considerably reduced.[54] The combination of a beta-blocker and a dihydropyridine calcium antagonist is particularly effective in patients with hypertension and angina pectoris.[53] Another well-studied example is the combination of the dihydropyridine calcium antagonist, felodipine, and the cardioselective beta-blocker, metoprolol (Logimax). Recent studies have demonstrated that adequate blood pressure reduction can be achieved in a greater percentage of patients with the combination compared with monotherapy with either component alone.[55]

Conversely, the combination of a beta-blocker and a phenyl alkylamine such as verapamil should be avoided, since the risk of atrioventricular conduction abnormalities will increase, particularly in patients with ischemic heart disease.[56] This adverse effect also occurs to a lesser extent with diltiazem.

ACE Inhibitors and Calcium Antagonists

Based on the effectiveness and favorable influence on cardiovascular risk profiles of the individual drugs, the recent development of fixed-dose combinations of ACE inhibitors and calcium antagonists is likely to provide a particularly attractive treatment option for a broad range of hypertensive patients and is generating increasing interest in the antihypertensive field.[2,57] In addition to their broad profiles of neutral or beneficial effects on cardiovascular risk factors (Table 1), both drug classes maintain physical, mental and sexual activity.[57]

When used in combination, the antihypertensive effects of the two classes are additive, as can be shown in factorial design trials (Figure 2). This is achieved by several mecha-

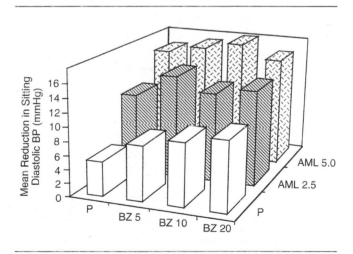

Figure 2. *Mean reduction in sitting diastolic blood pressure with the combination of amlodipine and benazepril at various doses.(AML 2.5 – amlodipine 2.5 mg; AML 5 = amlodipine 5 mg; BZ 5 = benazepril 5 mg; BZ 10 = benazepril 10 mg; BZ 20 = benazepril 20 mg; DBP = diastolic blood pressure; P = Placebo). (Reproduced with permission from Kuschnir et al. Clin Ther 1996;18:1213–1224.)*

nisms: Both ACE inhibitors and calcium antagonists lower blood pressure by vasodilatation and both classes have a natriuretic effect; however, their mechanisms of action are distinctly different and may therefore complement each other in producing an antihypertensive response. While ACE inhibitors are more effective in patients with high renin levels, calcium antagonists may be more effective in those with low renin levels; therefore, combination therapy ensures reliable treatment in both conditions.[2,7] Conceivably, the negative sodium balance induced by calcium antagonists may be responsible for facilitating the antihypertensive effects of an ACE inhibitor.

Conversely, ACE inhibition offsets the stimulatory effects of calcium antagonists on the renin-angiotensin and sympathetic nervous systems, counter-regulatory mechanisms that limit the antihypertensive efficacy of calcium antagonists.[7] By this mechanism, the edema and reflex tachycardia that may result from monotherapy with calcium antagonists, particularly with the dihydropyridine molecules, is diminished (Figure 3). Despite a similar antihypertensive effect, the combination of amlodipine/benazepril elicits considerably less peripheral edema than amlodipine 5 mg or amlodipine 10 mg once a day.[58] The Joint National Committee has recognized this synergistic effect by stating that "combinations of a dihydropyridine calcium antagonist and an ACE inhibitor induce less pedal edema than does the calcium antagonist alone."[59a]

Finally, one can argue that the reduced angiotensin II levels achieved with ACE inhibition should also increase the antihypertensive effect of the calcium antagonists, since it has been demonstrated that the activity of the renin-angiotensin system is inversely proportional to the level of blood pressure reduction achievable with calcium antagonists therapy.[60]

Antihypertensive Efficacy. The potent antihypertensive efficacy of ACE inhibitor/calcium antagonist combinations

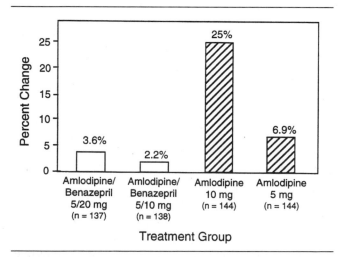

Figure 3. Incidence of edema (pedal edema including dependent, generalized leg, periorbital and peripheral edema) with amlodipine/benazepril versus amlodipine alone in double-blind, multicenter US clinical trials.

is particularly valuable in patients with hypertension who are uncontrolled by monotherapy.[61–62] The positive results of recent multicenter studies involving the new combination trandolapril plus verapamil SR further illustrate the advantages of these combinations.[63–65] Similarly impressive antihypertensive efficacy has been documented in a combination of amlodipine and benazepril (Figure 2).[58]

End Organ Protection. Combined renoprotective effects have also been demonstrated with ACE inhibitor/calcium antagonists combinations. Both ACE inhibitors and heart rate lowering calcium antagonists have been reported to exert renoprotective effects. In the kidney, the vasodilatory effect of the ACE inhibitors occurs primarily at efferent glomerular arterioles. In contrast, all calcium antagonists dilate afferent arterioles independently of the renin-angiotensin system. However, the three groups of calcium antagonists do not have identical intrarenal effects. The dihydropyridine compounds, such as nifedipine, predominantly lower afferent resistance. Thus, glomerular pressure remains elevated, and the albumin excretion rate tends to increase. Verapamil SR and diltiazem, on the other hand, lower both afferent and efferent arteriolar resistance. Consequently, these agents may exert protective effects on the diabetic kidney by lowering glomerular pressure and albumin excretion rate.

When an ACE inhibitor is combined with verapamil, the beneficial effects on nephropathy in diabetic patients appear to be additive. Over 1 year, combination therapy with trandolapril and verapamil SR in patients with established diabetic nephropathy resulted in a significantly greater reduction in urinary albumin excretion than with either agent administered alone[59] (Figure 4) and slowed the decline in glomerular filtration rate. In another study, hypertensive insulin-dependent diabetic patients treated with cilazapril plus verapamil had a greater reduction in albumin excretion rate than those who received monotherapy with either agent,[66] although there were no differences in arterial blood pressure between the three groups.

The benefits of both ACE inhibitors and calcium antagonists on reversal or on prevention of ventricular remodeling associated with hypertension and ischemic heart disease are well established,[67,68] and ACE inhibitors appear to be superior to other antihypertensive treatments in this respect.[68] Furthermore, heart rate lowering calcium antagonists, particularly verapamil SR, seem to be more effective than dihydropyridine agents for reversing left ventricular mass, independently of duration of treatment and degree of blood pressure reduction.[67,69] The cardioprotective benefits of verapamil have been demonstrated in a double-blind, placebo-controlled clinical study involving 1775 patients with acute myocardial infarction, in which the calcium antagonist produced a significant reduction of 29% in reinfarction rate compared with placebo.[70] ACE inhibitors have produced similar reductions in post-infarction morbidity; indeed, their cardioprotective properties have resulted in significant mortality reduction in patients who have suffered a myocardial infarction.[71] In a very provocative pilot study, Fischer Hansen et al.[72] have recently

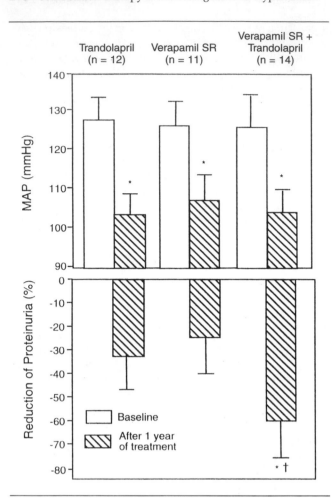

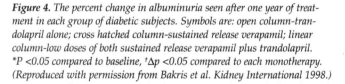

Figure 4. The percent change in albuminuria seen after one year of treatment in each group of diabetic subjects. Symbols are: open column-trandolapril alone; cross hatched column-sustained release verapamil; linear column-low doses of both sustained release verapamil plus trandolapril. *P <0.05 compared to baseline, †Δp <0.05 compared to each monotherapy. (Reproduced with permission from Bakris et al. Kidney International 1998.)

shown that the addition of verapamil SR to trandolapril in patients after myocardial infarction who had clinical symptoms and signs of congestive heart failure resulted in an event-free survival that was significantly better than that on trandolapril alone. This is even more astonishing since, until now, verapamil has been considered to be contraindicated in patients with congestive heart failure. Conceivably, in post-MI patients the presence of an ACE inhibitor nullifies the negative inotropic effects of verapamil. Interestingly enough, in two other studies, one in patients after myocardial infarction and the other in hypertensive diabetic patients, the combination of an ACE inhibitor with a calcium antagonist proved to be more beneficial than either drug alone. This would indicate that the synergism of this combination may enhance the primary or secondary cardioprotective effects.

Clearly, reduction of reinfarction rate (secondary prevention) with a drug or a drug class thus by no means indicates that the same agent will achieve primary prevention.

Nevertheless, the beneficial effect of the ACE inhibitor and heart-rate-controlling calcium antagonists on left ventricular hypertrophy and on reinfarction rate makes this combination attractive for the patient with hypertensive heart disease and/or coronary artery disease.

Collectively, these and other considerations have culminated in the development of several ACE-inhibitor/calcium antagonist combinations. The first such combination approved in the United States is that of amlodipine with benazepril (Lotrel). This is the first time that the FDA has granted permission for fixed combinations of antihypertensive medications that do not involve a diuretic. In addition, the FDA has approved three additional fixed-dose combinations: enalapril and diltiazem (Teczem), enalapril and felodipine (Lexxel) and verapamil SR/trandolapril (Tarka).

Combination of Two Different Calcium Antagonists

Since calcium antagonists are a very heterogeneous drug class (as opposed to the ACE inhibitors), some attempts have been made recently to combine two different calcium antagonists to enhance antihypertensive efficacy. Thus, heart-rate-controlling calcium antagonists, such as verapamil and diltiazem, have been combined with calcium antagonists that have little if any negative inotropic effects, such as amlodipine and felodipine. There is no carefully controlled study available to assess the efficacy of these combinations. Nevertheless, preliminary findings indicate that these combinations are well tolerated and possess impressive antihypertensive efficacy.

CONCLUSION

The most common rationale for combining antihypertensive drugs is enhanced efficacy in terms of reducing blood pressure. Enhancing tolerability and reducing or limiting side effects are additional attributes that assume additional relevance at a time when we are focusing on improving patient compliance. An additional exciting and novel concept is the possibility of enhancing salutary effects on target organ by combination therapy over and above the effect expected from the fall in arterial pressure alone. This approach could become a desirable therapeutic goal, provided such benefits are documented rigorously by carefully conducted morbidity and mortality studies.

REFERENCES

1. Oster JR, Epstein M. Fixed-dose combination medications for the treatment of hypertension: a critical review. J Clin Hypertens 1987;3:278–293.

2. Epstein M, Bakris G. Newer approaches to antihypertensive therapy: use of fixed dose combination therapy. Arch Intern Med 1996;156:1969–1978.

3. Sever P. The heterogeneity of hypertension: why doesn't every patient respond to every antihypertensive drug? J Hum Hypertens 1995;9:S33–S36.

4. Materson BJ, Reda DJ, Cushman WC, et al., for the Department of Veterans Affairs Cooperative Study Group on Antihypertensive Agents. Single-drug therapy for hypertension in men. A comparison

of six antihypertensive agents with placebo. N Engl J Med 1993;328:914–921.

5. Attwood S, Bird R, Burch K, et al. Within-patient correlation between the antihypertensive effects of atenolol, lisinopril and nifedipine. J Hypertens 1994;12:1053–1060.

6. Epstein M. Calcium antagonists in the management of hypertension. In: Epstein M, Ed. Calcium Antagonists in Clinical Medicine. Philadelphia: Hanley & Belfus, 1992:213–230.

7. Ménard J, Bellet M. Calcium antagonists-ACE inhibitors combination therapy: objectives and methodology of clinical development. J Cardiovasc Pharmacol 1993;21(Suppl. 2):S49–S54.

8. Safar ME, Weiss YA, Corvol PL, Menard JE, London GM, Milliez PL. Anti-hypertensive adrenergic-blocking agents: effects on sodium balance, the renin-angiotensin system and haemodynamics. Clin Sci Mol Med Suppl 1975;2:93S–95S.

9. Lake CR, Ziegler MG, Coleman MD, Kopin IJ. Hydrochlorothiazide-induced sympathetic hyperactivity in hypertensive patients. Clin Pharmacol Ther 1979;26:428–432.

10. Gillmore E, Weil J, Chidsey C. Treatment of essential hypertension with a new vasodilator in combination with beta-adrenergic blockade. N Engl J Med 1970; 282:521–527.

11. Ruzicka M, Leenen FHH. Relevance of intermittent increases in sympathetic activity for adverse outcome on short-acting calcium antagonists. In Laragh JH, Brenner BM, eds: *Hypertension: Pathophysiology, diagnosis, and management.* Raven Press, New York,1995:2815–2825.

12. Grossman E, Messerli FH. Effect of calcium antagonists on plasma norepinephrine levels, heart rate, and blood pressure. Am J Cardiol 1997;80:1453–1458.

13. Epstein M. Calcium antagonists should continue to be used for first-line treatment of hypertension. Arch Intern Med 1995;155: 2150–2156.

14. Kailasam MT, Parmer RJ, Cervenka JH, et al. Divergent effects of dihydropyridine and phenylalkylamine calcium channel antagonist classes on autonomic function in human hypertension. Hypertension 1995;26:143–149.

15. Fagan TC. Remembering the lessons of basic pharmacology (editorial). Arch Intern Med 1994;154:1430–1431.

16. Frishman WH, Bryzinski BS, Coulson LR, et al. A multifactorial trial design to assess combination therapy in hypertension: treatment with bisoprolol and hydrochlorthiazide. Arch Intern Med 1994;154:1461–1468.

17. Fenichel RR, Lipicky RJ. Combination products as first-line pharmacotherapy. Arch Intern Med 1994;154:1429–1430.

18. Messerli FH. Combination therapy in hypertension. J Hum Hypertens 1992;6(Suppl. 2): S19–S21.

19. Epstein M, Oster JR: Hypertension: Practical Management. Miami: Battersea, 1988:128.

20. Isles CG, Walker LM, Beevers GD, et al. Mortality in patients of the Glasgow Blood Pressure Clinic. J Hypertens 1986;4:141–156.

21. Burt VL, Whelton P, Roccella EJ, et al. Prevalence of hypertension in the US adult population. Results from the Third National Health and Nutrition Examination Survey, 1988–1991. Hypertension 1995;25:305–313.

22. Frohlich ED. There's good news and not so good news (editorial). Hypertension 25:303–304, 1995.

23. Hosie J, Wiklund I. Managing hypertension in general practice: can we do better? J Hum Hypertens 1995; 9:S15–S18.

24. Ménard J, Chatellier G. Limiting factors in the control of BP: why is there a gap between theory and practice? J Hum Hypertens 1995; 9:S19–S23.

25. Cost to pharmacist for 1 year's/day's treatment, according to January 1996 Average Wholesale Price (AWP) listed in Medi-Span Prescription Pricing Guide.

26. Messerli FH, Michalewicz L: Cardiac effects of combination therapy. Am J Hypertens 1997;10:146S–152S.

27. Frohlich ED. The heart in hypertension: A 1991 overview. Hypertension 18(III):62–68, 1991.

28. Bakris GL, Frohlich ED: The evolution of antihypertensive therapy: An overview of four decades of experience. J Am Coll Cardiol 14:1595–1608, 1989.

29. Arita M, Horinaka S, Frohlich ED: Biochemical components in myocardial performance after reversal of left ventricular hypertrophy in spontaneously hypertensive rats. J Hypertens 11:951–959, 1993.

30. Münter K, Hergenröder S, Jochims K, Kirchengast M. Individual and combined effects of verapamil or trandolapril on attenuating hypertensive glomerulopathic changes in the stroke-prone rat. J Am Soc Nephrol 1996; 7:681–686.

30a. Epstein, M. The benefits of ACE inhibitors and calcium antagonists in slowing progressive renal failure: Focus on fixed-dose combination antihypertensive therapy. Renal Failure 1996; 813–832.

31. Enalapril and enalapril-hydrochlorothiazide in the treatment of essential hypertension. The Enalapril-Hydrochlorothiazide in Essential Hypertension Canadian Working Group. Clin Ther 1993; 15:364–373.

32. Vaisse B, Renucci JF, Delage Y, Madonna O, Gressin V, Poggi L. Evaluation of the antihypertensive efficacy of lisinopril and captopril associated with hydrochlorothiazide by ambulatory measurement of arterial pressure [Fr]. Ann Cardiol Angeiol (Paris) 1993;42: 566–572.

33. Chrysant SG: Antihypertensive effectiveness of low-dose lisinopril-hydrochlorothiazide combination. A large multicenter study. Lisinopril-Hydrochlorothiazide Group. Arch Intern Med 1994;154: 737–743.

34. Mayaudon H, Chanudet X, Janin G, Madonna O. Comparison of the efficacy of enalapril + hydrochlorothiazide and captopril + hydrochlorothiazide combinations in mild-to-moderate arterial hypertension by ambulatory measurement of blood pressure [Fr]. Ann Cardiol Angeiol (Paris) 1995; 44:235–241.

35. Opie LH. Choosing the correct drug for the individual hypertensive patient. Drugs 1992;44(Suppl. 1):147–155.

36. Andersen L, Weiner L, Svensson A, Hansson L. Enalapril with either a 'very low' of 'low' dose of hydrochlorothiazide is equally effective in essential hypertension. A double-blind trial in 100 hypertensive patients. J Hypertens 1993;1(Suppl. 2):384–386.

37. Johnston CI, Arnolda L, Hiwatari M. Angiotensin-converting enzyme inhibitors in the treatment of hypertension. Drugs 1984;27:271–277.

38. Costa FV, Borghi C, Ambrosioni E. Captopril and oxprenolol in a fixed combination with thiazide diuretics: comparison of their antihypertensive efficacy and metabolic effects. Clin Ther 1984;6:708–718.

39. Bilo HJ, Westerman RF, Nicolaas-Merkus AM, Donker AJ. Effects of enalapril with and without hydrochlorothiazide in hypertensive patients with non-insulin-dependent diabetes mellitus. Diabetes Res 1988;9:21–25.

40. Sheih SM, Sheu WH, Shen DD, et al. Improvement in metabolic

risk factors for coronary heart disease associated with cilazapril treatment. Am J Hypertens 1992;5:506–510.

41. Burnier M, Waeber B, Brunner HR. First-line pharmacological treatment of hypertension. J Intern Med 1992;232:381–388.

42. Dahlöf B, Hansson L. The influence of antihypertensive therapy on the structural arteriolar changes in essential hypertension: different effects of enalapril and hydrochlorothiazide. J Intern Med 1993;234:271–279.

43. Sica DA. Fixed-dose combination antihypertensive drugs. Do they have a role in rational therapy? Drugs 1994;48:16–24.

44. Veterans Administration Cooperative study group on antihypertensive agents. Racial differences in response to low-dose captopril are abolished by the addition of hydrochlorothiazide. Br J Clin Pharmacol 1982;14:97S–101S.

45. Bakris GL, Wilson DM, Burnett JC Jr. The renal, forearm, and hormonal responses to standing in the presence and absence of propranolol. Circulation 1986;74:1061–1065.

46. Kincaid-Smith P, Macdonald IM, Hua A, Laver MC, Fang P. Changing concepts in the management of hypertension. Med J Aust 1975;1:327–332.

47. Waeber B, Brunner HR. Main objectives and new aspects of combination treatment of hypertension. J Hypertens (Suppl.) 1995;13: S15–S19.

48. Safar ME, Tzincoca C. Pharmacological basis for a fixed association of hydrochlorothiazide, amiloride hydrochloride, and timolol maleate. Sem Hop 1979;55:1095–1099.

49. Geyskes GG, Stutterheim A, Boer P, Dorhout-Mees EJ. Comparison of the antihypertensive effect of propranolol and practolol combined with chlorthalidone. Eur J Clin Pharmacol 1975;9:85–90.

50. Burns DG, Pittaway D. Combination of timolol maleate, hydrochlorothiazide, and amiloride hydrochloride in the treatment of hypertension: A multicentre trial. S Afr Med J 1980;57:815–818.

51. Prisant LM, Weir MR, Papademetriou V, et al. Low-dose drug combination therapy: an alternative first-line approach to hypertension treatment. Am Heart J 1995;130:359–366.

52. Frishman WH, Burris JF, Mroszek WJ, et al. First-line therapy option with low-dose bisoprolol fumarate and low-dose hydrochlorothiazide in patients with stage I and stage II systemic hypertension. J Clin Pharmacol 1995;35:182–188.

53. Chalmers J. The place of combination therapy in the treatment of hypertension in 1993. Clin Exp Hypertens 1993;15:1299–1313.

54. Stanley NN, Thirkettle JL, Varma MP, Larkin H, Health ID. Efficacy and tolerability of atenolol, nifedipine and their combination in the management of hypertension. Drugs 1988;35(Suppl. 4):29–35.

55. Dahlöf B, Jönsson L, Borgholst O, et al. Improved antihypertensive efficacy of the felodipine-metoprolol extended-release tablet compared with each drug alone. Blood Press 1993;1(Suppl. 1):37–45.

56. Hansson L, Himmelmann A. Calcium antagonists in antihypertensive combination therapy. J Cardiovasc Pharmacol 1991;18(10): S76–S80.

57. Opie LH: Individualised selection of antihypertensive therapy. Drugs 1993;46(Suppl. 2):142–148.

58. Kuschnir E, Acuna E, Sevilla D, et al: Treatment of patients with essential hypertension: amlodipine 5 mg/benazepril 20 mg compared with amlodipine 5 mg, benazepril 20 mg, and placebo. Clin Ther 1996;18:1213–1224.

59. Bakris GL, Weir MR, DeQuattro V, McMahon FG. Effects of an ACE inhibitor/calcium antagonist combination on proteinuria in diabetic nephropathy. Kidney Int 1998;54:1283–1289.

59a. Joint National Committee. Report on the diagnosis and treatment of hypertension (JNC VI). Arch Intern Med 1997;157: 2413–2446.

60. Evans RR, Davis WR, Wallace JM, DiPette DJ, Holland OB. Humoral factors determining the blood pressure response to converting enzyme inhibition and calcium channel blockade. Am J Hypertens 1990;3:605–610.

61. Ferrier C, Ferrari P, Weidmann P, Keller U, Beretta-Piccoli C, Riesen WF. Antihypertensive therapy with CA^{2+}. Antagonist verapamil and/or ACE inhibitor enalapril in NIDDM patients. Diabetes Care 1991;14:911–914.

62. Heagerty AM, Swales JD. The combination of verapamil and captopril in the treatment of essential hypertension. Pharmatherapeutica 1987;5: 21–25.

63. Messerli F, Frishman WH, Elliott WJ, for the Trandolapril Study Group. Effects of verapamil and trandolapril in the treatment of hypertension. Am J Hypertens 1998;11:322–327.

64. Levine JH, Applegate WB, and the Trandolapril/Verapamil Study Group. Trandolapril and verapamil slow release in the treatment of hypertension: A dose-response assessment with the use of a multifactorial trial design. Current Therapeutic Research 1997;58: 361–374.

65. Viskoper RJ, Compagnone D, Dies R, Zilles P. Verapamil and trandolapril alone and in fixed combination on 24-hour ambulatory blood pressure profiles of patients with moderate essential hypertension. Current Therapeutic Research. 1997;58:343–351.

66. Fioretto P, Frigato F, Velussi M, et al. Effects of angiotensin converting enzyme inhibitors and calcium antagonists on atrial natriuretic peptide release and action and on albumin excretion rate in hypertensive insulin-dependent diabetic patients. Am J Hypertens 1992;5:837–846.

67. Cruickshank JM, Lewis J, Moore V, Dodd C. Reversibility of left ventricular hypertrophy by differing types of antihypertensive therapy. J Human Hypertens 1992;6:85–90.

68. Dahlöf B, Pennert K, Hansson L. Reversal of left ventricular hypertrophy in hypertensive patients. A meta-analysis of 109 treatment studies. Am J Hypertens 1992;5:95–110.

69. Nalbantgil I, Onder R, Kiliccioglu B, Atabay G. Regression of hypertensive left ventricular hypertrophy with different calcium antagonists. Br J Cardiol 1994;May:213–216.

70. The Danish Study Group on Verapamil in Myocardial Infarction. Effect of verapamil on mortality and major events after acute myocardial infarction. (The Danish Verapamil Infarction Trial II-DAVIT II). Am J Cardiol 1990;66:779–785.

71. Pfeffer MA, Braunwald E, Moye LA, et al. Effect of captopril on mortality and morbidity in patients with left ventricular dysfunction after myocardial infarction. Results of the survival and ventricular enlargement trial. The SAVE investigators [see comments]. N Engl J Med 1992;327:669–677.

72. Fischer-Hansen J, Hagerup L, Sigurd B, et al. Cardiac event rates after acute myocardial infarction in patients treated with verapamil and trandolapril versus trandolapril alone. Danish Verapamil Infarction Trial (DAVIT) Study Group. Am J Cardiol 1997;79:738–741.

CHAPTER 19

Hypertensive Emergencies and Urgencies

Ehud Grossman
A. Ironi
Franz H. Messerli

Hypertensive crisis is defined as a severe elevation in blood pressure, such as a diastolic blood pressure above 120 to 130 mm Hg, and is classified as either urgency or emergency. Hypertensive urgency is said to be present when severe elevation in blood pressure is not associated with end-organ injury. There is no scientific evidence that acute blood pressure lowering is beneficial in hypertensive urgency. To the contrary, rapid uncontrolled pressure reduction may be harmful because it can precipitate acute ischemic stroke or myocardial infarction.

Therefore, the appropriate approach for patients with hypertensive urgency is to lower the blood pressure more gradually over 24 to 48 hours with oral antihypertensive agents. Any drug that lowers blood pressure precipitously should be avoided. When the cause of transient blood pressure elevation is easily identified, such as pain or acute anxiety (as in panic disorders), the appropriate therapy is analgesic or anxiolytic medication. When the cause of blood pressure elevation is unknown, various oral antihypertensive agents are available. The efficacy of the various agents seems to be similar, and any of them can be used as a first choice to lower blood pressure. The underlying pathophysiologic and clinical findings, mechanism of drug action, and the potential adverse effects should be taken into consideration when choosing the appropriate agent. Nifedipine and other dihydropyridine calcium antagonists increase heart rate, whereas clonidine, beta-blockers and labetalol tend to decrease it. This is particularly important in patients with ischemic heart disease. Labetalol and beta-blockers should not be used in patients with bronchospasm and bradycardia or heart blocks. Clonidine should be avoided if mental acuity is desired. Captopril should be avoided in patients with bilateral renal artery stenosis or unilateral renal artery stenosis in patients with solitary kidney.

In contrast to a hypertensive urgency, a hypertensive emergency is relatively rare and said to be present only when blood pressure elevation confers an immediate threat to the integrity of the cardiovascular system. Patients with a hypertensive emergency require an immediate reduction in blood pressure to avoid further end-organ damage, generally by intravenous therapy in an intensive care setting. Several drugs are available for use in these cases. Sodium nitroprusside is the most popular agent for treatment of hypertensive emergency. Nitroglycerin is preferred in the management of hypertensive emergency associated with acute coronary insufficiency. Addition of a beta-blocker may be desirable in some patients. Loop diuretics, nitroglycerin and sodium nitroprusside, are effective in patients with hypertensive emergency associated with pulmonary edema. Enalaprilat is theoretically helpful in these cases, especially when the renin system might be activated. Initial treatment of aortic dissection begins with rapid, controlled titration of arterial pressure to normal levels by using a combination of intravenous sodium nitroprusside and beta-blocking agent. If there are contraindications to beta-blockers urapidil or trimethaphan camsylate is a reasonable alternative. Hydralazine remains the drug of choice for patients with eclampsia. Labetalol, urapidil, or calcium antagonists are possible alternative therapeutic approaches if hydralazine fails or is contraindicated. For patients with catecholamine-induced crises, an alpha-adrenergic blocking drug such as phentolamine should be given. An alternative to phentolamine would be labetalol or sodium nitroprusside with beta-blockers. Few if any comparative or randomized trials provide definitive conclusions about the efficacy and safety of comparative agents. Some investigators recommend decreasing the diastolic blood pressure to no less than 100–110 mm Hg. A reasonable approach for most patients with hypertensive emergencies is to lower the mean arterial pressure by 25% over the initial 2 to 4 hours with the most specific antihypertensive regimen.

DEFINITION OF HYPERTENSIVE CRISIS

Hypertensive crisis is defined as a severe elevation in blood pressure, such as a diastolic blood pressure above 120 to 130 mm Hg[1] and can be subclassified into either emergency or urgency.[2]

Hypertensive emergency is relatively rare and defined as such only when there is an immediate threat to the integrity of the cardiovascular system (Table 1). Patients with a hypertensive emergency require an immediate reduction in blood pressure to avoid serious end-organ damage, generally effected by means of intravenous therapy in an intensive care setting.

Unlike hypertensive emergency, patients with severe elevation in blood pressure who have no evidence of progressive end-organ injury are classified as having an urgent hypertensive crisis and require only a gradual reduction in blood pressure over a period of 24 to 48 hours.

According to a recent study the prevalence of hypertensive crisis in an emergency room in 1 year is 3% of total

TABLE 1. DEFINITION OF HYPERTENSIVE EMERGENCY.

Moderate to severe elevation of arterial pressure associated with:

1. Malignant hypertension*
2. Intracranial hemorrhage
3. Atherothrombotic cerebral infarction
4. Acute congestive heart failure
5. Acute coronary insufficiency
6. Acute renal insufficiency
7. Acute aortic dissection
8. Adrenergic crisis (pheochromocytoma crisis, clonidine withdrawal, food and drug interactions with monoamine oxidase inhibitors, amphetamine overdose).
9. Eclampsia

*Malignant hypertension: A syndrome characterized by elevated blood pressure accompanied by encephalopathy or nephropathy or by papilledema and/or microangiopathic hemolytic anemia.

patients, but 27% of all medical urgencies-emergencies.[3] Before it was possible to treat accelerated-malignant hypertension, survival was 20% and 1%, for 1 and 5 years, respectively.[4] During the last two decades survival improved, with 10 year survival rate of 67% and mean survival of 18 years being reported.[4] Therapy has dramatically reduced immediate deaths from hypertensive encephalopathy, acute renal failure, hemorrhagic strokes, and congestive heart failure.

GENERAL GUIDELINES

The initial goal of the antihypertensive therapy is *not to* rapidly normalize blood pressure but rather to prevent damage to target organs by gradually decreasing mean arterial pressure, while minimizing the risk of hypoperfusion.[5] Before discussing drug therapy for patients with hypertensive crisis, we would like to emphasize that outcome data attesting to benefits of acutely lowering blood pressure are not available. Thus, most interventions currently used to treat hypertensive crisis have never been vigorously scrutinized. Much of the therapy, therefore, is entirely empirical and based on an attempt to best match pathophysiologic findings with pharmacologic properties of antihypertensive agents.

A number of pharmacological agents are available in the management of hypertensive crisis.[6] Those agents can be divided by mechanism of action and route of administration (parenteral vs oral or sublingual).

Drug selection should be based on the severity of the crisis and on the specific hypertensive case. Emergency situations should be aggressively treated typically using intravenous medication in units with monitoring facilities.[7]

PARENTERAL AGENTS

Several parenteral agents are available for the treatment of hypertensive emergencies (Table 2).

Sodium Nitroprusside

Sodium nitroprusside is the most popular agent for treatment of hypertensive emergency. It is a short acting direct vasodilator, requiring a constant intravenous infusion, that can decrease blood pressure in all patients irrespective of its severity. The drug is light sensitive and should be shielded from light to prevent degradation. Initial recommended infusion rate is 0.25 µg/kg/min and may be increased by 0.25 µg/kg/min every 5 to 10 minutes. Sodium nitroprusside dilates both the arteriolar resistance and the venous capacitance vessels, thereby decreasing peripheral resistance without causing an increase in venous return.[8] The drug does not have any direct negative inotropic or chronotropic effects on the heart. By reducing the preload and afterload, sodium nitroprusside improves left ventricular function in patients with congestive heart failure and low cardiac output, and reduces myocardial oxygen demand in patients with ischemic heart disease.

Interaction of sodium nitroprusside with sulfhydryl groups in erythrocytes and tissues generates cyanide ions that are converted to thiocyanate by rhodanese in the liver and then excreted by the kidney. However, with prolonged administration of sodium nitroprusside, or in patients with hepatic impairment or renal insufficiency, free cyanide may accumulate and interfere with aerobic metabolism, resulting in metabolic acidosis. Cyanide also interferes with the vasodilator action of sodium nitroprusside and may eventually lead to tachyphylaxis. Therefore, thiocyanate levels should be monitored periodically and maintained below 10 mg/100 ml in patients with hepatic impairment or renal insufficiency and in those receiving high dosages of sodium nitroprusside (3 µg/kg/min) or a prolonged infusion (>24–48 hours). Thiocyanate toxicity includes fatigue, nausea, headache, disorientation, psychotic behavior, skin rashes, anorexia, convulsions, unexplained cardiopulmonary arrest, coma, diffuse encephalopathy and even death.[9] When cyanide toxicity is diagnosed it can be treated by the administration of amyl nitrate, sodium nitrate and sulfhydryl compound such as sodium thiosulfate. In case of failure to respond to such therapy, hyperbaric oxygen therapy, hemodialysis or charcoal hemoperfusion may prove beneficial; however there is limited experience with this modes of therapy.[10]

The advantages of sodium nitroprusside in controlling hypertensive crisis in cardiac patients have been studied extensively. Kaplan and Jones[11] compared the effects of sodium nitroprusside and intravenous nitroglycerin in 20 patients during elective coronary artery surgery. Both regimens were effective in reducing intraoperative blood pressure. However, nitroglycerin improved electrocardiographic ST segment depression in 8 of 10 patients, whereas sodium nitroprusside made the ST segment depression more pronounced in 3 of 10 patients. Decreased coronary perfusion pressure and intracoronary steal syndrome may be involved in the worsening of ischemia seen in patients receiving sodium nitroprusside. Flaherty et al.[12] found that sodium nitroprusside increased intrapulmonary shunting whereas nitroglycerin decreased it, thus making nitroglycerin more useful

TABLE 2. PARENTERAL AGENTS FOR TREATMENT OF HYPERTENSIVE EMERGENCIES.

Drug	Dosage	Onset of Action	Duration of Action	Adverse Effects
Sodium nitroprusside	0.25–10 µg/kg/min	Immediate	1–2 min after infusion stopped	Nausea, hypotension, thiocyanate and cyanide toxicity, methemoglobinemia (rare)
Nitroglycerin	5–100 µg/min	1–5 min	3–5 min	Headache, nausea, tachycardia, vomiting, tolerance with prolonged use
Diazoxide	50–150 mg over 5 min, or 75–150 mg every 5 min, or 10–30 mg/min for 15–30 min	1–5 min	4–12 h	Increased cardiac output and heart rate, precipitate ischemia, sodium retention, hyperglycemia, postural hypotension
Hydralazine	10–20 mg i.v., or 10–50 mg i.m. repeat every 4–6 h	5–30 mg	3–9 h	Increased cardiac output and heart rate, headache, angina
Nicardipine	5–15 mg/h	5–15 min	30–40 min	Hypotension, tachycardia, nausea, vomiting, flushing
Trimethaphan	1–15 mg/min	1–10 min	3–10 min after infusion stopped	Hypotension, tachyphylaxis, orthostatic effect, sympathetic blockade, respiratory arrest

Labetalol	20–80 mg every 10–15 min, or 2–4 mg/min	5–10 min	3–6 h	Nausea, fornication, bronchospasm, bradycardia, heart block
Urapidil	12.5–25 mg bolus followed by infusion of 5–40 mg/h	3–5 min	4–6 h	Hypotension, headache, dizziness
Phentolamine	5–10 mg bolus	1–2 min	3–5 min	Tachycardia, flushing, headache, angina
Esmolol	0.5–1 µg/kg followed by 50–300 µg/kg/min	1–2 min	10–20 min	Hypotension, nausea
Enalaprilat	0.625–1.25 mg	15 min	4–12 h	Hypotension, renal failure
Fenoldopam	0.1–1.6 µg/kg/min	5–40 min	60 min	Headache, flushing, hypotension

for managing patients with large intrapulmonary shunt or pulmonary hypertension.

Fremes et al.[13] found that nitroglycerin caused a greater reduction in myocardial oxygen demand and consumption than sodium nitroprusside in hypertensive patients after elective coronary bypass surgery. Therefore, if one suspects perioperative myocardial ischemia in the setting of postoperative hypertension, nitroglycerin may be a better antihypertensive agent.

The efficacy of sodium nitroprusside was compared with fenoldopam[14,15] and with diazoxide and hydralazine[16] in hypertensive crises, and was found to be effective in 100% of the cases.

In spite of the fact that sodium nitroprusside can increase intracranial pressure, the fall in systemic pressure seems to block the rise in cerebral blood flow. It is therefore still recommended for management of some patients with encephalopathy and cerebrovascular accidents.[1,17] Despite its effectiveness as an antihypertensive agent, sodium nitroprusside has not been used widely in pregnancy because of negative outcomes in animal experiments.[18]

Nitroglycerin

Nitroglycerin is an antianginal as well as antihypertensive agent that dilates peripheral capacitance and resistance vessels. By diminishing preload, nitroglycerin decreases left ventricular end diastolic volume and pressure and myocardial wall tension, thus reducing myocardial oxygen consumption. These changes favor redistribution of coronary blood flow to the subendocardium, which is more vulnerable to ischemia. Nitroglycerin may dilate epicardial coronary vessels and their collaterals and increase blood supply to ischemic regions. At higher doses nitroglycerin dilates arteriolar smooth muscle, thereby reducing peripheral resistance and afterload. Continuous intravenous nitroglycerin is effective in decreasing the incidence of myocardial ischemia in patients with coronary artery disease undergoing cardiac and noncardiac surgery.[19] Nitroglycerin is a better vasodilator of coronary conductance arteries than sodium nitroprusside and for that reason is preferred in the management of hypertensive crisis associated with acute coronary insufficiency.[17] Intravenous nitroglycerin infusion also has been used in controlling hypertensive crisis during pregnancy. Snyder et al.[20] reported the successful use of intravenous nitroglycerin in controlling hypertension during anesthesia for cesarean section, without neonatal depression or hypotension. The usual initial dose is 5–15 µg/min and can be titrated upward to a desired therapeutic endpoint. Dose as high as 200–300 µg/min may be required to achieve an adequate response.[21] Onset of action is almost immediate with a very short duration of action of approximately 3–5 minutes.[22] Prolonged use of nitroglycerin is not associated with toxicity, but tolerance to its hemodynamic effects has been reported.[23] The main adverse effects are headache and hypotension. The drug can also be used sublingually in selected patients.

Diazoxide

Diazoxide is a direct rapid-acting vasodilator that decreases total peripheral resistance with a reflex increase in heart rate and cardiac output. The compensatory increase in cardiac output and heart rate can be blocked by concomitant beta-blocker therapy. Since it does not cross the blood brain barrier, diazoxide has no direct effects on cerebral circulation, but of course cerebral blood flow will fall if systemic pressure is reduced below the lower limit of autoregulation.[24] In the past diazoxide was initially given as a rapid bolus of 300 mg. However, the standard rapid intravenous bolus administration may cause profound hypotension with subsequent myocardial ischemia and cerebrovascular insufficiency.[25] The safer course is to give the drug either by slow infusion of 15 to 30 mg/min over 15 to 30 minutes or by smaller bolus doses of 75 to 100 mg intravenously, every 5 to 10 minutes These methods are equally effective and are associated with fewer adverse effects.[26] The side effects of diazoxide include fluid retention, nausea, flushing dizziness and hyperglycemia.[8] When using diazoxide, one must be aware of significant adverse effects such as postural hypotension, maternal and fetal hyperglycemia and cessation of gestational labor that results from relaxation of the uterine smooth muscle. Diazoxide is contraindicated in patients with severe angina, acute myocardial infarction, dissecting aneurysm, and congestive heart failure.

Hydralazine

Hydralazine is a direct arteriolar vasodilator, with little effect on venous capacitance vessels, that produces a rapid blood pressure decrease with diastolic pressure reduced more than systolic.[9] Its administration results in activation of baroreceptor reflexes leading to increase in heart rate, myocardial contractility and cardiac output and augmenting renal blood flow. Hydralazine can be given intravenously or intramuscularly in initial dose of 10–50 mg. The drug should not be diluted with solutions containing dextrose or other sugars, because of its ability to form potentially toxic hydrazones.[9] The drug reduces systemic vascular resistance and blood pressure in severe hypertension of pregnancy[27] without a significant change in uteroplacental blood flow.[28]

Although hydralazine easily crosses the placenta, its relative safety and efficacy combined with the extensive clinical experience have made it the most widely used antihypertensive agent in pregnancy-induced hypertension.[9] The major drawbacks of hydralazine are its side effects that include reflex tachycardia, salt and water retention, intense flushing, headache, nausea, vomiting, myocardial ischemia, and increased intracranial pressure. Therefore, the use of hydralazine is limited to patients with pre-eclampsia or eclampsia.

Nicardipine

Nicardipine is a dihydropyridine calcium antagonist that can be administered intravenously.[29] It is an effective antihypertensive agent that decreases afterload by reducing total peripheral resistance without reducing cardiac output. Nicardipine improves left ventricular ejection fraction and pumping activity, both in normal and failing hearts.[30] The drug dilates more selectively the coronary arteries than the remainder of the arterial tree, without changing the heart rate.[31] It may preserve tissue perfusion, and therefore may be advantageous in patients with ischemic disorders, such as coronary, cerebrovascular, and peripheral vascular disease. The drug is given as a continuous infusion at a starting dose of 5 mg/h followed by increments of 2.5 mg/h every 5 minutes until either reaching a maximal dose of 15 mg/h or achieving the desired reduction in blood pressure.

Nicardipine has been used for the treatment of postoperative hypertension.[32-38] Floyd et al.[33] used intravenous nicardipine in the treatment of acute hypertension in 11 patients undergoing coronary artery bypass grafting. Administration of 10 to 15 mg/h of nicardipine decreased blood pressure by more than 15% within 25 minutes, without a significant change in heart rate or cardiac index. In a double blind study intravenous nicardipine was compared with placebo in 123 patients with blood pressure over 213/126 mm Hg.[32] Of 73 patients who were treated with nicardipine, 67 achieved the therapeutic goal. Several side effects were reported; 30 patients had headache, 7 patients had hypotension, and 7 patients experienced nausea. The pharmacodynamics of nicardipine are comparable to sodium nitroprusside in terms of onset, duration and offset of action. Halperen et al.[36] and David et al.[38] found that nicardipine was as effective as sodium nitroprusside in patients with severe postoperative hypertension. Patients receiving intravenous nicardipine can then be easily switched to oral medication.

Labetalol

Labetalol produces selective antagonism at the postsynaptic alpha-adrenoreceptors and nonselective antagonism at the beta-adrenoreceptors. The drug can be given intravenously either by repeated bolus of 0.25-0.5 mg/kg every 10–15 minutes or by a continuous infusion of 2–4 mg/min. Alternatively the drug can be given in a bolus injection of 100 mg followed by an infusion of 2–4 mg/min. The average effective total dose is 200 mg. The response rate in patients with hypertensive emergencies is about 80–93%[39,40] The drug was found to be effective and safe in patients with myocardial infarction,[41] in patients with acute postoperative hypertension after aortocoronary bypass surgery[42] or surgery requiring general anesthesia,[43] in neurovascular surgical patients, in children with hypertensive crises and in hypertensive crisis complicating pregnancy.[9,44] Caution is needed to avoid postural hypotension if patients are allowed out of bed. Nausea, itching, tingling of the skin, and beta blockade side effects may be noted. Transition to oral therapy with the same drug is not difficult.

Urapidil

Urapidil is a selective post-synaptic alpha$_1$ adrenoreceptor antagonist with strong vasodilating properties. The fact that it also antagonizes the pre-synaptic 5HT1A (hydroxytrypta-mine) receptors explains the lack of reflex tachycardia in response to peripheral vasodilatation. Urapidil has a rapid onset of action, with a response rate it of 81%–100% in hypertensive emergencies.[45-47] Urapidil is given as an intravenous bolus at a dose of 12.5 to 25 mg followed by a continuous infusion at a rate of 5–40 mg/h. It has no effect on coronary sinus blood flow, myocardial oxygen consumption and myocardial lactate extraction, and it does not increase intracranial pressure. Adverse effects occur in 2% of all patients and include hypotension, headache, dizziness. Urapidil is safe and efficient in intraoperative hypertensive crisis. In a recent study the drug was given to 42 patients with intraoperative hypertensive crises. A significant reduction in blood pressure was observed within 10 minutes in 81% of the patients.[48] Indeed, the drug is not commonly used, but it can be used in intraoperative hypertensive crisis.

Phentolamine

Phentolamine is a parenteral nonspecific alpha adrenergic blocking agent with rapid onset and short-lasting hypotensive effect. It is given intravenously in a bolus of 5 to 10 mg, and repeated administration may be necessary. Adverse effects include tachycardia, vomiting and headache. In patients with coronary artery disease phentolamine may induce angina pectoris or myocardial infarction. It is specifically useful in treatment of catecholamine mediated hypertensive crises.[26] However, it is not consistently effective in other types of hypertensive emergencies.

Esmolol

Esmolol is an ultra-short acting beta$_1$-selective adrenergic blocker. The duration of action is extremely short, about 30 minutes, because of its rapid metabolism by a specific plasma esterase. This characteristic provides a significant advantage over similar agents such as propranolol because it is possible to titrate esmolol easily to the desired effect.[6] The drug can be administered either as a bolus injection or as a continuous intravenous infusion. The recommended loading dose is 0.5 to 1 mg/kg followed by an infusion of 50 to 300 µg/kg/min. Esmolol is frequently combined with direct vasodilators to provide a more desirable hemodynamic profile. The negative chronotropic effect produced by esmolol may be beneficial in patients with ischemic heart disease. Recently esmolol has been used successfully with sodium nitroprusside in a few cases of hypertensive crises.[49-52] Further prospective studies are required before esmolol can be recommended for routine use in the treatment of hypertensive crisis.

Enalaprilat

Enalaprilat is the only available angiotensin converting enzyme (ACE) inhibitor that can be administered intravenously, although in one report captopril was given intravenously to treat hypertensive crises.[53] Enalaprilat rapidly lowers blood pressure within minutes in patients with severe hypertension, without causing excessive hypotension or adverse reactions. The initial recommended dose for enalaprilat is 0.625 to 1.25 mg administered over 5 minutes. The maximal single dose should not exceed 5 mg for patients receiving diuretics and 1.25 mg for patients with renal impairment.[54] The initial dose can be repeated after 1 hour if clinical response is inadequate. The total daily dose should not exceed 20 mg. In patients with severe renal insufficiency the dose should be decreased because the compound is excreted primarily by the kidney.

African Americans seem to respond poorly to enalaprilat, possibly because of their low renin levels. Because enalaprilat does not impair cerebral blood flow, it may be useful for hypertensive patients at risk for cerebral hypotensive episodes.[9] In patients with hypertensive emergency the response rate is about 65%. Hirschl et al.[55] evaluated prospectively the efficacy and safety of various doses of parenteral enalaprilat in patients with hypertensive crises. Sixty-five consecutive patients with hypertensive crises (urgency or emergency) were randomly allocated to receive different doses of enalaprilat (0.625, 1.25, 2.5, and 5 mg). In 41 (63%) of 65 patients the treatment goal was achieved, with a similar response rate for all enalaprilat doses. Thus, 0.625 mg may be adequate as initial dose in the treatment of hypertensive crisis. In another study enalaprilat was compared with intravenous urapidil and sublingual nifedipine in the management of hypertensive crisis.[56] Only 70% of the patients in the enalaprilat group achieved goal blood pressure versus 96% and 71% in the urapidil and nifedipine groups, respectively.

Enalaprilat may be an alternative treatment for hypertensive crisis in patients with congestive heart failure. The most common adverse effect is hypotension. The risk for hypotension increases in patients with evidence of renal hypertension, volume depleted patients, and patients with prior use of diuretics. Enalaprilat is contraindicated in patients with evidence of bilateral renal artery stenosis or in patients with unilateral stenosis of a single kidney.[26] Thus, enalaprilat is an effective antihypertensive agent in acute situations,[57] and can be easily replaced by oral enalapril for long-term maintenance therapy.

Fenoldopam

Fenoldopam is a selective post-synaptic dopaminergic (DA_1) receptor agonist with weak alpha$_2$ antagonistic properties.[14] Fenoldopam is a natriuretic agent that has a potent vasodilative action affecting primarily the renal vasculature.[14,58] Several clinical trials recently showed the effectiveness of intravenous fenoldopam in the treatment of severe hypertension and hypertensive crisis.[14,15,58,59] Bodmann et al.[59] studied the hemodynamic effects of intravenous fenoldopam in 12 patients with hypertensive crisis. At a dose of 0.2–0.5 µg/kg/min fenoldopam decreased blood pressure to desired levels within 5 to 40 minutes in all patients. Hemodynamically the drug induced a decrease in total peripheral resistance and in pulmonary vascular resistance with a slight elevation in heart rate. No adverse events were reported, and in none of the patients did rebound hypertension occur upon termination of the drug. In another open, controlled, randomized, parallel trial intravenous fenoldopam was compared with sodium nitroprusside in 18 patients with severe hypertension and mild renal failure.[14] Both antihypertensive medications were infused at a maximal dose increment of 0.2 µg/kg/min (fenoldopam) and 1 µg/kg/min (sodium nitroprusside) with a maximal infusion rate of 1.5 µg/kg/min for fenoldopam or 8 µg/kg/min for sodium nitroprusside. Both antihypertensive agents successfully controlled blood pressure in all patients. The rate of side effects was similar in both groups of patients. However, in 2 patients treated with sodium nitroprusside toxic levels of thiocyanate were detected. Thus, fenoldopam may be superior to sodium nitroprusside for the control of hypertensive crisis in patients with decreased renal function. Gretler et al.[15] compared the electrocardiographic changes in 21 patients with hypertensive emergencies treated with either fenoldopam or sodium nitroprusside. Both drugs reduced blood pressure significantly in all patients. New T-wave inversion occurred in 2 patients treated with fenoldopam and in 4 patients treated with sodium nitroprusside. It seems that fenoldopam is comparable to sodium nitroprusside, but further studies are required to confirm its efficacy and safety.

TREATMENT OF SPECIFIC HYPERTENSIVE EMERGENCIES

There is a multiplicity of disorders or diseases accompanying elevated blood pressure that constitute a hypertensive crisis; and there is broad spectrum of pharmacological agents that may be selected for treatment of these cases. Some agents that are useful for one hypertensive emergency may actually be contraindicated for another.[60] The recommended therapeutic approach for specific conditions is summarized in Table 3.

Hypertensive Encephalopathy

When mean arterial pressure reaches a critical level (around 180 mm Hg), the previously constricted vessels are unable to withstand the pressure, counterregulation fails and generalized vasodilatation ensues. Such a breakthrough of cerebral blood flow (CBF) leads to hyperperfusing the brain under high pressure and results in cerebral edema and the clinical syndrome of hypertensive encephalopathy.[8] This scenario occurs at a much higher blood pressure in patients with chronic hypertension than in previously normotensive persons. If untreated, the clinical picture progressively worsens, culminating in coma and death. Hypertensive encephalopathy is often indistinguishable from other acute neurological complications of hypertension, i. e., cerebral infarction, subarachnoidal bleeding or intracerebral hemorrhage. The only definite criterion to confirm diagnosis of hypertensive encephalopathy is a prompt improvement in the patient's condition in response to antihypertensive therapy.[61] First choice drug for this condition includes intravenous sodium nitroprusside, labetalol, urapidil or nicardipine.

TABLE 3. PREFERRED AGENTS FOR SPECIFIC HYPERTENSIVE EMERGENCY.

Emergency Condition	Preferred Agent	Comments
Hypertensive encephalopathy	Sodium nitroprusside, labetalol, nicardipine, urapidil	Avoid methyldopa and diazoxide
Cerebrovascular accident	Sodium nitroprusside, labetalol, urapidil, esmolol, nimodipine	Benefit from acute lowing of blood pressure is uncertain
Dissecting aortic aneurysm	Sodium nitroprusside with ß-blocker (propranolol or esmolol), labetalol, trimethaphan, urapidil	Titrate blood pressure to the lowest possible level. Avoid hydralazine, diazoxide
Acute left ventricular failure	Sodium nitroprusside, nitroglycerin, enalaprilat, urapidil, furosemide, morphine	Avoid labetalol, esmolol, diazoxide,
Coronary insufficiency	Nitroglycerin, sodium nitroprusside, labetalol, nicardipine, esmolol	Blood pressure should be reduced gradually. Avoid hydralazine, diazoxide
Perioperative hypertension	Sodium nitroprusside, nitroglycerin, isradipine, nicardipine	Nitroglycerin is preferred in managing postcoronary bypass hypertension
Eclampsia	Hydralazine, labetalol, urapidil	Avoid diuretics, trimethaphan, sodium nitroprusside, ACE inhibitor
Catecholamine excess	Phentolamine, labetalol	Avoid diuretics
Renal insufficiency	Hydralazine, labetalol, fenoldopam, nicardipine	Avoid beta-blockers

Cardiovascular Accidents

Intracerebral hemorrhage. As a result of intracerebral hemorrhage, intracerebral pressure rises and higher intraarterial pressure is required to perfuse the brain adequately. In this condition, hypertension may be a result of increased intracerebral pressure and may resolve spontaneously within in 48 hours.[61] Rapid reduction in blood pressure may indeed prevent further bleeding, but at the risk of cerebral hypoperfusion.[1] There is no consensus with regard to the advisability of reducing blood pressure in patients with this condition.[17] In any event the reduction should not exceed 20% of pretreatment blood pressure level.[62] If blood pressure is extremely elevated (diastolic pressure greater than 140 mm Hg) and lasts more than 20 min, intravenous treatment is recommended.[63] First drug of choice for this condition include intravenous sodium nitroprusside, labetalol or urapidil. Recently it was reported that nimodipine has improved the outcome of patients with aneurysmal subarachnoid hemorrhage.[64]

Acute ischemic stroke. Cerebral infarction causes an impairment in the autoregulation of CBF; thus elevated blood pressure will accentuate perfusion through the damaged tissue, leading to edema and compression of normal brain tissue. This provides evidence for carefully reducing blood pressure in hypertensive patients with stroke.[8] Conversely, because of local vasoconstriction, high arterial blood pressure is required to perfuse jeopardized brain tissue around the infarcted area. This provides evidence against reducing blood pressure in acute ischemic stroke. Moreover, chronic hypertension and cerebral vascular disease move the autoregulation curve of CBF to the right so that a decrease in CBF occurs at a higher blood pressure level than in normal individuals. Therefore, cerebral hypoperfusion may appear at levels of blood pressure that are still above the upper limit of normal. Brott and Reed[63] recommended no antihypertensive treatment if blood pressure is less than 180/105 mm Hg. If blood pressure is higher than 230/120 mm Hg and persists more than 20 min, intravenous treatment is recommended. The target blood pressure should be 160–170/95–100 mm Hg for previously normotensive patients and 180–185/105–110 mm Hg for previously hypertensive patients. Although Brott and Reed[63] suggested a treatment regimen in acute stroke based on level of the blood pressure, Powers[65] pointed out that the benefits to be derived from acutely lowering blood pressure in patients with acute stroke of any kind remain conjectural and unsupported by good clinical or experimental studies. Sodium nitroprusside is the agent of choice whenever the blood pressure is to be reduced for patients with acute ischemic stroked.[1] Nimodipine is being used investigationally in this condition with equivocal results so far. Gelmers et al.[66] reported improved survival for men but not women and a better neurological outcome in patients treated with nimodipine compared with those given a placebo. Martinez-Vila et al.[67] reported no benefit on survival or neurologic outcome except for those patients who had mild deficits at the onset, who did seem to achieve greater recovery in the nimodipine group.

Acute Aortic Dissection

Most untreated patients with acute aortic dissection die within 1 year, and most of the deaths occur within 2 weeks.[61] Once diagnosis is suspected, attempts should be made to decrease the shear stress to the aortic wall with suitable agents.[61] Blood pressure should be reduced within 15–30 minutes to the lowest tolerated level that preserves adequate organ perfusion.[17,26] It has to be kept in mind that the force and velocity of ventricular contractions and pulsatile flow determine the shear stress on the aortic wall.[26] Drugs such as diazoxide, hydralazine, and nifedipine that reflexively stimulate sympathetic activity and increase the shear stress on the aortic wall are contraindicated. Initial treatment should consist of a combination of intravenous sodium nitroprusside and an intravenous beta-blocking agent, most commonly propranolol. Used alone, sodium nitroprusside increases the velocity of ventricular contraction so that simultaneous beta-blockade is obligatory.[26]

Acute Left Ventricular Failure

Severe hypertension may precipitate acute left ventricular failure.[65] Prompt reduction of blood pressure decreases the work load of the failing myocardium and improves cardiac function.[61]

Immediate decrease of afterload with a balanced vasodilating agent such as sodium nitroprusside is indicated in this circumstance.[26] Nitroglycerin is a reasonable alternative that has less afterload reducing capability, but may increase myocardial blood flow to ischemic areas in patients with acute myocardial ischemia. As urapidil has no influence on heart rate and myocardial oxygen consumption, it is a potential alternative to sodium nitroprusside and nitroglycerin if blood pressure is insufficiently reduced. Concomitant therapy with oxygen diuretics or opioids may enhance efficacy of antihypertensive agents.[26] Although the ACE inhibitors, may be useful in this situation,[54] there is paucity of clinical experience concerning the therapeutic response to ACE inhibition in patients with acute left ventricular failure.[61] Drugs that cause reflex tachycardia (diazoxide, hydralazine) or decrease myocardial contractility (labetalol) should be avoided in this setting.[26]

Ischemic Heart Disease

Reduction of systemic blood pressure by intravenous nitroglycerin reduces cardiac work, wall tension, and oxygen demand and therefore has became the drug of choice for this crisis. Flaherty[68] found that infarct size was limited and left ventricular ejection fraction was higher in a group of patients receiving intravenous nitroglycerin shortly after the onset of myocardial infarction than in a control group. However, there was no statistically significant difference in 3-month mortality between the groups. Intravenous vasodilators, mainly sodium nitroprusside and nitroglycerin, have been tested in 11 trials involving 2170 patients with acute myocardial infarction and have reduced mortality by 43%.[69] Cautious treatment of hypertension in patients with acute myocardial infarction is likely to be beneficial. Conversely, unnecessary reduction in blood pressure could compromise an already unstable situations, and therefore blood pressure should be reduced gradually until symptoms subside or until the diastolic blood pressure is approximately 100 mm Hg.[1] Rapid reduction of blood pressure with any drug may cause electrocardiographic changes.[15,69] These changes, observed during infusion of sodium nitroprusside[15] and after oral nifedipine,[70] are usually not accompanied by left ventricular wall motion abnormalities.

Initial treatment of patients with angina pectoris and severe hypertension includes sublingual nitroglycerin, beta-blockers, and morphine, followed by intravenous nitroglycerin if treatment is not successful. Nifedipine should not be used in this crisis, as it causes a reflex tachycardia, increases myocardial oxygen demand and may aggravate myocardial ischemia.[71]

Perioperative Hypertension

Most of the time, perioperative hypertension is not an emergency in the usual sense, but parenteral agents are frequently used to control blood pressure because patients are unable to receive medications orally. Severe hypertension may occur in some patients in the postoperative period, especially after open heart and carotid artery surgery. The etiology of this severe hypertension is multifactorial-withdrawal of antihypertensive drugs, pain, volume overload, and sympathetic activations.[61] In this setting hypertension, even of moderate severity, may jeopardize the integrity of the fresh vascular suture lines. Therapy should be individualized, and in some situations immediate lowering of the blood pressure is warranted.[61] Hypotension is to be avoided in patients who have fresh vascular suture lines because of the danger of thrombosis.[17] Sodium nitroprusside is usually the agent of choice, provided the patient is in an intensive care environment. Nitroglycerin administered intravenously may be the drug of choice for managing postcoronary bypass hypertension.[19]

Eclampsia

Pre-eclampsia occurring in pregnancy is the syndrome of hypertension, edema and proteinuria. Some patients with this condition may progress to eclampsia, which is associated with seizures and end-organ damage (cerebral hemorrhage, renal failure, microangiopathic hemolytic anemia).[72] The important part of safe treatment is to control hypertension, keeping in mind the risk that reducing blood pressure may further impair placental blood flow. Hydralazine administered intravenously has been the drug of choice in recent years when diastolic blood pressure is over 115 mm Hg or when eclampsia supervenes; it is effective and does not decrease placental blood flow. Labetalol, urapidil, or calcium antagonists are possible alternative therapeutic approaches if hydralazine is ineffectively.[17,26] Diuretics,

Trimethaphan camsylate, sodium nitroprusside and ACE inhibitors should be avoided. If convulsions are imminent or occur, magnesium sulfate should be administered parenterally.

Excessive Circulating Catecholamines

Catecholamine-induced crises are characterized by sudden increase in predominantly alpha-adrenergic tone. Plasma catecholamine levels are elevated in pheochromocytoma, in rebound hypertension following clonidine withdrawal, in hypertension associated with ingestion of sympathomimetics (cocaine hydrochloride, amphetamines, phencyclidine hydrochloride, lysergic acid diethylamide, and diet pills), and in the drug interaction of monoamine oxidase inhibitors with tyramine rich food (certain beers, cheese, wine, chicken liver).[73] When this condition is suspected, the alpha adrenergic blocking drug phentolamine should be given. An alternative to phentolamine would be labetalol or sodium nitroprusside with beta-blockers. A beta-blocking drug may be needed if the patient has a concomitant tachycardia or ventricular ectopy. Administration of beta-blocking agent should always be preceded by alpha-blockade to prevent unopposed alpha-mediated peripheral vasoconstriction.[1,65]

Renal Insufficiency

Deterioration of renal function in the face of elevated blood pressure is considered a hypertensive emergency and requires lowering the blood pressure.[26] Therapy should reduce systemic vascular resistance without compromising the renal blood flow or glomerular filtration.[1] Sodium nitroprusside is elective in these cases, but because the risk of thiocyanate toxicity is increased, dose adjustment and close thiocyanate levels monitoring are needed. Labetalol, calcium antagonists and fenoldopam are effective and well tolerated alternative.[1] beta-blockers reduce the renal plasma flow and the glomerular filtration rate and should therefore be used with caution if at all.

TREATMENT OF HYPERTENSIVE URGENCY

The ideal oral drug to treat hypertensive crisis should be one that has a rapid and smooth onset of action, few adverse effects, does not cause excessive hypotension, is convenient to monitor and can be easily converted to a maintenance therapy.[74] The Fifth Joint National Committee (JNC V) recommends the use of captopril, clonidine, labetalol, and nifedipine for the treatment of hypertensive urgency and emergency.[2] *However, the use of oral agents should be limited to hypertensive urgency.*

The optimal approach in patients with hypertensive urgency is to lower the blood pressure more gradually over 24 to 48 hours. When the cause of transient blood pressure elevations is easily identified, such as pain or acute anxiety (as in panic disorders)[7,75] the appropriate therapy is analgesic or anxiolytic medication. When the cause of blood pressure elevation is unknown, various oral antihypertensive agents are available. In the absence of any data comparing long-term outcome with the various agents, the choice of therapy should be based on efficacy and safety data. The efficacy of the various oral antihypertensive agents seems to be similar,[22,39,76-84] and it ranges in controlled trials between 96–98% for nifedipine, 79–100% for clonidine, 90–95% for captopril, 68–94% for labetalol, 65%–91% for nicardipine, 66%–82% for nitrendipine and 85% for nitroglycerin. Acute lowering of blood pressure may compromise cardiac and cerebral blood flow, especially in the elderly, and therefore may be associated with serious side effects.[71,85-93] We have recently published a review of serious adverse effects following oral or sublingual administration of nifedipine capsule in hypertensive emergencies and pseudoemergencies.[94] Given the potential seriousness of adverse events and the lack of any clinical documentation attesting to a benefit in rapid lowering blood pressure, nifedipine capsules and any drug that lowers blood pressure acutely to unpredictable levels should not be used in hypertensive crisis. Of note oral agents should be used only in hypertensive urgency, and not emergency, and in this condition a slower reduction of blood pressure over a period of hours to several days is more appropriated.[4]

One should be careful not to be too aggressive in lowering blood pressure and to use the right agent for the right condition. When considering the appropriate agent, the mechanism of action and the profile of adverse effects should be considered. Nifedipine and to lesser degree captopril tend to increase heart rate, and clonidine and labetalol tend to decrease it. This is particularly important in patients with ischemic heart disease. Other limitations are the use of labetalol in patients with bronchospasm and bradycardia and second and third degree heart blocks. Clonidine should be avoided if mental acuity is desired. Captopril should not be used in patients with bilateral renal artery stenosis or unilateral renal artery stenosis of a solitary kidney. All agents should be used carefully in volume depleted patients.

SPECIAL CONSIDERATIONS IN THE ELDERLY

In general, older persons have a lower blood volume, lower plasma renin activity, and increased peripheral vascular resistance[95] that affect the pharmacokinetics of some antihypertensive agents. With age the decrease in glomerular filtration rate and blunted baroreceptor reflexes increase the risk of overdose and orthostatic hypotension. If supine hypertension is treated too vigorously, older patients may experience presyncope or actual syncope. The increase in systolic blood pressure associated with age is actually atherosclerotic-related decrease in aortic distensibility. In this setting small changes in stroke volume can result in greater changes in systolic blood pressure. Rapid reduction of blood pressure is especially dangerous in elderly patients and can cause transient ischemic attacks, strokes, angina, myocardial infarction, and syncope;[9] therefore a low dose of antihypertensive agents should be used.

CONCLUSIONS

Hypertensive emergency is relatively rare and said to be present only when blood pressure elevation confers an immediate treat to the integrity of the cardiovascular system. In this setting immediate reduction in blood pressure is required generally by intravenous therapy in an intensive care unit. Unlike emergency, a hypertensive urgency is said to be present when severe elevation in blood pressure is not associated with end-organ injury. Outcome data attesting to benefits of acutely lowering blood pressure in this condition are not available.

Clearly, patients with hypertensive crisis are not good candidates for prospective randomized trials. Therefore, the accepted approach for patients with hypertensive urgency is to lower the blood pressure more gradually over 24 to 48 hours with oral antihypertensive agents. Any drug that lowers blood pressure precipitously should be avoided. The efficacy of nifedipine, captopril, clonidine, labetalol, nicardipine, nitrendipine, and nitroglycerin seems to be similar. Choice of the appropriate agent should be based on the underlying pathophysiologic and clinical findings, mechanism of action, and the potential adverse effects.

REFERENCES

1. Calhoun DA, Oparil S. Treatment of hypertensive crisis. N Engl J Med 1990; 323:1177-1183.

2. Joint National Committee on the Detection, Evaluation, and Treatment of Blood Pressure. The 1992 Report of the Joint National Committee on the Detection, Evaluation, and Treatment of Blood Pressure (JNC-V). Arch Intern Med 1993;153:154-183.

3. Zampaglione B, Pascale C, Marchisio M, Cavallo-Perin P. Hypertensive urgencies and emergencies. Prevalence and clinical presentation. Hypertension 1996;27:144-147.

4. Kaplan NM. Management of hypertensive emergencies. Lancet 1994; 344:1335-1338.

5. Varon J, Fromm RE Jr: Hypertensive crises. The need for urgent management. Postgrad Med 1996;99:189-191.

6. McKindley DS, Boucher BA. Advances in pharmacotherapy: treatment of hypertensive crisis. J Clin Pharm Ther 1994;19:163-180.

7. Phillips RA, Krakoff LR. Topics in hypertension: Hypertension emergencies, true and false. The American Society of Hypertension 1997;3-10.

8. Kaplan NM. Hypertensive crisis, in Clinical hypertension, Kaplan NM, ed. Maryland, Williams and Wilkins, 1995:281-297.

9. Abdelwahab W, Frishman W, Landau A. Management of hypertensive urgencies and emergencies. J Clin Pharmacol 1995;35:747-762.

10. Dabney BJ, Zelamey PT, Hall AH. Evaluation and treatment of patients exposed to systemic asphyxiants. Emergency Care Quarterly 1990;6:65-80.

11. Kaplan JA, Jones EL. Vasodilator therapy during coronary artery surgery. Comparison of nitroglycerin and nitroprusside. J Thorac Cardiovasc Surg 1979;77:301-309.

12. Flaherty JT, Magee PA, Gardner TL, et al. Comparison of intravenous nitroglycerin and sodium nitroprusside for treatment of

acute hypertension developing after coronary artery bypass surgery. Circulation 1982; 65:1072-1077.

13. Fremes SE, Weisel RD, Mickle DAG, et al. A comparison of nitroglycerin and nitroprusside. I. Treatment of postoperative hypertension. Ann Thorac Surg 1985;39:53-60.

14. Reisin E, Huth MM, Nguyen BP, Weed SG, Gonzalez FM. Intravenous fenoldopam versus sodium nitroprusside in patients with severe hypertension. Hypertension 1990;15(Suppl. 2):I59-I62.

15. Gretler DD, Elliott WJ, Moscucci M, et al. Electrocardiographic changes during acute treatment of hypertensive emergencies with sodium nitroprusside or fenoldopam. Arch Intern Med 1992;152: 2445-2448.

16. Deal JE, Barratt TM, Dillon MJ. Management of hypertensive emergencies. Arch Dis Child 1992;67:1089-1092.

17. Gifford RW Jr. Management of hypertensive crises. JAMA 1991; 266:829-835.

18. Cunningham FG, Lindheimer MD. Hypertension in pregnancy. N Engl J Med 1992;326:927-932.

19. Kaplan JA, Dunbar RW, Jones EL. Nitroglycerin infusion during coronary-artery surgery. Anesthesiology 1976;45:14-21.

20. Snyder SW, Wheeler AS, James FM III. The use of nitroglycerin to control severe hypertension of pregnancy during cesarean section. Anesthesiology 1979;51:563-564.

21. Charash B, Scheidt S. Nitroglycerin. In: *Cardiovascular Drug Therapy*. Messerli FH (ed). Philadelphia:W.B. Saunders 1990:871-880.

22. Bussman WD, Kenedi P, von Mengden HJ, et al. Comparison of nitroglycerin with nifedipine in patients with hypertensive crisis or severe hypertension. Clin Investig 1992;70:1085-1088.

23. Cottrell JE, Turndorf H. Intravenous nitroglycerin. Am Heart J 1978;96:550-553.

24. Barry DI, Strandgaard S, Graham DI, et al. Effect of diazoxide-induced hypotension on cerebral blood flow in hypertensive rats. Eur J Clin Invest 1983;13:201-207.

25. Kumar GK, Dastoor FC, Robayo JR, Razzaque MA. Side effects of diazoxide. JAMA 1976;235:275-276.

26. Hirschl MM. Guidelines for the drug treatment of hypertensive crises. Drugs 1995;50:991-1000.

27. Cotton DB, Gonik B, Dorman KF. Cardiovascular alterations in severe pregnancy-induced hypertension seen with an intravenously given hydralazine bolus. Surg Gynecol Obstet 1985;161:240-244.

28. Lunell NO, Lewander R, Nylund L, et al. Acute effect of dihydralazine on uteroplacental blood flow in hypertension during pregnancy. Gynecol Obstet Invest 1983;16:274-282.

29. Clifton GG, Cook ME, Bienvenu GS, Wallin JD. Intravenous nicardipine in severe systemic hypertension. Am J Cardiol 1989;64:16H-18H.

30. Rousseau MF, Etienne J, Van Mechelen H, et al. Hemodynamic and cardiac effects of nicardipine in patients with coronary artery disease. J Cardiovasc Pharmacol 1984;6:833-839.

31. Lambert CR, Hill JA, Nichols WW, et al. Coronary and systemic hemodynamic effects of nicardipine. Am J Cardiol 1985;55:652-656.

32. Wallin JD, Fletcher E, Ram CV, et al: Intravenous nicardipine for the treatment of severe hypertension. A double-blind, placebo-controlled multicenter trial. Arch Intern Med 1989;149:2662-2669.

33. Floyd J, Komer C, Frishman W, et al. Treatment of acute hypertension post-coronary artery bypass grafting with intravenous nicardipine (abstract). Crit Care Med 1989;17:S11.

34. Halpern NA, Sladen RN, Goldberg JS, et al. Nicardipine infusion for postoperative hypertension after surgery of the head and neck. Crit Care Med 1990;18:950-955.

35. IV Nicardipine Study Group. Efficacy and safety of intravenous nicardipine in the control of postoperative hypertension. Chest 1991;99:393-398.

36. Halpern NA, Goldberg M, Neely C, et al. Postoperative hypertension: a multicenter, prospective, randomized comparison between intravenous nicardipine and sodium nitroprusside. Crit Care Med 1992;20:1637-1643.

37. Clifton GG, Wallin JD. Intravenous nicardipine: an effective new agent for the treatment of severe hypertension. Angiology 1990;41:1005-1009.

38. David D, Dubois C, Loria Y. Comparison of nicardipine and sodium nitroprusside in the treatment of paroxysmal hypertension following aortocoronary bypass surgery. J Cardiothorac Vasc Anesth 1991;5:357-361.

39. McDonald AJ, Yealy DM, Jacobson S. Oral labetalol versus oral nifedipine in hypertensive urgencies in the ED. Am J Emerg Med 1993;11:460-463.

40. Dunn FG, Oigman W, Messerli FH, et al. Hemodynamic effects of intravenous labetalol in essential hypertension. Clin Pharmacol Ther 33:139-143, 1983.

41. Wilson DJ, Wallin JD, Vlachakis ND, et al. Intravenous labetalol in the treatment of severe hypertension and hypertensive emergencies. Am J Med 1983; 75(4A):95-102.

42. Morel DR, Forster A, Suter PM. I.v. labetalol in the treatment of hypertension following coronary-artery surgery. Br J Anaesth 1982;54:1191-1196.

43. Leslie JB, Kalayjian RW, Sirgo MA, et al. Intravenous labetalol for treatment of postoperative hypertension. Anesthesiology 1987;67:413-416.

44. Mabie WC, Gonzalez AR, Sibai BM, Amon E. A comparative trial of labetalol and hydralazine in the acute management of severe hypertension complicating pregnancy. Obstet Gynecol 1987;70:328-333.

45. Hirschl MM, Seidler D, Zeiner A, et al. Intravenous urapidil versus sublingual nifedipine in the treatment of hypertensive urgencies. Am J Emerg Med 1993;11:653-656.

46. Giuntoli F, Gabbani S, Natali A, et al. Treatment of hypertensive emergencies with urapidil. Curr Ther Res 1991;49:296-299.

47. Nagy RM, Wang AL. Nifedipine: bite-and-swallow administration. Am J Psychiatry 1991;148:1759.

48. Fontana F, Allaria B, Brunetti B, et al. Cardiac and circulatory response to the intravenous administration of urapidil during general anaesthesia. Drugs Exp Clin Res 1990;16:315-318.

49. Zakowski M, Kaufman B, Berguson P, et al. Esmolol use during resection of pheochromocytoma: report of three cases. Anesthesiology 1989;70: 875-877.

50. Mohindra SK, Udeani GO. Intravenous esmolol in acute aortic dissection. DICP 1991;25:735-738.

51. Fenner SG, Mahoney A, Cashman JN. Repair of traumatic transection of the thoracic aorta: esmolol for intraoperative control of arterial pressure. Br J Anaesth 1991;67:483-487.

52. Mihm FG, Sandhu JS, Brown MD, Rosenthal MH. Short-acting beta-adrenergic blockade as initial drug therapy in pheochromocytoma. Crit Care Med 1990;18:673-674.

53. Savi L, Montebelli MR, Mazza A, et al. A new therapy for hypertensive emergencies: intravenous captopril. A preliminary report. Curr Ther Res 1990;47:1073-1081.

54. Gavras H. The role of angiotensin converting enzyme inhibitors in the management of urgent hypertensive situations: a review. Cardiovasc Drug Rev 1992;10:117-124.

55. Hirschl MM, Binder M, Bur A, et al. Clinical evaluation of different doses of intravenous enalaprilat in patients with hypertensive crises. Arch Intern Med 1995;155:2217-2223.

56. Hirschl MM, Seidler D, Mullner M, et al. Efficacy of different antihypertensive drugs in the emergency department. J Hum Hypertens 1996;10:143-146.

57. Passmore J, Loomis JH. The role of IV enalaprilat in lowering blood pressure. Hospital Formulary 1993;28:173-179.

58. SK&F (Smith, Kline, & French) Fenoldopam Working Group. Effects of intravenous fenoldopam (SK&F 82526-J) on blood pressure in severe hypertension (letter). Cardiovasc Drugs Ther 1992;6:445-446.

59. Bodmann KF, Troster S, Clemens R, Schuster HP. Hemodynamic profile of intravenous fenoldopam in patients with hypertensive crisis. Clin Invest 1993; 72:60-64.

60. Frohlich ED. American College of Chest Physicians' Consensus Panel on Hypertensive Emergencies. Chest 1990;98:785-786.

61. Ram CVS. Immediate management of severe hypertension. Cardiol Clin 1995;13:579-591.

62. Lavin P. Management of hypertension in patients with acute stroke. Arch Intern Med 1986;146:66-68.

63. Brott T, Reed RL. Intensive care for acute stroke in the community hospital setting. The first 24 hours. Stroke 1989;20:694-697.

64. Wong MCW, Haley EC Jr. Calcium antagonists: stroke therapy coming of age. Stroke 1990;21:494-501.

65. Powers WJ. Acute hypertension after stroke: the scientific basis for treatment decisions (editorial). Neurology 1993;43:461-467.

66. Gelmers HJ, Gorter K, de Weerdt CJ, Wiezer HJ. A controlled trial of nimodipine in acute ischemic stroke. N Engl J Med 1988;18:203-207.

67. Martinez-Vila E, Guillen F, Villanueva JA, et al. Placebo-controlled trial of nimodipine in the treatment of acute ischemic cerebral infarction. Stroke 1990;21:1023-1028.

68. Flaherty JT. Comparison of intravenous nitroglycerin and sodium nitroprusside in acute myocardial infarction. Am J Med 1983;74:53-60.

69. Lau J, Antman EM, Jimenez-Silva J, et al. Cumulative meta-analysis of therapeutic trials for myocardial infarction. N Engl J Med 1992;327:248-254.

70. Phillips RA, Goldman ME, Ardeljan M, et al. Isolated T-wave abnormalities and evaluation of left ventricular wall motion after nifedipine for severe hypertension. Am J Hypertens 1991;4:432-437.

71. O'Mailia JJ, Sander GE, Giles TD. Nifedipine-associated myocardial ischemia or infarction in the treatment of hypertensive urgencies. Ann Intern Med 1987;107:185-186.

72. Lindheimer MD, Katz AI. Hypertension in pregnancy. N Engl J Med 1985; 313:675-680.

73. Grossman E, Messerli FH. High blood pressure. A side effect of drugs, poisons, and food. Arch Intern Med 1995;155:450-460.

74. Gales MA. Oral antihypertensives for hypertensive urgencies. Ann Pharmacol 1994; 28:352-358.

75. White WB, Baker LH. Ambulatory blood pressure monitoring in patients with panic disorder. Arch Intern Med 1987;147:1973-1975.

76. Komsuoglu B, Sengun B, Bayram A, Komsuoglu SS. Treatment of hypertensive urgencies with oral nifedipine, nicardipine, and captopril. Angiology 1991;42:447-454.

77. Pascale C, Zampaglione B, Marchisiti M. Management of hypertensive crisis: nifedipine in comparison with captopril, clonidine, and furosemide. Curr Ther Res 1992;51:9-18.

78. Pastorelli R, Ferri C, Santucci A. New therapeutic possibilities in hypertensive emergencies. Curr Ther Res 1991;50:857-868.

79. Ceyhan B, Karaaslan Y, Caymaz O, et al. Comparison of sublingual captopril and sublingual nifedipine in hypertensive emergencies. Jpn J Pharmacol 1990;52:189-193.

80. Rohr G, Reimnitz P, Blanke P. Treatment of hypertensive emergency. Comparison of a new dosage form of the calcium antagonist nitrendipine with nifedipine capsules. Intensive Care Med 1994;20: 268-271.

81. Just VL, Schrader BJ, Paloucek FP, et al. Evaluation of drug therapy for treatment of hypertensive urgencies in the emergency department. Am J Emerg Med 1991;9:107-111.

82. Panlilio AG, Vilela GC, San Vicente FG. Randomized single-blind parallel study of the short-term blood pressure response to sublingual clonidine and sublingual nifedipine in hypertensive emergencies. Philippine Journal of Internal Medicine 1990;28:447-456.

83. Savi L, Montebelli MR, D'Alonzo S, et al. Sublingual nicardipine to treat hypertensive urgencies. Int J Clin Pharmacol Ther Toxicol 1992;30:41-45.

84. Angeli P, Chiesa M, Caregaro L, et al. Comparison of sublingual captopril and nifedipine in immediate treatment of hypertensive emergencies. A randomized, single-blind clinical trial. Arch Intern Med 1991;151:678-682.

85. Nobile-Orazio E, Sterzi R. Cerebral ischaemia after nifedipine treatment. Br Med J 1981;283:948.

86. Schwartz M, Naschitz JE, Yeshurun D, Sharf B. Oral nifedipine in the treatment of hypertensive urgency: cerebrovascular accident following a single dose (letter). Arch Intern Med 1990;150:686-687.

87. Wachter RM. Symptomatic hypotension induced by nifedipine in the acute treatment of severe hypertension. Arch Intern Med 1987;147:556-558.

88. Zangerle KF, Wolford R. Syncope and conduction disturbances following sublingual nifedipine for hypertension. Ann Emerg Med 1985;14:1005-1006.

89. Nifedipine, hypotension and myocardial injury (letter). Ann Intern Med 1988;108:305-306.

90. Shettigar UR, Loungani R. Adverse effects of sublingual nifedipine in acute myocardial infarction. Crit Care Med 1989;17:196-197.

91. Cheng TO. Adverse effects of sublingual nifedipine in acute myocardial infarction (letter). Crit Care Med 1989;17:1364.

92. Aromatorio GJ, Uretsky BF, Reddy PS. Hypotension and sinus arrest with nifedipine in pulmonary hypertension. Chest 1985;87:265-267.

93. Impey L. Severe hypotension and fetal distress following sublingual administration of nifedipine to a patient with severe pregnancy induced hypertension at 33 weeks. Br J Obstet Gynaecol 1993;100:959-961.

94. Grossman E, Messerli EH, Grodzicki T, Kowey P. Should a moratorium be placed on sublingual nifedipine capsules given for hypertensive emergencies and pseudoemergencies? JAMA 1996;276:1328-1331.

95. Messerli FH, Sundgaard-Riise K, Ventura HO, et al. Essential hypertension in the elderly: haemodynamics, intravascular volume, plasma renin activity, and circulating catecholamine levels. Lancet 2:983-986, 1983.

96. Thacker HL, Jahnigen DW. Managing hypertensive emergencies and urgencies in the geriatric patient. Geriatrics 1991;46:26-30.

CHAPTER 20

The Elderly

John B. Kostis
Kevin O'Malley
Eoin O'Brien

The elderly population, arbitrarily defined here as age 65 and older, is increasing and in many parts of the world (for example, in Sweden and the United States) approaches or exceeds 20%. The major cause of morbidity and mortality in older persons is cardiovascular disease and, as in younger persons, raised blood pressure is a potent risk factor.

In this chapter, we examine the impact of hypertension as a cardiovascular risk factor, the results of the major intervention trials, and the special features of hypertension in the elderly as they pertain to diagnosis and management.[1]

EPIDEMIOLOGY AND CLINICAL TRIALS

The relationship between blood pressure and cardiovascular morbidity and mortality has been clearly documented for the elderly in various publications including those from the Framingham Heart Study, the Multiple Risk Factor Intervention Trial (MRFIT), and others. The key findings are that raised blood pressure, particularly systolic hypertension, is positively related to coronary artery disease, stroke, and heart failure. Apart from age itself, raised blood pressure is the most powerful predictor of cardiovascular end-organ damage and its associated morbidity and mortality. Despite this strong evidence, there has been a reluctance to assertively treating raised blood pressure in the elderly mainly because of concerns, not scientifically quantified, that drug treatment results in an unacceptable burden of adverse drug reactions in the elderly. With the advent of six major intervention studies,[2–12] the results of which have been published over the past 15 years, this position is no longer tenable. The results of these studies are summarized in Table 1.

TABLE 1. RISK REDUCTION TO SEVERAL EVENTS BY ACTIVE TREATMENT IN PLACEBO-CONTROLLED STUDIES OF HYPERTENSION IN OLDER ADULTS.

	Stroke	Heart Failure	Cardiac Ischemic Events	Total Mortality
Australian[2]	34	NR	19	23
HDFP[11]	50	NR	11	17
EWPHE[3]	36	16	11	8
MRC[8]	24	NR	18	3
STOP-Hypertension[7]	45	NR	10	43
SHEP[5]	35	53	26	12
STONE[12]	57	68	68	44
Coope & Warrender[4]	42	32	-2	3
SYST-EUR[10]	42	32	26	14
All (CI)*	38 (30–45)	39 (26–50)	17 (8–26)	13 (6–20)

NR = not reported
HDFP = Hypertension Detection and Follow-Up Program
EWPHE = European Working Party on Hypertension in the Elderly
MRC = Medical Research Council
STOP = Swedish Trial in Old Patients with Hypertension
SHEP = Systolic Hypertension in the Elderly Program
STONE = Shanghai Trial of Nifedipine in the Elderly
SYST-EUR = Systolic Hypertension in Europe Trial
*Metaanalysis using Mantel Haentzel

Despite differences in study design, entry criteria, and drug regimens, there is a remarkable degree of agreement across these studies. Thus, strokes (fatal or non-fatal) were reduced by between 24% to 50%, cardiac ischemic events were reduced by 10% to 68%, and heart failure by 16% to 67%. In most case, diuretics or beta-blockers were used as first-line drugs and unquestionably the efficacy of diuretics in terms of blood pressure reduction, approximately 20/10 mm Hg, was impressive, as was the reduction in morbid events. In one study, the Medical Research Council (MRC) trial, atenolol and hydrochlorothiazide were compared, and the latter was found to be superior in reducing study endpoints. In another study, the Systolic Hypertension in the Elderly Program (SHEP),[5] raised systolic pressure alone (isolated systolic hypertension) was specifically studied and, again, a diuretic-based regimen was found to be effective in reducing the complications associated with raised blood pressure.

These studies were not designed to test the hypothesis that drug treatment of hypertension in the elderly reduces overall mortality and did not have the statistical power to demonstrate an effect on mortality. In the Swedish Trial in Old Patients with Hypertension (STOP-Hypertension) trial,[7] a statistically significant reduction of 43% was observed. This outcome may be related to high mean entry blood pressure (195/102 mm Hg) or to the play of chance. Metaanalysis of eight trials (Table 1) indicates a 13% decrease in mortality, 37% decrease in stroke, 16% decrease in cardiac ischemic events and a 44% decrease in heart failure.

The value of treating raised blood pressure in the elderly is particularly impressive. While the percentage reduction in complications is similar to that seen in treated young hypertensives, the background incidence of cardiovascular complications is much greater in the elderly, so a similar percentage reduction translates into a substantially greater ab-solute prevention of cardiovascular complications. Thus, in young patients with mild hypertension, one cardiovascular event may be prevented per 1,000 patient years of treatment, whereas in the elderly this figure may be as low as 50 patient years. Among patients with isolated systolic hypertension and a prior history of myocardial infarction, the number needed to treat to prevent one heart failure event was 15 patient years.[6] Such considerations not only justify but demand an assertive approach to the management of hypertension in the elderly.

The adverse reactions observed in these various studies were qualitatively predictable but in terms of clinical burden were seen to be acceptable and in no way excessive compared with that observed in younger persons. This outcome is in part due to the fact that relatively low doses of diuretics (usually 12.5 or 25 mg chlorthalidone or hydro-chlorothiazide) were used or, alternatively, potassium-sparing diuretics were combined with thiazides. Clinically significant metabolic sequelae of diuretic therapy such as hypokalemia, hyperglycemia, and hyperuricemia were relatively uncommon and rarely translated into clinical problems.

DIAGNOSIS OF HYPERTENSION IN THE ELDERLY

Taking into account all the available data, it is probably reasonable to take 140/90 mm Hg as the cutoff pressures for definition of hypertension in the elderly.[13] Combined systolic and diastolic hypertension should be treated above these levels, as should isolated systolic hypertension; that is, a systolic pressure greater than 160 and diastolic pressure less than 90 mm Hg. Again, diastolic values greater than 90 mm Hg should also be considered for treatment. There is no unanimity on the use of drug therapy for isolated systolic hypertension between 140 mm Hg and 159 mm Hg, and, though the likelihood is that treatment is beneficial, usually non-drug therapy is recommended for these patients. In the SYST-EUR clinical trial of patients with isolated systolic hypertension defined as systolic blood pressure between 160 and 219 mm Hg with a diastolic blood pressure lower than 95 mm Hg, drug therapy with the calcium antagonist nitrendipine with the possible addition of enalapril and hydrochlorothiazide resulted in 42% reduction in total stroke and 26% reduction in all fatal and nonfatal cardiac end points.

Two problems may arise in interpreting blood pressure levels in the elderly. First, in some patients with high or, indeed, very high blood pressure levels, there may be little evidence of end-organ damage, and the question of pseudo-hypertension arises wherein indirect blood pressure is substantially greater than direct pressure, the latter being "normal." If suspicion to this effect is strong, it may be worthwhile to carry out direct and indirect blood pressure measurements. White coat hypertension may be excluded by ambulatory blood pressure measurements. The second clinical problem is postural hypertension, which is not uncommon in the elderly; it is important to ascertain its presence because drug treatment may exacerbate matters.

In addition to hypertension, other cardiovascular risk factors pertain in the elderly as in the young. These include hypercholesterolemia, cigarette smoking, hyperglycemia, obesity, and left ventricular hypertrophy, usually a sequela of hypertension. As with raised blood pressure, the impact of these risk factors is compounded by the presence of concomitant diseases. For example, in the European Working Party on Hypertension in the Elderly study,[3] those with lowest cholesterol had higher complication rates than did those with high cholesterol. This presumably is due to the presence of one or more additional variables. However, although in epidemiologic studies it is clear that increased cholesterol is a risk factor in the elderly, there are to date few data on which to base intervention for primary prevention. However, lipid-lowering treatment is used in elderly patients with clinical evidence of cardiovascular disease.

MANAGEMENT

Nonpharmacologic Treatment

There is increasing evidence that a variety of nonpharmacologic measures lower blood pressure in the elderly. These include weight reduction in the obese, reduction in salt intake, exercise, and moderation of alcohol intake. These various strategies should be considered, as in younger patients, since their successful adoption may obviate the need for drug treatment. In the Trial of Nonpharmacologic Interventions in the Elderly (TONE), weight loss (in obese participants), sodium restriction and especially their combination were proven successful in the long term control of hypertension after discontinuation of drug therapy.[14]

Choosing a Drug

As indicated, in most cases the intervention studies to date employ a diuretic as a first-line drug and, in three, the addition of a beta-blocker. Thus, most data on the impact of drug treatment on cardiovascular complications have been derived from studies employing these two drug classes as first-line treatment. Information is emerging that other drug classes such as angiotensin-converting enzyme (ACE) inhibitors and calcium channel blockers lower cardiovascular events in hypertension. Significantly lower rates of mortality, heart failure and cardiac ischemic events were observed with the ACE inhibitor enalapril in hypertensive patients with left ventricular dysfunction in SOLVD; and in SYST-EUR a lower rate of stroke was observed with the calcium-channel blocker nitrendipine with or without HCTZ.[9–10] In the MRC trial,[8] a diuretic was clearly superior to atenolol, the latter failing to statistically alter the key event rates. Beta-blockers were effective in the Coope and Warrender study[4] and in the STOP-Hypertension trial.[7] These observations raise the possibility that there are true and important differences among drug classes in their impact on clinical outcome. We do know that all the major drug classes effectively lower blood pressure in the elderly, and therefore *a priori* they should reduce morbidity and mortality. We must consider all five major drug groups as candidate agents in the treatment of hypertension in the elderly. In so doing, a paramount consideration is the frequency with which older patients present with concomitant disease. Thus, some drug classes would be considered suitable because the patient has a condition that may benefit, as an example the hypertensive patient with heart failure for whom a diuretic or an ACE inhibitor would be appropriate. In others, the presence of complications will exclude drugs from choice. For example, in a patient with bronchospasm, beta-blockers would be contraindicated. The move from stepped care, evident in the past five years, is being generally accepted, and in no group is this more appropriate than in the elderly in whom individualization of choice (and dose) must be the approach (Table 2).

Diuretics

Diuretics have been the mainstay of antihypertensive drug treatment for decades, and the use of lower doses and potassium-sparing diuretics yields clinical results that are impressive both in terms of pressure-lowering efficacy and in the level of adverse drug reactions. Indeed, the diuretic group is the standard against which other antihypertensive drugs must be compared. As shown in the SHEP trial, low-dose (12.5 mg to 25 mg per day) chlorthalidone, a thiazide-like diuretic, is effective as monotherapy in a large proportion of patients. There is little to choose between chlorthalidone and

TABLE 2. SELECTION OF ANTIHYPERTENSIVE DRUG TREATMENT ACCORDING TO COEXISTING DISEASE.

Coexisting Disease	Diuretic	Beta-Blocker	Calcium Blocker	ACE Inhibitor or A-II Antagonist	Alpha-Blocker
None	++	+	+	+	+
Heart Failure	++	#	-*	++	+
Angina	+	++	++	+	+
Asthma or chronic obstructive airways disease	++	-	+	+	+
Peripheral vascular disease	+	-	++	-*	++
Gout	-	+	+	+	+
Diabetes	-	-	+	++	+

++ = First-line drug
+ = Suitable alternative drug
- = Usually contraindicated
* = High proportion of patients with peripheral vascular disease will have occult renovascular disease
ACE = Angiotensin-Converting Enzyme
# = Recently completed clinical trials have shown that cautious use of beta-blockers may improve outcome of patients with heart failure
Modified from Beard K, Bulpitt C, Mascie-Taylor H, et al. Management of elderly patients with sustained hypertension. Br Med J 1992;304:412–416.

the thiazides, but higher doses or loop diuretics should be used only in heart failure. In the elderly, important adverse effects include postural hypotension and hypokalemia. Diuretics should be avoided in diabetes. The adverse effects on lipids, whereby low-density lipoprotein (LDL) cholesterol tends to rise and high-density lipoprotein (HDL) cholesterol to fall, may attenuate in part the benefit of reducing blood pressure. Clearly, however, the net benefit observed outweighs this theoretical shortcoming.

Beta-Blockers

The efficacy of beta-blockers in decreasing blood pressure, as well as adverse clinical events, has been determined in major intervention trials. The results of the Coope and Warrender study[4] were impressive and consonant with those of the diuretic-based studies. However, the direct comparison of atenolol with hydrochlorothiazide in the MRC trial pointed to an advantage of diuretics over beta-blockers. Confirmation of this finding would have important implications. Beta-blockers should be used with great caution in those with congestive heart failure, peripheral vascular disease, diabetes, and respiratory disorders; but they would be particularly suitable for those with angina or a previous myocardial infarction. Side effects include depression, fatigue, cold extremities, and bradycardia. A beta-blocker with partial agonist activity such as pindolol may be tried when bradycardia becomes a problem.

ACE Inhibitors

ACE inhibitors have been shown to be effective in reducing blood pressure in the elderly and to have few adverse drug reactions. While concern has been expressed about their potential to cause problems in patients with renal artery stenosis, quantitative data on this aspect are lacking. Hypotension might also be seen in rare instances, and, therefore, low initial doses, withdrawal of diuretics, and initiation of treatments under careful monitoring seem wise. ACE inhibitors may be particularly suitable in the elderly because of the frequent occurrence in this group of congestive heart failure and diabetes mellitus as they have been found to produce clinical benefits in patients with these conditions. Furthermore, contraindications are rare. Angiotensin II antagonists have been shown to control blood pressure alone or in combination with low dose diuretics with a very favorable side effect profile, and they do not cause cough, a side effect of ACE inhibitors.

Calcium Antagonists

These agents are effective in lowering blood pressure in the elderly as well as in younger persons. Side effects relate to their vasodilatory action, such as flushing, headaches, palpitations, and ankle edema. Constipation due to verapamil may be bothersome to some older patients. Some of these effects are reduced with control-release or long-acting formulations that provide for lower peak plasma levels and prolonged apparent half-life. As with ACE inhibitors, there are few contraindications. Concern has been voiced about the safety of these agents, especially the short-acting dihydropyridines because of an apparent increase in myocardial infarction (and potentially in cancer and hemorrhage) in uncontrolled studies.[15] On the other hand, in the controlled SYST-EUR, a decreased rate of stroke and cardiac events was seen with therapy based on nitrendipine.[10]

Alpha-Blockers

Like calcium antagonists, alpha-blockers (the most extensively studied of which is doxazosin) act as vasodilators but with a decreased proclivity to cause reflex tachycardia. Concern about postural hypotension does not appear to be realized in the elderly, though a priori this important side effect must be considered. In patients with prostatic hypertrophy, these agents may provide an additional benefit. Beneficial effects on lipid profile with these drugs, which include a decrease in LDL and an increase in HDL cholesterol, raise the possibility of an enhanced effect on morbidity and mortality over that realized with other drug groups; for example, diuretics. We await the relevant clinical studies.

WHEN TO START AND STOP TREATMENT

The evidence for treating raised blood pressure up to age 80 is convincing, and data from two studies[5-7] support treatment thereafter, to approximately the mid-eighties (Figure 1). We are on less sure footing with the very old, and even the epidemiologic data are confusing in that, in some studies, the conventional relationship between raised blood pressure and risk appears to reverse in the ninth and tenth decades. In the hypertension optimal treatment (HOT) randomized trial, intensive lowering of blood pressure was associated with low rate of cardiovascular events.[16] As mentioned previously, additional variables compound matters, but it may well be that in

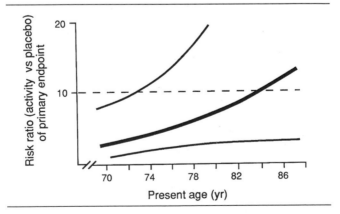

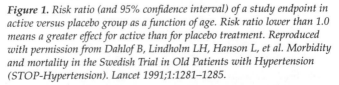

Figure 1. Risk ratio (and 95% confidence interval) of a study endpoint in active versus placebo group as a function of age. Risk ratio lower than 1.0 means a greater effect for active than for placebo treatment. Reproduced with permission from Dahlof B, Lindholm LH, Hanson L, et al. Morbidity and mortality in the Swedish Trial in Old Patients with Hypertension (STOP-Hypertension). Lancet 1991;1:1281–1285.

otherwise healthy individuals high blood pressure confers risk irrespective of age and, therefore, such very old persons are suitable candidates for both pharmacologic and non-pharmacologic management. In an open perspective randomized blind end point assessment trial of treating hypertension in patients older than 80, the average orthostatic fall in blood pressure was 10 mm Hg in the average and more than 20 mm Hg in 16% of the patients. This may affect tolerance to treatment.[17] Ambulatory blood pressure measurement is useful in the elderly to identify patients with "white coat hypertension," especially since in certain instances isolated systolic hypertension only occurs in the physician's office. It is also useful in evaluating variability of blood pressure and in selection of an appropriate antihypertensive medication, taking into account the diurnal blood pressure pattern and evaluating overtreatment causing hypotension at night.[18]

As more and more old patients are starting on antihypertensive drug treatment, the question will often arise as to whether drugs can or should be stopped. A trial period off medication with careful monitoring of blood pressure may be reasonable, particularly with predominantly diastolic hypertension, as there is a tendency for diastolic blood pressure to fall in later decades. This strategy is more likely to succeed after a non-drug therapy program has been instituted.[14]

CONCLUSION

The epidemiologic evidence that raised blood pressure is a potent risk factor for cardiovascular disease in the elderly is incontrovertible. Major intervention studies have demonstrated the value of treating raised blood pressure, both isolated systolic hypertension and combined systolic and diastolic hypertension, in this age group. As the absolute benefit is far greater than in the young, an assertive approach to the detection and management of raised blood pressure in the elderly is required. Diuretics and beta-blockers reduce morbidity and mortality with acceptable levels of adverse drug reactions. Recent data suggest that ACE inhibitors and calcium antagonists share this potential. The choice of drug prescribed is based on a global evaluation of each patient and will often be decided on the presence and nature of concomitant disease, which are particularly prevalent in the elderly.

REFERENCES

1. Beard K, Bulpitt C, Mascie-Taylor H, O'Malley K, Sever P, Webb S. Management of elderly patients with sustained hypertension. Br Med J 1992;304:412–416.

2. Management Committee. Treatment of mild hypertension in the elderly. Med J Aust 1981;3:398–402.

3. Amery A, Birkenhager WH, Brixko P, Bulpitt C, Clement D, Deruyttere M, et al. Mortality and morbidity results from the European Working Party on High Blood Pressure in the Elderly trial. Lancet 1985;1:1349–1354.

4. Coope J, Warrender TS. Randomised trial of treatment of hypertension in elderly patients in primary care. Br Med J 1986;293: 1145–1151.

5. SHEP Cooperative Research Group. Prevention of stroke by anti-hypertensive drug treatment in older persons with isolated systolic hypertension. JAMA 1991;265:3255–3264.

6. Kostis JB, Davis BR, Cutler J, et al. For the SHEP Cooperative Research Group. Prevention of heart failure by antihypertensive drug treatment in older persons with isolated systolic hypertension. JAMA 1997;278:212–216.

7. Dahlof B, Lindholm LH, Hanson L, Schersten B, Ekbom T, Wester PO. Morbidity and mortality in the Swedish Trial in Old Patients with Hypertension (STOP-Hypertension). Lancet 1991;338: 1281–1285.

8. Medical Research Council Working Party. MRC trial of treatment of hypertension in older adults: Principal results. Br Med J 1992;304:405–412.

9. Kostis JB. The effect of enalapril on mortal and morbid events in patients with hypertension and left ventricular dysfunction. Am J Hypertens 1995;8:909–914.

10. Staessen JA, Fagard R, Thijs L, Celis H et al. Randomised double-blind comparison of placebo and active treatment for older patients with isolated systolic hypertension. Lancet 1997;350:757–764.

11. Stamier J. Risk factor modification trials: implications for the elderly. Eur Heart J 1988;9(Suppl. D):9–53.

12. Gong L, Zhang W, Zhu Y, et al. Shanghai trial of nifedipine in the elderly (STONE). J Hypertension 1996;14:1237–1245.

13. Joint National Committee. The sixth report of the joint national committee on prevention, detection, evaluation, and treatment of high blood pressure (JNC VI). Arch Intern Med 1997;157:2413–2446.

14. Appel LJ, Espeland M, Whelton PK, Dolecek T, Kumanyika S, Applegate WB, Ettinger Jr WH, Kostis JB, Wilson AC, Lacy C, Miller ST. Trial of nonpharmacologic intervention in the elderly (TONE) design and rationale of a blood pressure control trial. Ann Epidemiol 1995;5:119–129.

15. Pahor M, Guralnik JM, Ferrucci L, Corti MC, Salive ME, Cerhan JR, Wallace RB, Havlik RJ. Calcium-channel blockade and incidence of cancer in aged populations. Lancet 1996; 348(9062):493–497.

16. Hansson L, Zanchetti A, Carruthers SG, et al. Effects of intensive blood presure lowering and low-dose aspirin in patients with hypertension: principal results of the Hypertension Optimal Treatment (HOT) randomised trial. HOT Study Group. Lancet 1998;351(9118): 1755–1762.

17. Bulpitt CJ, Connor M, Fletcher AE on behalf of the HYVET Investigators. Orthostatic fall in blood pressure in the very elderly hypertensive (pilot trial results from the Hypertension in the Very Elderly Trial [HYVET]) J Hypertens 1997;15(4):S50.

18. O'Brien E. Aging and blood pressure rhythms. Ann NY Acad Sci 1996;783:186–203.

CHAPTER 21

The Patient with Congestive Heart Failure

Bashar A. Shala
Jay M. Sullivan

The only cardiovascular disorder that is increasing in frequency in the United States is congestive heart failure (Figure 1). This has been attributed to two factors: (1) The aging of the population as the prevalence of hypertension increases with age. (2) Inadequate control of hypertension. (3) Increased survival after acute coronary syndromes. The development of congestive heart failure has long been observed in patients with hypertension. However, the NHANES III (Phase 2) Survey revealed that only 27% of hypertensive patients have their blood pressure controlled to levels beneath 140/90 mm Hg. In the Framingham Study, hypertension was present in 70% of patients that developed heart failure. This study also observed that levels of systolic blood pressure of only 140 to 160 mm Hg were associated with an increased risk of congestive heart failure and stroke. As cardiovascular death remains the leading cause of mortality in the United States, congestive heart failure becomes a major public health concern. Prevention and treatment of cardiac failure

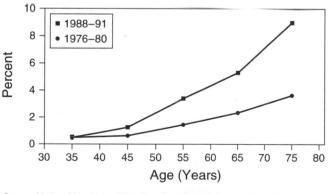

Source: National Health and Nutrition Examination Survey (1976–80 and 1988–91), National Center for Health Statistics.

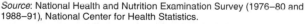

Figure 1. *Prevalence of heart failure by age, 1976–1980 and 1988–1991.*

emerges as a cornerstone in treating patients. Furthermore, overall mortality has been strongly linked to the development and progression of left ventricular dysfunction.

CAUSES AND ETIOLOGY

Hypertension and the rise of vasculare resistance cause increase in afterload and pressure overload on the myocardium. In response to these hemodynamic changes, the ventricular wall thickens without an increase in radius, to maintain wall stress within normal limits, giving rise to concentric ventricular hypertrophy and impaired diastolic relaxation.

With persistent and severe pressure overload, myocardial contractility becomes depressed, at which point ventricular dilatation provides the circulatory compensation necessary to maintain normal wall stress. Cardiac output may still be normal at rest but falls with stress.

As contractility becomes more depressed, cardiac output decreases further with significant increase in left ventricular end diastolic volume, and pressure and overt congestive heart failure dominates the clinical picture.

Another mechanism by which hypertension causes clinical "heart failure" is impaired ventricular relaxation or diastolic dysfunction. As concentric hypertrophy develops, the myocardium does not lengthen sufficiently in early diastole to allow rapid filling of the ventricle. This causes inappropriate change in diameter (or volume) to a given change of force (or pressure) and implies a reduction in ventricular compliance, i.e, the ventricle "stiffens."

Diastolic dysfunction may coexist with systolic dysfunction as a result of fibrosis, cellular disarray and ischemia. The presence of diastolic dysfunction often complicates the clinical picture in patients with congestive heart failure and may worsen overall prognosis.

CLINICAL FEATURES

The presence of congestive heart failure significantly changes the quality of life for hypertensive patients. The clinical course tends to be progressive and the severity of symptoms correlates well with prognosis (Figures 2 and 3). The New York Heart Association has classified patients into four classes based on degree of activity tolerance and functional capacity (Table 1).

Symptoms

Patients become dyspnic (DOE, PND, and orthopnia) and have a low threshold for fatigue and lethargy. In more advanced cases pulmonary edema and excessive fluid overload result in frequent hospitalization.

Physical Examination

Cardiovascular examination in patients with hypertension and congestive heart failure is characterized by signs of vol-

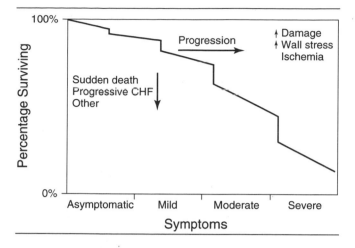

Figure 2. The natural history of congestive heart failure, with progression of symptomatic failure and mortality increases. From Cheitlin, MD (ed.). Dilemmas in Clinical Cardiology. Philadelphia:FA Davis, 1990;256.

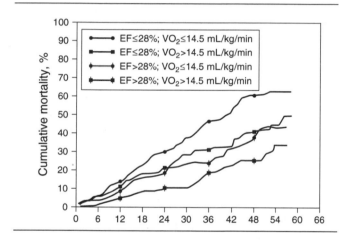

Figure 3. Multivariate analysis of survival in the V-HEFT studies shows increased mortality with worsening ejection fraction and decreased peak exercise oxygen consumption. From Rector TS and Cohn JN.Prognosis, use of prognostic variables, and assessment of therapeutic responses. In Colucci, WS (ed.). Heart Failure: Cardiac Function and Dysfunction.

ume expansion and low cardiac output in addition to signs of hypertension.

Signs of venous congestion may include distended jugular veins, hepatomegaly, hepatojugular reflex and dependent pitting edema.

Cardiac examination may reveal a laterally displaced and diffuse apical impulse, which is a sign of cardiomegaly. A third or fourth heart sound or gallop may indicate decreased myocardial compliance and deteriorating systolic function. Murmurs of mitral regurgitation and aortic insufficiency may be present in hypertensive heart failure. Pulsus alternans indicates severe left ventricular systolic dysfunction. Pulmonary examination may reveal rales as signs of pulmonary congestion.

TABLE 1. NEW YORK HEART ASSOCIATION FUNCTIONAL
CLASSIFICATION.

Class	Classification
I	Patients with cardiac disease but without resulting limitations of physical activity. Ordinary physical activity does not cause undue fatigue, palpitation, dyspnea, or anginal pain.
II	Patients with cardiac disease resulting in slight limitation of physical activity. They are comfortable at rest. Ordinary physical activity results in fatigue, palpitation, dyspnea, or anginal pain.
III	Patients with cardiac disease resulting in marked limitation of physical activity. They are comfortable at rest. Less than ordinary physical activity causes fatigue, palpitation, dyspnea, or anginal pain.
IV	Patient with cardiac disease resulting in inability to carry on any physical activity without discomfort. Symptoms of cardiac insufficiency or of the anginal syndrome may be present even at rest. If any physical activity is undertaken, discomfort is increased.

Chest x-ray. Chest x-ray films may show cardiomegaly and signs of pulmonary congestion such as pulmonary edema with bronchial cuffing, alveolar filling , and Kerley B lines. A "batwing" appearance is characteristic of cardiac pulmonary edema. Pleural effusions may be present.

Echocardiogram. Echocardiographic examination of the failing hypertensive heart may reveal increased chamber dimensions, diffuse hypokinesis, or the presence of regional wall motion abnormalities in the case of ischemia. Wall thickness may be increased in concentric or eccentric hypertrophy or decreased in severe dilated cardiomyopathy. Plethoric and dilated inferior vena cava could indicate systemic venous congestion. Furthermore, diastolic dysfunction may be assessed using Doppler interrogation of transmitral and pulmonary venous flows.

Nuclear cardiology. Radionuclide ventriculograms, using the multigated acquisition scan (MUGA) method, have been used to estimate ejection fractions accurately utilizing blood pool imaging. Recently, perfusion imaging techniques such as gated single photon emission computed tomography (Gated-SPECT) are being used to assess myocardial perfusion and function simultaneously.

Laboratory. Congestive heart failure is associated with neurohumoral changes that are detectable by laboratory measurements. Decreased cardiac output activates the sympatho-adrenal and renin-angiotensin-aldosterone systems and results in higher levels of renin, angiotensin II and aldosterone. Activation of the sympathetic nervous system is evident by higher levels of circulating cathecholamines.

Hyponatremia may be present due to increased vasopressin and atrial natriuretic hormone levels and indicate severe failure. Worsening renal function and prerenal azotemia may indicate decreased renal perfusion.

ACUTE HEART FAILURE

Hypertensive patients may occasionally present with acute development of signs and symptoms of left-sided heart failure, mainly acute or "flash" pulmonary edema. This syndrome is usually associated with severe hypertension and constitutes a hypertensive emergency where afterload reduction is the main therapeutic intervention. Intravenous therapy is often necessary, using sodium nitroprusside or other agents, to acutely decrease afterload. Other etiologies for acute heart failure should be ruled out, especially myocardial ischemia and aortic dissection.

TREATMENT

Treatment strategies in hypertensive patients with failing ventricles aim at improving survival, controlling symptoms and slowing the progression of cardiac disease.

The Sixth Report of the Joint National Committee on Prevention, Detection, Evaluation and Treatment of High Blood Pressure (JNC-6) outlined the management of patients with cardiac failure based on evidence derived from multiple clinical trials.

Lifestyle modifications is a cornerstone of initial management. Dietary change with decreased sodium intake to prevent fluid retention is essential. Weight reduction for obese patients, and a low-cholesterol, low-fat diet for patients with coronary artery disease and hyperlipidemia are also very important. Regular aerobic exercise, especially in supervised cardiac rehabilitation programs, has been shown to improve activity tolerance and quality of life in patients with congestive heart failure.

Several advances in pharmacologic treatment have been achieved in the last decade, with survival data playing a major role in drug selection. Classes of agents used in congestive heart patients are discussed below.

Angiotension Converting Enzyme (ACE I) Inhibitors

This class of drugs has become first line therapy for heart failure. Several large scale clinical trials have shown reduction of mortality with ACE inhibitors when compared to placebo or other treatment of congestive heart failure.

The Veterans Administration Cooperative Vasodilator Heart Failure Trial (VcHeFT-2) compared captopril to a combination of hydracazine and isosorbide dinitrate and showed reduction in mortality in the captopril arm; however, there was greater improvement in ejection fraction and exercise capacity in the hydralazine-nitrate arm. This mortality reduction was also evident when enalapril was used in the SOLVD (Studies of Left Ventricular Dysfunction Trial) and CONSENSUS-1 (Cooperative New Scandinavian Enalapril Survival Study).

Furthermore, in patients with heart failure who had suffered myocardial infarction, ACE inhibitors have shown survival benefit. This was evident with captopril in SAVE (Survival and Ventricular Enlargement), ramipril in AIRE (The Acute Infarction Ramipril Efficacy) and trandolapril in TRACE (Trandolapril Cardiac Evaluation). ACE inhibitors reduce afterload by lowering blood pressure and vasculare resistance, and reduce preload by decreasing sodium and fluid retention. Other mechanisms on cellular and molecular levels are under extensive investigation.

Renal function should be monitored closely initially upon starting ACE inhibitors and less frequently thereafter if function remains stable. Special precautions should be taken in patients with severe hypertension who underwent excessive diuresis, as renal perfusion may be dependent on the renin-angiotensin-aldosterone system. Concomitant use of NSAIDs may lead to exaggerated deterioration of renal function due to constriction of afferent arterioles during prostaglandin inhibition.

Hyperkalemia may occur and could be significant especially in combinations with potassium-sparing diuretics.

Chronic cough has been associated with ACE I use due to bradykinin accumulation and may lead to discontinuation of the drug. A rare, but important, side effect is angioedema which could be life-threatening when involving upper respiratory airways. In this particular case, all ACE I should be discontinued and patients should be switched to a different class of drugs (i.e., combination of hyralazine and nitrate or possibly angiotensin II receptor-blocking agents).

Angiotensin II Receptor Blockers

This class of drugs work directly by blocking angiotensin II type I receptor sites and does not cause activation and accumulation of bradykinin and kallikenin. Chronic cough should not be a major concern with this class, and angioedema has been reported rarely.

In the ELITE Study (Evaluation of Losartan in the Elderly), losartan was compared to captopril to assess safety profile; however, a secondary analysis showed survival benefit in the losartan group. Further studies are underway to test survival advantages of this class compared with ACE inhibitors.

Diuretics

Different types of diuretics have been used in congestive heart failure to decrease cardiac preload and manage fluid retention.

Thiazide diuretics have been used in hypertensive patients with mild congestive failure to prevent volume expansion and to enhance blood pressure control at the same time. Combinations of thiazides and potassium-sparing diuretics are commonly used.

Loop diuretics are used chronically in more advanced failure stages or acutely to manage pulmonary edema or venous congestion. In patients with severe cardiac failure or renal failure, a distally-acting agent, such as metolazone, could be added to loop diuretics and often results in effective diuresis.

Dehydration may occur with diuretic therapy, especially in elderly patients. Clinical signs of overdiuresis and prerenal azotemia should be followed to adjust treatment.

Hypokalemia and hypomagnesemia are common problems with diuretics. Hypokalemia may occur despite use of potassium-sparing diuretics. Electrolyte monitoring is important in patients on diuretics and diuretic combinations because potassium or magnesium depletion can result in cardiac arrhythmias. The concomitant use of potassium-sparing diuretics and ACE inhibitors can cause hyperkalemia in certain individuals.

Diuretic "sliding scales" have been used in compliant patients who monitor their weight and volume status and adjust diuretic dose accordingly.

Digoxin

Digitalis group cardiac glycosides are among the earliest drugs used in the treatment of heart failure. At the cellular level, digoxin inhibits the sodium-potassium ATPase pump which causes sodium to accumulate in the cell, increased sodium-calcium exchanges and higher concentration of intracellular calcium available to activate actin and myocin molecules, thereby enhancing contractility. Aside from this positive inotropic action, digoxin has vagomimetic properties that are responsible for the depression of the SA node and prolonged conduction in AV node. In higher levels, digoxin increases sympathetic outflow which enhances atrial and ventricular automaticity.

The Digitalis Investigation Group (DIG) recently examined the effects of digoxin on morbidity and mortality in heart failure patients in a large scale multicenter trial. The results indicated that digoxin therapy, in patients with congestive heart failure and ejection fraction less than 45%, was associated with lower overall hospitalization rates and less hospitalization due to worsening of heart failure. However, there was no difference in mortality between the digoxin and placebo groups.

Digoxin levels should be monitored in patients on therapy, and levels higher than 1.5–2 should be avoided because this may lead to increased sympathetic discharge and digoxin toxicity.

Beta-Blockers

It has been observed that patients with the highest circulating cathecholamines have the worst prognosis in congestive heart failure. These findings suggested that beta-blockers might be useful in decreasing the effects of sympathetic activation in heart failure patients and possibly improve prognosis.

Several beta-blockers have been investigated. The Metopolol in Dilated Cardiomyopathy (MDC) Study showed that metopolol was well tolerated, reduced clinical deterioration, and improved cardiac function, but no reduction in mortality was noted. Similar findings were shown using bisoprolol in CIBIS (The Cardiac Insufficiency Bisoprolol Study).

A number of studies used carvedilol, which is a nonselective beta-blocker with alpha-1 blocking and antioxidant properties. PRECISE (Prospective Randomized Evaluation of Carvedilol on Symptoms and Exercise) showed that carvedilol improved exercise capacity, symptoms, treadmill time, and NYHA Class. Two additional studies showed that in symptomatic congestive heart failure patients (Carvedilol Heart Failure Study) and mildly symptomatic patients (US Carvedilol Heart Failure Study) carvedilol reduced overall mortality, congestive heart failure mortality, and hospitalization in patients who were receiving treatment with ACE I, diuretics, and digoxin. Furthermore, the MOCHA Study (Multicenter Oral Carvedilol Heart Failure Assessment) showed that in subjects with mild to moderate failure, carvedilol resulted in dose-related improvement in LV function and reduction in mortality and hospitalization rates.

Currently, recommendations are to start with low doses (3.125 mg–6.25 mg BID) and gradually advance every two weeks to a large dose (25–50 mg BID). Initial worsening of symptoms can be expected; however, most patients tolerate the drug well eventually. Other studies examining the effect of different beta-blockers are in progress. It is important to note that beta-blockers are useful in the long-term treatment of stable patients, but are of no value in treating decompensated congestive heart failure patients.

Calcium-Channel Blockers

From the hypothesis that the vasodilator properties of these drugs may be beneficial in reducing afterload and improving heart failure hemodynamics, multiple drugs have been tested in this class.

Diltiazem, in the Dilated Cardiomyopathy Trial (DiDi) showed that diltiazem improved cardiac function, exercise capacity, and subjective status without deleterious effects on transplant-free survival. In PRAISE (Prospective Randomized Amlodepine Survival Evaluation Trial) amlodepine was not associated with increased mortality or morbidity among patients with severe congestive heart failure, and it was associated with better outcome in patients with non-ischemic cardiomyopathy.

Inotropic Agents

Different inotropic agents have been used in intensive and acute care settings for management of acute decompensation of heart failure.

Several intravenous agents are widely used, for example, dobutamine, which is an adrenergic and dopaminergic agonist, and milrinone and amrinone, which are phosphodieolerase inhibitors, for short term therapy. Long term inotropic use has been shown to be detrimental to morbidity and mortality as in PROMISE Trial using Milrinone (Prospective Randomized Milrinone Survival Trial). Several oral inotropic agents have failed survival trials as well.

Antiarrhythmic Therapy

Since sudden cardiac death due to ventricular arrhythmias is common in patients with heart failure, the use of routine antiarrhythmic therapy has been advocated. However, with the discouraging results of increased mortality of CAST (Cardiac Arrhythmic Suppression Trial) using class 1-C agents and SWORD using D-Sotalol, routine administration of antiarrhythmic therapy has not been implemented.

Amiodarone has been shown to be safe and to reduce mortality in congestive heart failure patients in the GESICA Trial. However, survival benefit was present only in non-ischemic cardiomyopathy in another trial (Amiodarone in Patients with Congestive Heart Failure and Asymptomatic Ventricular Arrhythmia). Additionally the EMIAT (European Myocardial Infarct Amiodarone Trial had patients with congestive heart failure who were included in the study as infarct survivors, and no change in mortality was noted.

Given the data available to us at this point, it is probably most appropriate to use amiodarone as the antiarrhythmic of choice if such therapy is indicated in heart failure patients. Routine use of these agents is not standard practice at this time.

OTHER MANEUVERS AND TREATMENTS

Surgical techniques have been used for treatment of severe congestive heart failure. Two of these techniques are cardiac reduction surgery (Batista's procedure) and myoplasty using latissimus dorsi. Ultimately, cardiac transplant has been a widely used treatment for appropriate candidates with end-stage disease. This practice is limited by the sparse availability of heart donors. Also, several ventricular-assist devices have been used as a "bridge" to transplant in selected patients.

Automatic defibrillators have been shown to decrease mortality over conventional antiarrhythmic therapy in patients with low ejection fraction in MADIT (Multicenter Automatic Defibrillator Implantation Trial) and in patients who had ventricular events while receiving Amiodarone or Sotalol in the AVID Trial (Antiarrhythmics versus Implanted Defibrillators).

CONCLUSION

Overall, the treatment of heart failure in hypertensive patients should be individualized to patients' needs and medical history. Patients' education and involvement in treatment, with emphasis on compliance issues, is essential for successful management.

REFERENCES

The Sixth Report of the Joint National Committee on Prevention, Detection, Evaluation and Treatment of High Blood Pressure. Arch Intern Med 1997;157:2413–2446.

Braunwald, E. *Heart Disease: A Textbook of Cardiovascular Medicine*, 5th ed. Phila.: W.B. Saunders, 1997:421–533.

Williams JR Jr, Griston MR, Fowler MB, et al. Guidelines for the evaluation and management of heart failure. Report of the American College of Cardiology/American Heart Association Task Force on Practical Guidelines (Committee on Evaluation and Management of Heart Failure). J Am Coll Cardiol 1995;26:1376.

CONSENSUS Trial Study Group. Effects of enalapril on mortality in severe congestive heart failure. Results of the Cooperative North

Scandinavian Enalapril Survival Group (CONSENSUS). N Engl J Med 1987;316:1429.

SOLVD Investigators. Effect of enalapril on mortality and the development of heart failure in asymptomatic patients with reduced left ventriculare ejection fractions. N Engl J Med 1992;327:685.

Acute Infarction Ramipril Efficacy (AIRE) Study Investigators. Effect of ramipril on mortality and morbidity of survivors of acute myocardial infarction with clinical evidence of heart failure. Lancet 1993;312:821.

Gruppo Italiano per lo Studio della sopravvivenza nell'Infarto Mocardico, GISSI-3 Investigators. Effects of lisinopril and transdermal glyceryl trinitrate singly and together on a 6-week mortality and ventricular function after acute myocardial infarction. Lancet 1994;343:1115.

Cohn JN, Johnson G. Zeische S, et al. A comparison of enalapril with hydralazine-isosorbide dinitrate in the treatment of chronic congestive heart failure. N Engl J Med 1991;325:303–310.

Pitt B, Martinez FA, Meurers GG, et al. Randomised trial of losartan versus captopril in patients over 65 with heart failure (Evaluation of Losartan in the Elderly Study, ELITE). Lancet 1997;349:747–752.

The Digitalis Investigation Group. The Effect of digoxin on mortality and morbidity in patients with heart failure. N Engl J Med 1997;336:525–533.

Australia/New Zealand Heart Failure Research Collaborative Group. Randomized, placebo-controlled trial of carvedilol in patients with congestive heart failure due to ischaemic heart disease. Lancet 1997;349:375–380.

Waagstein F, Bristo MR, Swedberg K, et al. Beneficial effects of metoprolol in idiopathic dilated cardiomyopathy. Lancet 1993;342: 1441–1446.

CIBIS Investigators and Committees. A randomized trial of b-blockade in heart failure. The Cardia Insufficiency Bisoprolol Study (CIBIS). Circulation 1994;90:1765.

Packer M, Bristow MR, Cohn JN, et al. The effect of carvedilol on morbidity and mortality in patients with chronic heart failure. N Engl J Med 1996; 334:1349–1355.

Bristow MR, Gilbert EM, Abraham WT, et al. Carvedilol produces dose-related improvements in left ventricular function and survival in subjects with chronic heart failure. Circulation 1996;94:2807–2816.

Colucci WS, Packer M, Bristow MR, et al. Carvedilol inhibits clinical progression in patients with mild symptoms of heart failure. Circulation 1996;94:2800–2906.

Packer M, O'Connor CM, Ghali JK, et al. Effect of amlodipine on morbidity and mortality in severe chronic heart failure. N Engl J Med 1996;335:1107–1114.

Figulla HR, Gietzen F, Zeymer U, et al. Diltiazem improves cardiac function and exercise capacity in patients with idiopathic dilated cardiomyopathy. Results of the diltiazem in dilated cardiomyopathy trial. Circulation 1996;94:346–352.

The Cardiac Arrhythmia Suppression Trial (CAST) Investigators. CAST mortality and morbidity. Treatment versus placebo. N Engl J Med 1991;324:791.

Doval HC, Nul DR, Grancelli HO, et al. Randomized trial of low-dose amiodarone in severe congestive heart failure. Lancet 1994;344:493–498.

Packer M, Carver JR, Rodeheffer RJ, et al. Effect of milrinone on mortality in severe chronic heart failure. N Engl J Med 1991;325:1468–1475.

CHAPTER 22

The Patient with Coronary Heart Disease

Peter Sleight

Hypertension is one of the well-known risk factors for coronary heart disease (CHD), increasing the risk of CHD some twofold to threefold. The majority of hypertensive subjects will die of CHD, not stroke or renal failure. CHD is a common cause of congestive heart failure, as well as sudden death, angina, or myocardial infarction.

Until recently, it had been generally believed that the treatment of hypertension was very effective in preventing stroke, but, in contrast, the incidence of CHD was little affected by drug treatment of hypertension. Some felt that this was because the drugs that in the past had been used to lower blood pressure—mainly the thiazide diuretics—might have adverse effects on lipids and thereby increase the risk of atheroma.[1] Thiazides also reduce serum potassium and might additionally increase the risk of sudden arrhythmic death.[2]

A recent meta-analysis[3] suggested that this view was mistaken. More recent randomized trials have reinforced these data. It now seems more likely that coronary disease can be reduced by antihypertensive treatment, particularly in elderly patients,[4,5] and, paradoxically, thiazide diuretics rather than beta-blockers are the agents of choice.

Despite this, drug treatment has less effect on CHD than it does on stroke.[6] This realization and the recent recognition of the frequent association among hypertension, hyperlipidemia, and insulin resistance (the so-called syndrome X or metabolic syndrome) have place new emphasis on a "holistic" approach to the hypertensive patient.[7] This underlines the importance of intervening to change some of these other risk factors in addition to lowering blood pressure.

THE RELATION BETWEEN BLOOD PRESSURE AND CHD RISK IS CONTINUOUS IN THE WHOLE POPULATION

MacMahon and colleagues[8] carried out a meta-analysis of the long-term observational data from nine large studies totaling 420,000 persons followed for a mean of ten years (range 6 to 25 years). During this time, approximately six coronary events occurred for each stroke event (4,856 CHD events versus 843 strokes). Over the whole range of diastolic pressures encountered in these populations (70 mm Hg to 110 mm Hg), the risks of both stroke and CHD were continuously related to the usual diastolic pressure. This curvilinear relationship becomes absolutely linear when a doubling ordinate scale of risk is used (Figure 1). Even when the bottom quintile (76 mm Hg) is divided into two equal halves, the risk still separates as before; that is, there is no evidence of any threshold for the increased risk associated with raised pressure, even in these normotensive subjects. Similar data from less-developed countries suggests that Western levels of normality for blood pressure, like values for "normal" cholesterol, are biologically abnormal.

The linearity of the plots in Figure 1 suggests that the proportional benefit of lowering pressure is equal whether one goes from the fifth (top) quintile of pressure to the fourth (105 mm Hg to 98 mm Hg) or from the second to the first (84 mm Hg to 76 mm Hg). Because of the doubling scale, the absolute benefit is, of course, greater at the higher levels. However, if the patient has a high risk of CHD because of family history, smoking, diabetes, or cholesterol, the *absolute* benefit of reducing pressure may be worthwhile even at borderline levels of pressure. This has not yet been tested, but the concept is useful because it underlines the importance of considering not only the level of blood pressure but also the presence of other risk factors in the decision to lower blood pressure.

Figure 1 also illustrates a further important general concept. The size of the squares in Figure 1 is proportional

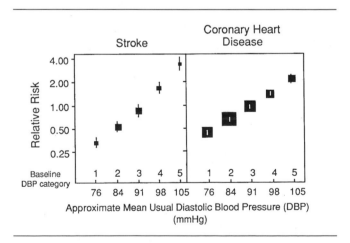

Figure 1. *Relative risks of stroke and of coronary heart disease, estimated from combined results. Estimates of the usual diastolic blood pressure (DBP) in each baseline DBP category are taken from mean DBP values four years post-baseline in the Framingham study. Solid squares represent disease risks in each category relative to risk in the whole study population; sizes of squares are proportional to number of events in each DBP category; and 95% confidence intervals for estimates of relative risk are denoted by vertical lines. Modified from MacMahon S, Peto R, Collins R. Blood pressure, stroke and coronary heart disease. Lancet 1990;335:765–774.*

to the number of events. Thus, although the absolute risk is greater for the top quintile of blood pressure in the population, the vast majority of the pressure-related CHD events are occurring at diastolic pressures ranging from 76 mm Hg to 91 mm Hg.

In these observational studies (epidemiology, not trials), the long-term effects of quite modest differences in usual blood pressure are striking. Differences of 5 mm Hg, 7.5 mm Hg, and 10 mm Hg in diastolic blood pressure are associated with differences of at least 34%, 46%, and 56%, respectively, in risk of stroke and differences of 21%, 29%, and 37% in CHD.

EVIDENCE ON THE BENEFIT FOR CHD FROM LOWERING BLOOD PRESSURE

In a companion paper, Collins et al.[3] examined the evidence from 14 properly randomized trials in 37,000 hypertensive patients. On average, in these trials, diastolic blood pressure was lowered by 5 mm Hg to 6 mm Hg. Because few trials lasted longer than five years, the average time to a CHD event was half this—just 2 to 3 years. Despite this short time (short relative to the slow progression of atheroma), CHD events were significantly reduced by about 14%—not significantly different from the 20% to 25% reduction expected from the much longer epidemiologic studies[8] (Figure 2). This reduction of 14% increases to 16% when the 1990 overview is updated by more recent data from the U.S. Systolic Hypertension in the Elderly Program (SHEP),[4] the Swedish Scandinavian Trial in Older Patients (STOP),[5] and the British Medical Research Council (MRC)[6] trial of elderly hypertensives.

The most surprising fact in this overview is not so much that hypotensive therapy produces about two thirds of what one might expect from the epidemiology, but rather that the benefit occurs extraordinarily rapidly. This suggests that the

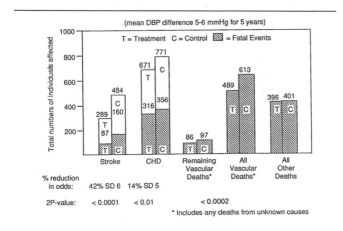

Figure 2. Summated results of the events (fatal—hatched, nonfatal—open) in the nonconfounded trials of blood pressure lowering by hypotensive drugs. From Collins R, Peto R, MacMahon S, et al. Blood pressure, stroke and coronary heart disease. Lancet 1990;335:827–838.

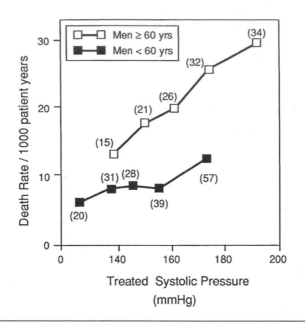

Figure 3. *Mortality from CHD per 1,000 patient years (age adjusted) in men in the U.K. Department of Health Hypertension Care Computing project. Modified from Bulpitt CJ, Palmer AJ, Fletcher AE, et al. Relation between treated blood pressure and death from ischaemic heart disease at different ages: A report from the Department of Health Hypertension Care Computing Project. J Hypertens 1992;10:1273–1278.*

mechanism of benefit for CHD is not just through regression of atheroma (which would be rather slow) but rather through some other mechanism, perhaps by prevention of plaque rupture. Many acute CHD events occur as a result of a crack or fissure in an atheromatous plaque. These cracks occur at the edges of a lesion, where macrophages die and release proteolytic enzymes. When a fissure appears, it is powerfully attractive to platelets and causes a platelet thrombus, which then initiates fibrin thrombus that may occlude or partially occlude the coronary lumen. Such fissures are initiated by wall stress, which, in turn, is pressure dependent. It is clear from a number of studies that on-treatment blood pressure is more important for prognosis than pretreatment blood pressure. This suggests that such mechanical factors may be more important than the amount of atheroma existing as a result of long-term pressure elevation (Figure 3).[9]

THE SIGNIFICANCE OF THE J-SHAPED CURVE: A MARKER OF EXISTING VASCULAR DISEASE

It is now well accepted that the relation between baseline blood pressure and future risk in patients—as opposed to the population data cited—is not always a steady increase. Particularly in patients with evidence of preexisting vascular disease (e.g., abnormal initial electrocardiogram), there may be a paradoxical increase in risk at the lowest levels of diastolic pressure, so that the blood pressure–mortality curve is J shaped, with the lowest risk at diastolic blood pressure of approximately 80 mm Hg. In such instances, the risk increases not only with increasing diastolic blood pressure above this, as would be expected, but it also increases with lower pressures, below 80 mm Hg, producing a "hockey stick" or J curve. The earlier explanation for this curve was the harmful effects of reducing coronary perfusion pressure (largely determined by diastolic blood pressure), particularly if coronary stenoses already existed. It is argued, therefore, that treatment might be dangerous in these patients. It seems equally likely (and data support this view) that, as arteries become sclerosed (and, hence, stiffer), the pulse pressure widens because the "Windkessel" effect of diastolic elastic recoil is absent or diminished. So the adverse prognosis is not due to the lower diastolic pressure measured but rather to the fact that the low diastolic pressure is an artifact caused by stiff and diseased vessels. This marker naturally identifies subjects at increased risk.

Subjects with stiff arteries are, therefore, characterized by isolated systolic hypertension. Such subjects are likely to be elderly. The SHEP[4] trial and the SYST-EUR trial[10] (Figure 4) have shown that CHD in such subjects is *reduced* by hypotensive drugs. A previous meta-analysis had shown a striking and significant reduction in CHD mortality (26%) by treatment of hypertension in the elderly.[11] Therefore, it now

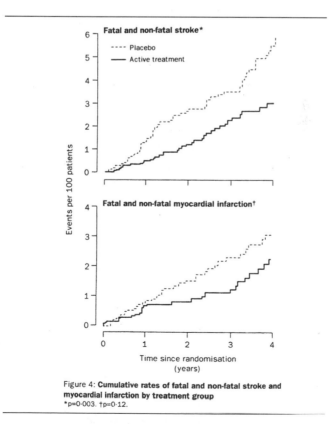

Figure 4: **Cumulative rates of fatal and non-fatal stroke and myocardial infarction by treatment group**
*p=0·003. †p=0·12.

Figure 4. Cumulative rates of fatal and non-fatal stroke and myocardial infarction by treatment group (*p = 0.003; †p - 0.12).[10]

seems particularly inappropriate to reduce or withhold treatment for patients with isolated systolic hypertension who have low diastolic blood pressure.

THE RISK WHEN A HYPERTENSIVE PATIENT HAS A MYOCARDIAL INFARCTION

Hypertension not only increases the risk of vascular damage from hyperlipidemia, diabetes, smoking, and other risk factors, but it may also accelerate the risk of an acute clinical event by provoking rupture or fissuring of these atheromatous plaques. Epidemiologic studies also show that the subsequent mortality from myocardial infarction is substantially and significantly higher in hypertensives than in normal subjects (Figure 5).[12] This may be because of the diminished coronary flow reserve in hypertensive patients with left ventricular hypertrophy.

TREATING ACUTE MYOCARDIAL INFARCTION IN HYPERTENSION

In general, the treatment of acute myocardial infarction (AMI) is the same for hypertensive as for normotensive patients, but with some changes of emphasis because of the high pressure and increased risk of cerebral hemorrhage from some thrombolytics such as tPA.

Aspirin

In the short term, I would use immediate aspirin—160 mg to 300 mg, chewed for quick absorption—and then swallowed

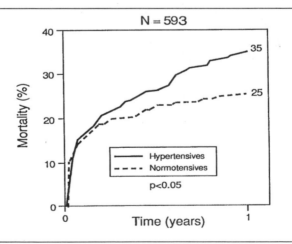

Figure 5. One-year mortality from acute myocardial infarction (AMI) in 324 unselected hypertensive patients in Gothenberg (continuous line) is significantly higher (p <0.05) than in the 593 normotensive subjects with AMI. (This may be due to the reduction in coronary flow reserve seen in patients with left ventricular hypotrophy.) Modified from Herlitz J, Karlson BW, Richter A, et al. Prognosis in hypertensives with acute myocardial infarction. J Hypertens 1992;10:1265–1271.

daily for at least one month at a dose of 75 mg to 160 mg. The use of long-term aspirin seems prudent but is not well proven in hypertensives by trials. The use of prophylactic aspirin before AMI in a patient who only has hypertension as a risk factor is even less well proven. There is a slight risk of cerebral bleeding. It is likely that the prophylactic benefit for AMI will outweigh this risk; aspirin is currently being tested in trials of antihypertensive treatment (see recent HOT study, Lancet 1998).

Thrombolysis

Hypertension increases the risk of cerebral bleeding and is thus a relative contraindication for thrombolysis at pressures over 200 mm Hg systolic and 110 mm Hg diastolic. Nevertheless, if a patient is at high risk, I would still use lytic treatment after the pressure has been reduced by drugs such as intravenous beta-blockade (see next section), intravenous nitrates, or both.

The risk of cerebral hemorrhage increases steadily with systolic blood pressure over 125 mm Hg to 175+ mm Hg. The increased risk is much steeper for tissue plasminogen activator (tPA) than with streptokinase. Streptokinase is, therefore, the treatment of choice for the hypertensive, particularly the elderly hypertensive.

Intravenous Beta-Blockade

Intravenous beta-blockade has been shown to reduce the risk of cardiac rupture, which is increased by hypertension. If the hemodynamic state is favorable (Killip 1 or 2), I would use intravenous beta-blockade, 5 mg to 10 mg of atenolol or 5–15 mg of metoprolol. In practice, up to 50% of patients with AMI tolerated this in the Gruppo Italiano per lo Studio della Streptochinasi nell'infarto miocardico (GISSI-2) trial[13] simultaneously with thrombolysis.

ACE Inhibitors and Angiotensin II Receptor Blockers

Early ACE inhibition is now accepted treatment for the majority of patients after the first few hours of circulatory instability.[14-16] The drug should not be given to patients who are hypotensive (say SBP<100–105 mm Hg) or who are on a high dose of diuretic (>80 mg furosemide daily) when angiotensin levels are high. It should be started in low doses (6.25 mg captopril, or 2.5–5 mg lisinopril), both of which have been tested in large randomized studies.[15,16] If LV function remains normal, the drug can be stopped just before hospital discharge. It is likely, but not yet proven, that A II blockers would have a similar benefit.

MULTIPLE RISK FACTOR INTERVENTION IN HYPERTENSION TO REDUCE THE RISK OF CHD

Life-Style Changes

Encourage Exercise. This has several synergistic benefits. First, exercise lowers blood pressure and can usefully augment blood pressure lowering drugs.[17] Second, exercise may reduce obesity and not only lower blood pressure by weight reduction but also favorably affect lipids. Third, sedentary habits are associated with increased CHD risk, regardless of whether the other risk factor studied was smoking, hyperlipidemia, or genetic predisposition to diabetes. Exercise also reduces insulin resistance.

Discourage Smoking. The serious adverse interaction of smoking has long been known in men, but it has recently been reinforced by the U.S. Nurses' Health study.[18] This interaction appears to be mediated by many factors including increased vascular and endothelial damage, and an increased thrombotic tendency due to raised fibrinogen and platelet stickiness.

Reduce Serum Lipids. Serum lipids should be reduced by diet or, where necessary, by drugs. Lipids appear to have a "permissive" effect on the prevalence of CHD. In Japan and China, where serum lipids have been low, cigarette smoking causes lung cancer but not CHD. Hypertension causes strokes but is less associated with CHD, as occurs in the West. The distribution curves for serum lipids in China and Japan scarcely overlap those in the West. Most Western cholesterol values are abnormal. The preoccupation with the possible hazards of low cholesterol seems dangerously overdone. It seems likely that the relation seen in some studies is related to confounding with other diseases, such as cancer or hepatitis virus carrier state, both of which can have much longer latencies than generally thought.

It is notable that the longest (ten years) and greatest (about 25%) reduction in cholesterol (achieved in the Program on the Surgical Control of the Hyperlipidemias [POSCH][19] trial of partial ileal bypass in middle-aged men, post AMI) showed no increase in cancer, suicide, or violent death.

Drug Treatment: What Therapy Is Best for the Hypertensive Patient in Order to Reduce CHD?

Thiazide Diuretics. For the elderly, the best-proven treatment is low-dose thiazide diuretics. These are cheap, effective against both stroke and CHD, and massively well proven in large randomized trials despite adverse effects on lipids and glucose metabolism. For the middle-aged hypertensive, both thiazide diuretics and beta-blockers are well proven.

Beta-Blockers. Cardioselective beta-blockers such as atenolol and metoprolol seem effective in both smokers and nonsmokers and have lesser adverse effects on triglycerides and HDL cholesterol than do nonselective beta-blockers. The newer vasodilating beta-blockers, such as carvedilol and celiprolol, have favorable effects on lipids but have not been adequately tested in mortality trials.

New Agents: ACE Inhibitors and Calcium Channel Blockers. One of the intriguing findings in the recent trials of

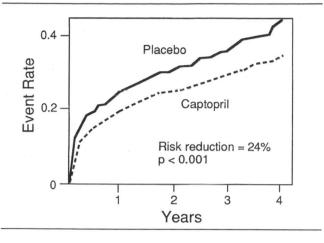

Figure 6. Life-table analysis of the 25% reduction in recurrent MI in survivors of a first MI treated with captopril (only patients who had an ejection fraction <35% after the index MI were eligible for the SAVE trial). From Pfeffer MA, Braunwald E, Moyé LA, et al. Effect of captopril on mortality and morbidity in patients with left ventricular dysfunction after myocardial infarction. N Engl J Med 1992;323:669–677. Reproduced with permission.

angiotensin-converting enzyme (ACE) inhibitors (captopril and enalapril) in the trials post AMI (such as the Survival and Ventricular Enlargement [SAVE] trial)[20] and in patients with left ventricular dysfunction (such as the Studies of Left Ventricular Dysfunction [SOLVD] trials),[21] has been the unexpected reduction in ischemic events, as well as the expected reduction in heart failure (Figure 6). This may be the result simply of the reduction in blood pressure, but it may also be due to beta-blockade of the production of angiotensin II, a growth factor for vascular smooth muscle.

It has also been claimed (from a meta-analysis of uncontrolled data)[22] that ACE inhibitors are superior to other agents in regression of left ventricular hypertrophy. However, in direct comparison with a calcium channel antagonist in a randomized, controlled trial in Belgium, there was no significant difference.

None of the trials involving calcium channel antagonists had addressed the question of long-term mortality in hypertensive patients until very recently. In stable angina, calcium antagonists control symptoms but case control studies in hypertension had suggested the possibility of harm, particularly from dihydropyridines. The unreliability of such uncontrolled data has been recently shown by the STONE[23] and Syst Eur trials,[10] both of which showed clear benefit of two different dihydropyridine calcium blockers. In post-AMI patients, verapamil significantly lowers sudden death and recurrent AMI.[24] It is, therefore, a reasonable choice among the calcium blockers for hypertensive patients. It is not generally used with beta-blockade.

We will soon have further mortality studies in hypertensive patients with both ACE inhibitors and calcium channel blockers.

CONCLUSION

We now recognize the need to treat hypertension not only as a disease of pressure alone but also as a disease of life style, genes, and environment that requires a multifactorial approach in order to address one of its major lethal consequences, coronary heart disease.

REFERENCES

1. McInnes GT, Yeo WW, Ramsay LE, Moser M. Cardiotoxicity and diuretics: Much speculation—little substance. J Hypertens 1992;10: 317–335.

2. Beilin LJ. Epitaph to essential hypertension—a preventable disorder of known etiology. J Hypertens 1988;6:85–94.

3. Collins R, Peto R, MacMahon S, et al. Blood pressure, stroke and coronary heart disease. Lancet 1990;335:827–838.

4. SHEP Cooperative Research Group. Prevention of stroke by antihypertensive drug treatment in older persons with isolated systolic hypertension. JAMA 1991;265:3255–3264.

5. Dahlöf B, Lindholm LH, Hansson L, Scherstén B, Ekbom T, Wester P-O. Morbidity and mortality in the Swedish Trial of Old Patients with Hypertension (STOP-Hypertension). Lancet 1991;338: 1281–1285.

6. Medical Research Council Working Party. MRC trial of treatment of mild hypertension: Principal results. Br Med J 1985;219:97

7. Raij L. Hypertension, endothelium and cardiovascular risk factors. Am J Med 1991;91:2S–13S.

8. MacMahon S, Peto R, Collins R. Blood pressure, stroke and coronary heart disease. Lancet 1990;335:765–774.

9. Bulpitt CJ, Palmer AJ, Fletcher AE, et al. Relation between treated blood pressure and death from ischaemic heart disease at different ages: A report from the Department of Health Hypertension Care Computing Project. J Hypertens 1992;10:1273–1278.

10. Staessen JA, Fagard R, Thijs L, Celis H, Arabidze GG, Birkenhager WH, et al. Randomised double-blind comparison of placebo and active treatment for older patients with isolated systolic hypertension. The Systolic Hypertension in Europe (Syst-Eur) Trial Investigators. Lancet 1997;350:757–764.

11. Tijs L, Fagard R, Lijnen P, et al. A meta-analysis of outcome trials in early hypertensives. J Hypertens 1992;10:1103–1109.

12. Herlitz J, Karlson BW, Richter A, et al. Prognosis in hypertensives with acute myocardial infarction. J Hypertens 1992;10:1265–1271.

13. GISSI-2. A factorial randomised trial of alteplase versus streptokinase and heparin versus no heparin among 12,490 patients with acute myocardial infarction. Lancet 1990;336:65–71.

14. ACE-inhibitor Myocardial Infarction Collaborative Group. Indications for ACE-inhibitors in the early treatment of acute myocardial infarction: systematic overview of individual data from 100,000 patients in randomized trials. Circulation 1998;97–2202-12.

15. GISSI-3 (Gruppo Italiano per lo Studio della Streptochinasi nell'Infarction Miocardico). GISSI-3: effects of lisinopril and transdermal glyceryl trinitrate singly and together on 6-week mortality and ventricular function after myocardial infarction. Lancet 1994;343:1115–1121.

16. ISIS-4 (Fourth International Study of Infarct Survival) Collaborative Group. ISIS-4 a randomised trial comparing oral captopril versus placebo, oral mononitrate versus placebo, and intra-

venous magnesium sulphate versus control among 58,050 patients with suspected acute myocardial infarction. Lancet 1995;345: 669–687.

17. Sleight P. After the diagnosis of hypertension, is risk factor management important? Am J Cardiol 1992;69:1D–4D.

18. U.S. Nurses' Health Study. N Engl J Med 1991;325:756–762.

19. Program on the Surgical Control of the Hyperlipidemias (POSCH Trial). N Engl J Med 1990;323:946–955.

20. Pfeffer MA, et al. Effect of captopril on mortality and morbidity in patients with left ventricular dysfunction after myocardial infarction. N Engl J Med 1992;323:669–677.

21. The SOLVD Investigators. Effect of enalapril on survival in patients with reduced left ventricular ejection fraction and congestive heart failure. N Engl J Med 1991;325:293–302.

22. Dahlöf B, Pennert K, Hansson L. Reversal of left ventricular hypertrophy in hypertensive patients: A meta-analysis of long treatment studies. Am J Hypertens 1992;5:95–110.

23. Gong L, Zhang W, Zhu Y, Zhu J, Kong D, Page V, Ghadirian P, et al. Shanghai trial of nifedipine in the elderly (STONE). J Hypertens 1996;14:1237–1345.

24. The Danish Verapamil Infarction Trial II—DAVIT II.Effect of verapamil on mortality and major events after acute myocardial infarction (DAVIT II). Am J Cardiol 1990;66:779–785.

CHAPTER 23

Insulin Resistance Syndrome

M. Lester
S. Khoury
James R. Sowers
Franz H. Messerli

Evidence continues to accumulate that there is an association between insulin resistance, hyperinsulinemia hypertension, and accelerated atherosclerosis.[1-7] This association results from the fact that skeletal muscle and fat lead to compensatory hyperinsulinemia which, in turn, elicits responses of the sympathetic nervous system, the kidneys and the cardiovascular system.[4,6] This concept requires that insulin resistance be selective to specific tissues, but not other tissues. However, studies over the last several years indicate that insulin, per se, does not cause hypertension.[4,6] Acutely, insulin is a vasodilator in most vascular beds, and longtime insulin infusions in dogs reduces pressor responses to vasoconstrictors and lowers blood pressure.[6] Furthermore, epidemiologic studies have not shown a relationship between plasma insulin concentrations and hypertension in Pima Indians and Mexican-Americans. However, there are now considerable data that insulin resistance interacts with other pathophysiologic factors such as salt, heightened sympathetic nervous system activity and the renin angiotensin system to promote hypertension in certain populations.[1-6]

Resistance to the actions of insulin and insulin-like growth factor (IGF-1) may promote hypertension in insulin resistant states. Insulin and IGF-1 normally causes peripheral vasodilatation, in part, through stimulation of vascular nitric oxide (NO) production.[1] The ability of insulin and IGF-1 to stimulate vascular NO production appears to be decreased in states of insulin resistance, thereby contributing to the increased incidence of hypertension in obese persons, type II diabetics, and many persons with essential hypertension. Furthermore, resistance to the vascular actions of insulin is induced by administration of the NO synthesis inhibitor L-NMMN.[1]

There is also considerable evidence that altered divalent cation metabolism contributes to the relationship between insulin resistance and hypertension.[1,2] In insulin resistant states there are increased vasoconstrictor responses in parallel with increased vascular smooth muscle cell (VSMC) intracellular calcium [Ca^{2+}]i responses. Insulin normally regulates VSMC activity of the sodium-potassium ATPase (Na, K+-ATPase) pump, and VSMC pump activity is decreased in states of insulin resistance. Reduced activity of this pump contributes to increased [Ca^{2+}]i vis-a-vis alterations in Na+-Ca^{2+} exchanges. Elevated [Ca^{2+}]i is, in turn, associated with attenuated insulin-stimulated glucose transport in several insulin-sensitive tissues. Thus, abnormal [Ca^{2+}]i regulatory mechanism may be a fundamental abnormality that contributes to increased vasoconstriction and impaired insulin action in states of insulin resistance. Abnormalities of intracellular magnesium [Mg^{2+}]i metabolism may also contribute to hypertension in states of insulin resistance. Insulin normally increases cellular-uptake of Mg^{2+}, and in states of insulin resistance that is a reduction in [Mg^{2+}]i. Depletion of tissue [Mg^{2+}]i, in turn, has been shown to lead to increases in [Ca^{2+}]i and insulin resistance. Induced, oral Mg^{2+} supplementation has been reported to improve insulin sensitivity in type II diabetic patients. Thus, elevations in [Ca^{2+}]i and depletions in [Mg^{2+}]i may contribute to vasodilatory defect as well as the glucose uptake properties of insulin and thus contribute to the association of hypertension and insulin resistance (reviewed in references 1 and 2).

Hyperinsulinemia, in conjunction with insulin resistance, has been shown in four large prospective studies to be a predictor of coronary heart disease. A recent report of a prospective study of 2,103 middle aged men from Montreal clearly showed that high fasting insulin concentrations are an independent predictor of myocardial infarction.[7] Several recent studies also reported a relationship between carotid wall atherosclerotic lesions and insulin resistance. Thus, hyperinsulinemia appears to be a predictor for the development of coronary heart disease and stroke.[8-11]

ANTIHYPERTENSIVE THERAPY

The effect of various antihypertensive drugs and drug classes on insulin resistance is variable. Although differences have been well identified from one drug class to the other, it is not entirely clear to what extent such differences will have an effect on morbidity and mortality. For instance, diuretics have been well recognized to increase insulin resistance to some extent but nevertheless in the SHEP have been shown to have distinct benefits in the subgroup of hypertensive elderly patients with diabetes.[12] Clearly, in this study the beneficial effect of blood pressure lowering of the diuretics did override the potential detrimental effect on insulin resistance. All other factors being equal, it seems, however, that antihypertensive drugs that are neutral with regard to insulin resistance or even have a favorable effect should be preferred over drugs that have been shown to reverse the effect of this metabolic abnormality. Both beta-blockers and high-dose diuretics in general have been shown to be unfavorable in patients with insulin resistance syndrome. In contrast, long-acting calcium antagonists, ACE inhibitors, angiotensin receptor blockers (ARBs), and postsynaptic alpha adrenergic blockers seem to be either neutral or to have a favorable effect. In the SYST-EUR,[13] diabetic patients treated with a calcium blocker had significantly less morbidity and mortality than the diuretic strategy. Thus, while the hypertensive patient with insulin resistance and frank diabetes remains a primary indication for an ACE inhibitor, low-dose diuretics and calcium antagonists may be employed as well. This is an important point, as most diabetic, hypertensive patients will require at least several antihypertensive medications to achieve goal blood pressure of 130/85 mm Hg.

REFERENCES

1. Sowers JR. Insulin and insulin-like growth factor in normal and pathological cardiovascular physiology. Hypertension 1997;29: 691–699.

2. Kahn AM, Song T. Effects of insulin on vascular smooth muscle contraction. In: Sowers JR, ed. Endocrinology of the Vasculature. Totowa, NJ: Humana Press; 1996:215–223.

3. Baron AD, Steinberg HO. Vascular actions of insulin in health and disease. In: Sowers JR, ed. Endocrinology of the Vasculature. Totowa, NJ: Humana Press; 1996:95–107.

4. Sowers JR, Sowers PS, Peuler JD. Role of insulin resistance and hyperinsulinemia in development of hypertension and atherosclerosis. J Lab Clin Med 1994;123:647–652.

5. Walsh MF, Dominguez LJ, Sowers JR. Metabolic abnormalities in cardiac ischemia. Cardiol Clin 1995;13:529–538.

6. Hall JE, Coleman TG, Mizelle HL, Smith MJ Jr. Chronic hyperinsulinemia and blood pressure regulation. Am J Physiol 1990;258: F722–F731.

7. Despres J-P, Lamarche B, Mauriege P, et al. Hyperinsulinemia as an independent risk factor for ischemic heart disease. N Engl J Med 1996; 334:952–957.

8. Salomaa V, Riley W, Kark JD, Nardo C, Folsom AR. Non-insulin-dependent diabetes mellitus and fasting glucose and insulin concentrations are associated with arterial stiffness indexes: the ARIC study. Atherosclerosis Risk in Communities Study. Circulation 1995;91:1432–1443.

9. Agewall S, Fagerberg B, Attvall S, Wendelhag I, Urbanavicius V, Wikstrand J. Carotid artery wall intima-media thickness is associated with insulin-mediated glucose disposal in men at high and low coronary risk. Stroke 1995;26:956–960.

10. Shinozaki K, Suzuki M, Ikebuchi M, et al. Insulin resistance associated with compensatory hyperinsulinemia as an independent risk factor for vasospastic angina. Circulation 1995;92:1749–1757.

11. Shinozaki K, Naritomi H, Shimizu T, Suzuki M, Ikebuchi M, Sawada T, Harano Y. Role of insulin resistance associated with compensatory hyperinsulinemia in ischemic stroke. Stroke 1996;27:37–43.

12. SHEP Cooperative Research Group. Prevention of stroke by antihypertensive drug treatment in older persons with isolated systolic hypertension: Final results of the systolic hypertension in the elderly program (SHEP). JAMA 1991;265:3255–3264.

13. Staessen JA, Fagard R, Thijs L, et al. Randomised double-blind comparison of placebo and active treatment for older patients with isolated systolic hypertension. The Systolic Hypertension in Europe (Syst-Eur) Trial Investigators. Lancet 1997;350:757–764.

CHAPTER 24

Hypertension and Stroke

J. David Spence
Olaf B. Paulson
Svend Strandgaard

Hypertension affects nearly 40% of people in the United States by age 60,[1] and by age 70 there are approximately 1,000 stroke deaths per 100,000 population, costing more than a billion dollars per annum in the United States.[2]

Protection of the brain against stroke has been a major achievement of antihypertensive therapy. The picture of hypertensive stroke is changing dramatically with effective detection and treatment of hypertension.[3] These changes could be observed in London, Ontario, because the installation of the first computerized axial tomography (CAT) scanner at Victoria Hospital in 1976 was followed two years later by the initiation of a large hypertension detection and treatment program by the University of Western Ontario Department of Family Medicine.[4] In the mid 1970's, 500 patients per year were being admitted to that hospital with stroke. By 1977, with the improved diagnostic accuracy resulting from routine use of CAT scanning, it was apparent that half of the strokes were a consequence of hypertension; of these, approximately three quarters were due to lacunar infarction. In the Family Medicine study,[5] 34 physicians followed 32,124 patients for a period of five years, and special hypertension assistants were assigned to half the practices with a view to improving detection and treatment of hypertension, beginning 1978. By 1983, 94% of hypertensive patients in the London area were detected, 92% were on treatment, and 72% were well controlled. By 1984, despite an increase in the population by nearly one third from the late 1970s, and some aging of population, the number of stroke patients admitted to our hospital was down to 250 per year, and there had been a marked change in the composition of the stroke population: fewer than 10% of cases were now a consequence of hypertension. In contrast, strokes due to cerebral atherosclerosis (mainly extracranial carotid disease) had gone from 35% of 500 per year to 70% of 250 per year. That is, there had been no reduction in atherosclerotic stroke despite a dramatic decline in strokes due to hypertensive arteriolar disease.

To understand these events is to understand the nature of hypertensive stroke, as described by Pickering[6] and Russell,[7] who pointed out that strokes resulting from high blood pressure were due to hemorrhage and lacunar infarction caused by hypertensive arteriolar disease, and that treatment of hypertension should, therefore, prevent only that type of stroke.

The management of hypertension and stroke is critically based on understanding of two issues. First, as shown in Figure 1, the effects of blood pressure in the brain are predominantly on arterioles branching off the short, straight arteries perfusing the base of the brain (called the "vascular centrencephalon" by Hachinski and Norris).[8] Second, the physiology of cerebral vascular autoregulation dictates a special approach to the management of hypertensive encephalopathy. Furthermore, occasionally overzealous antihypertensive treatment may cause or aggravate cerebral ischemia. Thus, therapy may provoke the very event that it was meant to prevent.

THE CONCEPT OF AUTOREGULATION OF CEREBRAL BLOOD FLOW

Cerebral blood flow (CBF) is normally autoregulated; that is, within wide limits kept constant during variations in blood pressure or, more strictly, perfusion pressure (blood pressure minus intracranial pressure). There is a lower and an upper limit of autoregulation. Below a mean blood pressure of 60 mm Hg to 70 mm Hg, cerebral vasodilation is inadequate and CBF decreases. Above a mean blood pressure of around 150 mm Hg, autoregulatory vasoconstriction gives way to pressure-forced vasodilation.[9]

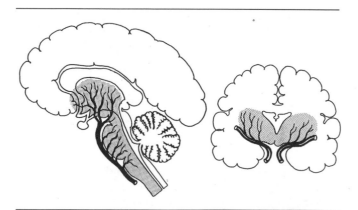

Figure 1. Vascular centrencephalon. The mesial and basal portions of the brain and brain stem are perfused by short, straight arteries from the ventral surface, penetrating in the dorsal direction; gradation between arterial and capillary pressure occurs over a short distance with few branches, so that pressures to which arterioles are exposed are not dissipated to the same extent as in the newer parts of the brain. Drawn from Hachinski VC. The acute stroke. *Philadelphia:FA Davis, 1985:2740.*

Hypertensive Adaptation of CBF Autoregulation

In chronic hypertension, the level of CBF is the same as in normotension, around 50 mL/100 g/min. Hypertension does, however, profoundly influence CBF autoregulation by shifting both the lower and upper limits toward high pressure (Figures 2 and 3).[9-11] This is presumably due to hyper-

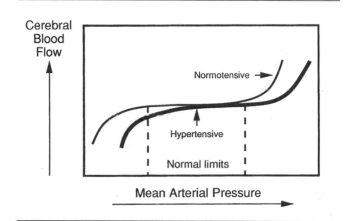

Figure 2. *Adaptation of the lower and upper limit of autoregulation of cerebral blood flow to chronic hypertension.*

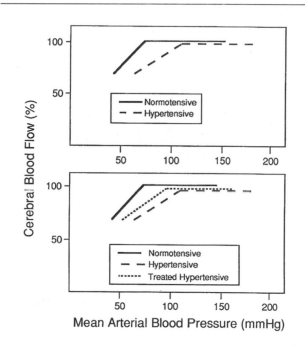

Figure 3. *Adaptation of the lower limit of autoregulation of cerebral blood flow to chronic hypertension and the effect of long-term antihypertensive treatment. From Strandgaard S,* Circulation *1976;53:720–727.*

tensive structural vascular adaptation and remodeling with arteriolar narrowing and vessel wall thickening. The shift of autoregulation on the one side impairs the potential for vasodilation and hence the patient's tolerance to blood pressure reduction; at the same time, this shift improves the patient's tolerance of acutely raised blood pressure.

HYPERTENSION AND INTRACRANIAL PRESSURE

Intracranial pressure is normally 10 mm Hg to 15 mm Hg. Perfusion pressure in the brain is the difference between blood pressure and intracranial pressure. Because intracranial pressure is normally quite low, it can be ignored when autoregulation is discussed. However, in malignant hypertension, intracranial pressure is frequently elevated, and perfusion pressure may differ somewhat from blood pressure. In hypertensive encephalopathy, brain edema is probably due to autoregulatory failure beyond the upper blood pressure limit, and intracranial pressure is elevated.[9-11] As discussed below, some antihypertensive drugs may increase intracranial pressure.

ATHEROSCLEROSIS, CBF, AND BLOOD PRESSURE

Atheroma frequently narrows the larger cerebral resistance vessels. Distal to a vascular stenosis, blood pressure may be low, and the cerebral arterioles react to this with autoregulatory dilation, thus maintaining normal blood flow. Even with a reduced local blood flow distal to a stenosis, the tissue may survive by extracting more oxygen from the blood, so-called "chronic threatening ischemia."[9] If systemic blood pressure is lowered by antihypertensive treatment, blood pressure distal to the stenosis may fall critically, and as autoregulation is exhausted in the resting state, focal cerebral ischemia may be the result. Atheroma is common in the cerebral arterial system, but most often it is not hemodynamically significant. Even if the atherosclerotic lesion in the single vessel is severe, blood pressure and flow distal to the lesion may still be adequate due to the presence of collateral circulation. This may explain why focal cerebral ischemia is so seldom provoked by treatment of mild-to-moderate hypertension.

Cerebral vasodilators may cause a "steal" of blood flow away from an area of chronic threatening or manifest ischemia even if they do not lower the blood pressure.[12] This is brought about by vasodilation of the surrounding, normally perfused brain tissue; the vasodilator is unable to further dilate the vessels and to increase blood flow distal to the stenosis in the area of chronic threatening or manifest ischemia.

ACUTE BLOOD PRESSURE LOWERING AND THE CEREBRAL CIRCULATION

When the blood pressure is lowered acutely by a drug, two kinds of response can be anticipated from the cerebral circulation. First, if blood pressure is lowered moderately, auto-regulation will tend to keep CBF constant. If the pressure is taken below the lower limit of autoregulation, CBF will fall. Second, this response may be modified by specific pharmacologic effects of the various antihypertensive drugs on the cerebral vessels.

Based on their cerebrovascular pharmacology, drugs used for emergency blood pressure lowering can be divided into the following groups.[11]

Cerebral Vasodilators

Dihydralazine, hydralazine and sodium nitroprusside are examples of cerebral vasodilators. When dihydralazine is injected intravenously in normotensive volunteers, a transient, rather marked rise in CBF is induced.[13] In neurosurgical patients with intracranial pressure monitoring, dihydralazine causes a rise in the already elevated intracranial pressure.[14] In the rat, the drug causes paralysis of autoregulation[15] (Figure 4). Thus continuous infusion of large doses of dihydralazine may cause headache and other more serious symptoms of raised intracranial pressure. Sodium nitroprusside may similarly cause impairment of CBF autoregulation and a rise in intracranial pressure.[16] Cerebral vasodilators should not be used in acute stroke, and should only be used

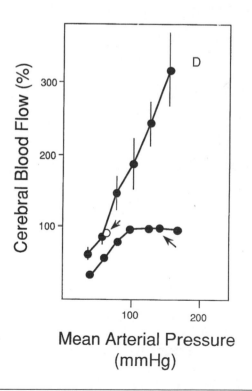

Figure 4. *Paralyzing effect of dihydralazine (D) on autoregulation of cerebral blood flow in spontaneously hypertensive rats. Normal curve is shown for comparison. Modified from Barry DI and Strandgaard S. Progr Appl Microcirc 1985;8:206–212.*

with the utmost care in a hypertensive cerebral crisis, where intracranial pressure may be high, as discussed below.

Calcium Antagonists

Calcium antagonists may cause some increase in intracranial pressure and some impairment of autoregulation.[17] This may explain why patients sometimes experience headache as a side effect. Generally, however, calcium antagonists have much less effect on the cerebral circulation than do other cerebral vasodilators. In ischemic stroke, calcium antagonists have the potential to cause a steal of blood flow away from ischemic tissue.[18] Thus, the beneficial effect of calcium antagonists reported in experimental stroke may by cytoprotective rather than hemodynamic. In clinical stroke the effect of calcium antagonists have been disappointing.

Angiotensin-Converting Enzyme (ACE) Inhibitors

ACE inhibitors have a unique effect on the cerebral circulation. They do not raise the level of CBF but appear to dilate the larger cerebral resistance vessels.[19] This large-vessel dilation is added to the autoregulatory dilation of the small arteries and arterioles. The net result is that the lower limit of autoregulation is shifted toward lower pressure, improving the patient's tolerance of hypotension (Figure 5). This effect probably explains why heart failure patients can tolerate surprisingly low blood pressures when treated with ACE inhibitors.

Angiotensin II Antagonists

These agents are increasingly used in the treatment of hypertension and heart failure. They appear to have the same beneficial effect in the cerebral circulation as the ACE-inhibitors.[20]

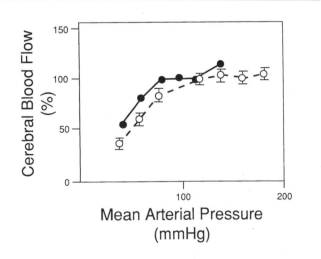

Figure 5. Captopril (solid line) shifts the lower limit of autoregulation toward lower pressure in spontaneously hypertensive rats. Modified from Barry DI, et al. Hypertens 1984;2:589-597.

Alpha-Adrenergic and Ganglionic Blocking Agents

These drugs abolish the weak constricting effect of the alpha-adrenergic perivascular nerves in the larger, "inflow tract" resistance vessels in the brain. This effect is similar to that of the ACE inhibitors. The alpha-blockers and the alpha-beta-blocker labetalol do not impair CBF autoregulation and do not cause an increase in intracranial pressure.[21]

Drugs without Pharmacologic Effects in the Cerebral Circulation

Diazoxide, which, to some extent, has gone out of clinical use, is the best studied of this group of drugs. It may be presumed that these agents are unable to penetrate the endothelial blood-brain barrier and reach the cerebral vascular smooth muscle cells.[22]

CHRONIC ANTIHYPERTENSIVE TREATMENT AND THE CEREBRAL CIRCULATION

When the blood pressure is lowered chronically by drugs, just as with acute pressure lowering, CBF may stay constant if the blood pressure remains above the lower limit of autoregulation; cerebrovascular pharmacologic effects of the drugs may modify this response. Chronic blood pressure lowering may also cause a partial or complete readaptation of CBF autoregulation to the reduced pressure (see Figure 3).[11] A group of well-treated hypertensive patients had values for the lower limit of CBF autoregulation overlapping both normotensive and uncontrolled hypertensive persons.[23] In animal studies, hypertensive cerebrovascular adaptation can be normalized during a two-month course of antihypertensive treatment.

The chronic effects of antihypertensive drugs in the cerebral circulation have not been studied as extensively as the acute effects described above. It has been shown, for instance, that treatment for a couple of weeks or months with a diuretic, an ACE inhibitor, or an alpha-blocker causes a modest fall in blood pressure and no change in CBF. In patients with heart failure, chronic ACE inhibitor treatment, as mentioned earlier, often causes very low blood pressure, which is well tolerated;[24] this presumably is caused by the dilatory effect on larger resistance vessels also seen in acute studies. The headache experienced by some patients during chronic treatment with calcium antagonists may be due to cerebral vasodilation and possibly a somewhat raised intracranial pressure.

HYPERTENSIVE ENCEPHALOPATHY

Giese[25] showed that during severe hypertensive crisis, the apparent vasospasm that can be observed experimentally is probably the normal response to markedly increased pressure, as part of autoregulation of blood flow to various tissues. As Giese showed, and Skinhoj, Strandgaard, Lassen, and others confirmed,[25-27] apparent areas of vasodilation are the injured part of the arteriole, while the "spastic" segments are normal. Hypertensive encephalopathy appears to be the result of forced vasodilation due to failure of cerebral autoregulation, markedly increased cerebral blood flow, engorgement of the brain, and cerebral edema. These changes are associated with areas of cerebral ischemia due to fibrinoid necrosis and occlusion of some small vessels. The occipital cortex appears to be particularly susceptible to edema, perhaps accounting for the cortical blindness and flashing lights that lead to the name of this syndrome when it is seen in association with pregnancy (eclampsia).

There are two sources of diagnostic confusion in the management of hypertensive encephalopathy. One is the belief that papilledema is a *sine qua non* of the diagnosis. This is untrue; the development of papilledema takes time, and patients with sudden elevation of blood pressure can present with hypertensive encephalopathy before the development of papilledema. A second confusion is the belief that for hypertensive encephalopathy to be present, the pressures must be very high (240/140 mm Hg or greater). This is untrue for patients who were previously normotensive; it is not uncommon for young women, whose pressures before and early in pregnancy were at levels such as 100/70 mm Hg, to develop hypertensive encephalopathy in the setting of eclampsia, with blood pressures as low as 160/100 mm Hg.

These patients illustrate an important point: The pressure at which cerebral autoregulation fails is determined by the pressure level to which the individual's arterioles have been exposed in the recent past. Thus, patients with premorbid pressures at a low normal level will experience failure of cerebral autoregulation at modestly elevated pressures, whereas patients with long-standing severe hypertension will tolerate much higher pressures, presumably because of structural adaptation of the arterioles to high pressure, as suggested by Folkow,[28] Baumbach and Heistad[29] and others. Thus, in the clinic of JDS, two patients have walked in, with no symptoms or signs of any significant problem, with blood pressures greater than 300/170 mm Hg.

Treatment of Severely Elevated Blood Pressure in the Patient without Symptoms

A patient with a diastolic blood pressure above around 115 mm Hg who is newly diagnosed should be evaluated quickly for target organ damage as well as for secondary hypertension, and treatment should be started gently with e.g., a thiazide diuretic or a calcium antagonist, followed later by other agents. The goal should be around 25 % reduction of the blood pressure in the initial phase of treatment. A patient with a blood pressure of 240/140 thus should be treated to a level of around 180/105. As a precaution against over-treatment, treatment should attempt to keep diastolic blood pressure above around 100 mm Hg. Over weeks to months, blood pressure can be lowered further, and ultimately may be normalized. Patients with severe hypertension should be carefully investigated for renal artery stenosis, pheochromocytoma or adrenocortical hypertension. A stimulated plasma renin level can be a very useful indicator of the underlying cause of hypertension: patients with abnormally low nonstimulable plasma renin usually have adrenocortical hyperplasia, whereas patients with renovascular hypertension will have a high stimulated level of plasma renin. Because of the risk of acute renal failure, ACE inhibitors and angiotensin II receptor antagonists should be used with caution if renovascular hypertension is suspected.

Patients with minimal or no symptoms of their very high blood pressure should under no circumstances be given emergency parenteral antihypertensive treatment. Sublingual or oral nifedipine, a popular treatment in many emergency rooms, should be avoided as it may cause uncontrollable hypotension leading to stroke or myocardial infarction.[30] One of the authors (JDS) is aware of three strokes caused by sublingual nifedipine. In fact, the use of the term "sublingual" is a misnomer for nifedipine, as absorption from the buccal mucosa is very slow; the drug has to be swallowed before it can be absorbed.[31] Over-treatment of the blood pressure with any drug may cause cerebral ischemia and provoke a stroke. Acute blindness seems to be a particularly common symptom following drastic blood pressure lowering. A diagnostic procedure such as angiography can also cause an additional dangerous fall in blood pressure in a patient with treated severe hypertension[33] (figures 6 and 7).

Treatment of Acute Hypertensive Encephalopathy

In the rare patients with acute hypertensive encephalopathy, the blood pressure should be controlled by parenterally given drugs. The first phase of treatment should aim for around 25 % reduction of blood pressure. Sublingual nifedipine should not be used for the reasons discussed above, and the start of oral antihypertensive treatment should wait till the patient has stabilized clinically.

We recommend parenteral treatment with the alpha-beta blocker labetalol, or with an infusion of diazoxide (without a bolus), for such patients. If there are signs of heart failure, a loop diuretic such as furosemide may also be given. Where beta-blockers are thought to be contra-indicated (heart failure, asthma) an infusion of diazoxide may be preferred. For patients with angina or aortic dissection, labetolol is preferred. Cerebral vasodilators such as dihydralazine and sodium nitroprusside may be used, but their paralyzing effect on CBF autoregulation should be kept in mind, and patients with hypertensive crises who are given these drugs should be observed carefully for signs of a rising intracranial pressure.

HYPERTENSIVE STROKES

The reader is referred to recent extensive reviews for illustrations and references in this area.[36,37] In brief, hypertension

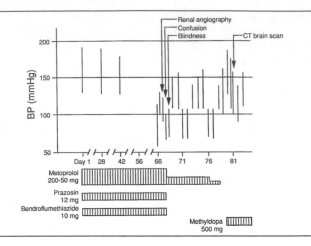

Figure 6. *Clinical course in a 28-year-old man with renovascular hypertension and treatment-related cerebral ischemia. During outpatient control, blood Pressure was high, possibly because of poor compliance with drug intake. Upon admission (day 66), blood pressure was normal. A few days later, renal angiography caused transient hypotension, leading to irreversible blindness. For result of computed tomography scan, see Figure 6. Modified from Strandgaard S, et al. Acta Med Scand 1984;216:417–422.*

leads to the sudden onset of focal neurologic dysfunction (stroke) in two ways, hypertensive intracerebral hemorrhage or lacunar infarction.

Hypertensive intracerebral hemorrhage is due to rupture of cerebral microaneurysms, while lacunar infarction is due to occlusion of arterioles or small arteries by fibrinoid necrosis and/or hyaline degeneration. Both kinds of event tend to be located in the thalamus, basal ganglia, pons, or cerebellum, corresponding to the distribution of the vascular centrencephalon.

The effective detection and treatment of hypertension has markedly reduced hypertensive intracerebral hemorrhage to the point that, in the practice of JDS, intracerebral hemorrhage is now less likely to be due to hypertension than to amyloid angiopathy, a condition of the elderly, sometimes associated with Alzheimer's disease.[38] These hemorrhages occur characteristically at the junction of cortex and white matter, often in the posterior lobes.[39]

In our opinion, the term *lacunar infarction* should be reserved for strokes due to hypertensive small vessel disease; unfortunately, because of the advent of brain imaging by CAT scanning and magnetic resonance imaging, there is an increasing tendency to label any small, deep lesion of the white matter seen on brain tomography as a lacune, whether or not the patient has significant hypertension, and whether or not there is another more likely cause of the focal ischemia, such as embolization from a known ipsilateral carotid stenosis.[40] This appears to be the most common diagnostic error in stroke. This trend is unfortunate because the appropriate management of stroke depends on diagnosis; for patients with true lacunar infarction, the appropriate management is effective control of hypertension, whereas

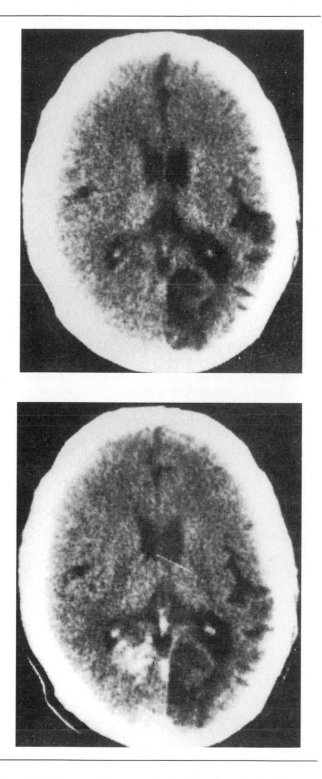

Figure 7. Brain computed tomography scan from the patient in Figure 5, obtained 17 days after hypotensive insult with loss of vision, before (top) and after (bottom) contrast injection. A huge infarct is seen in the right occipital lobe. Following contrast injection, linear enhancement is seen in the left occipital lobe, suggesting an infarct here as well. From Strandgaard S, et al. Acta Med Scand 1984;216:417-422.

for patients with symptomatic severe carotid stenosis, the appropriate management is endarterectomy.[41] For patients with symptomatic moderate stenosis the results will be known soon; for asymptomatic severe stenosis the benefit with surgery is only marginal in hospitals with excellent (low) complication rates of 3%, and is non-existent in hospitals with average complication rates.[42]

One possible confounding condition in diagnosis is leuko-airaiosis, described recently by Hachinski et al.[43] This condition may be related to hypertensive arteriolar thickening with reduced autoregulatory reserve, combined with episodes of relative hypotension. This concept is similar to one postulated by Floras,[44] in relation to nocturnal hypotension in patients with reduced myocardial reserve, as a possible explanation for the J-shaped curve of vascular risk.[45,46]

HYPERTENSION AND ATHEROSCLEROTIC STROKE

Now that the arteriolar complications of hypertension are largely being prevented by effective detection and treatment of hypertension, the remaining challenge is the prevention of atherosclerotic complications. Antihypertensive drugs have effects on many other factors besides pressure, which may influence the development of atherosclerosis and its complications, including effects on lipoproteins, flow disturbances, and platelets. The reader is referred to recent reviews for extensive discussion of these issues.[36,37] A particularly important area with respect to stroke prevention is hypertension in the elderly, as it has recently been shown that treatment of isolated systolic hypertension significantly reduces stroke and myocardial infarction.

Stamler[47] has recently reviewed the issue of hypertension in the elderly in the light of the Systolic Hypertension in the Elderly Program (SHEP) study,[48] saying "The optimal systolic blood pressure (SBP) for adults is a level under 118 mm Hg, and the relationship of systolic blood pressure to risk is continuous, strong, graded and exponential; risk is significantly increased for the 80% of the population who have SBP above optimal...and not just for those with frank hypertension."

As in the SHEP study, most experts would agree that small doses of thiazide (such as 12.5 mg daily of hydrochlorothiazide) would be the treatment of choice for systolic hypertension in the elderly; it is important to keep the dose low to minimize adverse effects such as potassium depletion, gout, glucose intolerance, and aggravation of hyperlipidemia. In a commentary on recent literature, Kaplan[49] suggested that a dose of hydrochlorothiazide of 10 mg to 12.5 mg should be about right," and speculated that doses as low as 6.25 mg may be suitable. Salt restriction also minimizes potassium depletion, and in patients with significant problems of potassium depletion it is useful to know the stimulated plasma renin status.[35,36,50]

Beta-adrenergic blockers, by reducing heart rate, may aggravate systolic hypertension because the increased stroke volume, in combination with a stiff vascular tree, widens pulse pressure. Therefore, addition of a vasodilator such as hydralazine or a dihydropyridine (e.g., amlodipine, felodipine,nifedipine) may be preferable to a beta-blocker without vasodilators in patients with high diastolic pressures who do not respond to a diuretic alone. This may be important if Christensen's finding[51] that reduction of pulse pressure is necessary to normalize small artery structure translates from rats to the human condition.

Elderly Hypertensive Patients

Over-treatment of hypertension may occur in elderly persons whose cerebral circulation does not readily readapt when the blood pressure is lowered. It is likely that the risk of over treating hypertension in the elderly is restricted to patients with postural hypotension, or those in whom apparent high blood pressure is due to stiffening of the artery wall.

A special problem in the management of hypertension in the elderly is the error in blood pressure measurement related to stiff arteries. Among patients over 60 who have high diastolic pressures but no signs of end-organ disease, approximately one half will have a false elevation of the diastolic pressure by 30 mm Hg or more. The problem of pseudohypertension, sometimes detected by the Osler maneuver,[52] has been reviewed recently.[53]

Pseudohypertension may account for a number of elderly patients who do not seem to tolerate reduction of blood pressure toward normal and who suffer symptoms suggesting hypotension at relatively normal pressures. For the most part, however, even elderly patients with hypertension can be successfully treated; the approach is to use small doses of medication, increase doses cautiously and conservatively, and consider the possibility of secondary hypertension in patients who are resistant to treatment.[50] Since the advent of balloon angioplasty, renovascular hypertension is a common, readily treatable cause of severe, resistant hypertension in the elderly.

MANAGEMENT OF THE PATIENT WITH HYPERTENSION AND A STROKE

High Blood Pressure in Acute Stroke

The presentation to the emergency room of a patient with a stroke and high blood pressure is a common conundrum. The key to management of acute stroke is diagnosis; this issue has been reviewed elsewhere.[54] It is often not immediately obvious whether the stroke was caused by the hypertension or whether the blood pressure is being aggravated by the autonomic reactions that sometimes attend large hemisphere infarctions or brain-stem infarctions.

About 70% of patients with acute stroke have high blood pressure when admitted to the hospital. In most cases, the blood pressure falls spontaneously, and four days later only about 50% of patients are hypertensive.[55] A few patients with acute stroke have very high blood pressures, 120 mm Hg diastolic or higher. It has been much debated whether these very high pressures should be treated acutely. Leaving the blood pressures untreated might cause hemorrhage into ischemic infarcts, or might aggravate edema secondary to ischemia. Conversely, lowering the blood pressure might further threaten the perfusion of ischemic but viable tissue around an infarct (Figure 8). Undoubtedly, in some cases, high blood pressure maintains collateral perfusion in ischemic tissue distal to a vascular occlusion, and can be understood as a homeostatic reaction (Figure 9).

Frequently, it is recommended that hypertension not be treated in the setting of cerebral ischemia because of concern that relative hypotension may aggravate the process and enlarge the stroke by imperiling the perfusion of the

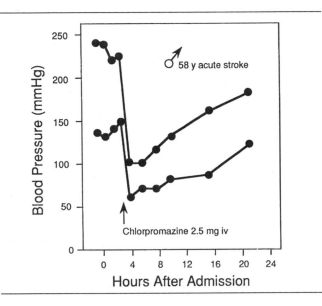

Figure 8. *Drastic fall in blood pressure in a patient with acute stroke following a small intravenous dose of chlorpromazine. No change in the patient's necrologic deficit was reported following the hypotensive episode.*

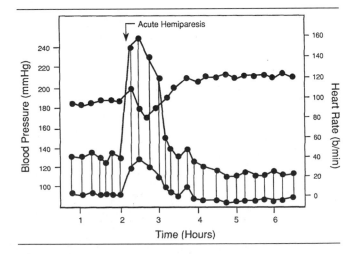

Figure 9. *Severely hypertensive response to an embolic stroke in a 57 year-old woman one week after myocardial infarction. Modified from Gottstein U. Med Welt 1965;15:715–726.*

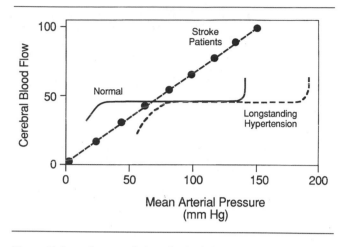

Figure 10. *Loss of autoregulation of crebral blood flow in acute stroke. In patients with long-standing severe hypertension, higher pressures are tolerated and normal pressures are less well tolerated than in normal subjects; in patients with cerebral ischemia, cerebral perfusion becomes dependent on perfusion pressure.*

ischemic penumbra—i.e., the area surrounding the infarction, in which autoregulation is precarious (see Figure 10)—and perfusion pressure is reduced because of increased tissue pressure from edema.

Counterarguments in favor of treating blood pressure judiciously in the setting of cerebral ischemia lie in two areas. First, associated conditions coexist with cerebral ischemia in a number of patients, mandating treatment of hypertension. These include aortic dissection, which can cause cerebral ischemia by picking off the origin of a carotid artery; myocardial ischemia and/or congestive heart failure, which will be aggravated by severe hypertension; and the presence of a known cerebral berry aneurysm, which may rupture if pressures are left too high.

Second, some aspects of the pathogenesis of progressive cerebral ischemia, related to cerebral edema in the ischemic zone and its surrounds, mandate that severe hypertension be controlled because edema will be aggravated by excess pressure in the zone of impaired autoregulation. For these reasons, to say that hypertension should not be treated in patients with cerebral ischemia is too simplistic; some patients with very high pressures must be treated. In those circumstances, the appropriate management is to carefully lower the pressure with intravenous drugs, as described for patients with hypertensive encephalopathy. Diuretics should probably only be given in cases of concomitant heart failure because many stroke patients are already somewhat dehydrated upon hospital admission.

There is a need for controlled clinical trials to settle this controversy, which until now is purely a matter of opinion.

REFERENCES

1. Stamler J. High blood pressure in the United States an overview of the problem and the challenge. In: Proceedings of the National

Conference on High Blood Pressure Education. National Heart and Lung Institute. U.S. Department of Health, Education and Welfare publication number (NIH) 73486, 1973:11.

2. Kurtzke JF. Epidemiology of cerebrovascular disease. In: McDowell FH, Caplan LR, eds. Cerebrovascular survey report, National Institute of Neurological and Communicative Disorders and Stroke, 1985:1–34.

3. Spence JD. Antihypertensive therapy and prevention of atherosclerotic stroke. Stroke 1986;17:808–810.

4. Bass MJ, McWhinney IR, Donner A. Do family physicians need medical assistants to detect and manage hypertension? Can Med Assoc J 1986;134:1247–1255.

5. Birkett NJ, Donner A. Prevalence and control of hypertension in an Ontario county. Can Med Assoc J 1985;132:1019–1024.

6. Pickering G. *Hypertension: Causes, consequences and management.* London: Churchill-Livingstone, 1974:4042.

7. Russell RWR. How does high blood pressure cause stroke? Lancet 1975;2:1283–1285.

8. Hachinski VC, Norris JW. The vascular infrastructure. In: Hachinski VC and Norris JW, eds. The acute stroke. Philadelphia: F.A. Davis, 1985 27–40.

9. Paulson OB, Strandgaard S, Edvinsson L. Cerebral autoregulation. Cerebrovasc Brain Metab Rev 1990;2:161–192.

10. Paulson OB, Waldemar G, Schmidt JF, Strandgaard S. Cerebral circulation under normal and pathologic conditions. Am J Cardiol 1989;63:2C–5C.

11. Paulson OB, Strandgaard S Hypertensive disease and the cerebral circulation. In: Laragh JH, Brenner BM, eds. *Hypertension. Pathophysiology, diagnosis and management.* 2nd ed. New York: Raven, 1995:448–463.

12. Paulson OB. Cerebral apoplexy (stroke). Pathogenesis, pathophysiology and therapy as illustrated by regional blood flow measurements in the brain. Stroke 1971;2:327–360.

13. Schroeder T, Sillesen H. Dihydralazine induces marked cerebral vasodilatation in man. Eur J Clin Invest 1987;17:214–217.

14. Overgaard J, Skinhøj E. A paradoxical cerebral haemodynamic effect of hydralazine. Stroke 1975;6:402–404.

15. Barry DI, Strandgaard S. Acute effects of antihypertensive drugs on autoregulation of cerebral blood flow in spontaneously hypertensive rats. Progr Appl Microcirc 1985;8:206–212.

16. McDowall DG. Drugs and cerebral autoregulation. Eur J Clin Invest 1982;12:377–378.

17. Schmidt JF, Albeck M, Gjerris F. The effect of nimodipine on intracranial pressure and cerebral blood flow in patients with normal-pressure hydrocephalus. Acta Neurochir 1990A;102:11–13.

18. Vorstrup S, Andersen A, Blegvad N, Paulson OB. Calcium antagonist (PY 108–068) treatment may further decrease flow in ischemic areas in acute stroke. J Cereb Blood Flow Metabol 1986; 6:222–229.

19. Paulson OB, Waldemar G, Andersen AR, Barry DI, Pedersen EV, Schmidt JF. Role of angiotensin in autoregulation of cerebral blood flow. Circulation 1988;77 (Suppl. I):I55–158.

20 Vraamark T, Waldemar G, Strandgaard S, Paulson OB. Angiotensin II receptor antagonist CV-11974 and cerebral blood flow autoregulation. J Hypertens 1995;13:755–761.

21. Olsen KS, Svendsen LB, Larsen F. S., Paulson O. B. Effect of labetalol on cerebral blood flow, oxygen metabolism and autoregulation in healthy humans. Brit J Anaest 1995;75:51–54.

22. Barry DI, Strandgaard S, Graham DI, Brændstrup O, Svendsen UG, Bolwig TG. Effect of diaxozide induced hypotension on cerebral blood flow in hypertensive rats. Eur J Clin Invest 1983;13:201–207.

23. Strandgaard S. Autoregulation of cerebral blood flow in hypertensive patients. The modifying influence of prolonged antihypertensive treatment on the tolerance to acute, drug- induced hypotension. Circulation 1976;53:720–727.

24. Paulson OB, Jarden J O, Godtfredsen J, Vorstrup S. Cerebral blood flow in patients with congestive heart failure treated with captopril. Amer J Med 1984;76:5B:91–95.

25. Giese J. Acute hypertensive vascular disease. 2. Studies on vascular reaction patterns and permeability changes by means of vital microscopy and colloidal tracer technique. Acta Pathol Microbiol Scand 1964;62:497–517.

26. Skinhoj E, Strandgaard S. Pathogenesis of hypertensive encephalopathy. Lancet 1973;1:461–462.

27. Strandgaard S, Olesen J, Skinhoj E, et al. Autoregulation of brain circulation in severe arterial hypertension. Br Med J 1973;1:507–510.

28. Folkow B. Structural factors: The vascular wall. Consequences of treatment. Hypertension. 1983;5(Suppl. 111):58–62.

29. Baumbach GL, Heistad DD. Adaptive changes in cerebral blood vessels during chronic hypertension. J Hypertens 1991;9:987–991.

30. Grossman E, Messerli FH, Grodzicki T, Kowey P. Should a moratorium be placed on sublingual nifedipine capsules given for hypertensive emergencies and pseudoemergencies? JAMA. 1996;276: 1328–1331.

31. van Harten J, Burggraaf K, Danhof M, et al. Negligible sublingual absorption of nifedipine. Lancet 1987;2:1363–1365.

32. Strandgaard S, Andersen GS, Ahlgreen P, Nielsen PE. Visual disturbances and occipital brain infarct following acute, transient hypotension in hypertensive patients. Acta Med Scand 1984;216:417–422

33. Levitt AD, Zweiffler AJ. Nifedipine, hypotension and myocardial injury. Ann Intern Med 1988;108:305–306.

34. Spence JD, Del Maestro RF. Hypertension in acute strokes. Treat Arch Neurol 1985;42:1000–1002.

35. Spence JD, Spence JD. Management of hypertensive emergencies. Can J Diagn 1992;9:72–93.

36. Spence JD, Hachinski VC. Neurological complications of hypertension. In: Goetz CG, Tanner CM, Aminoff MJ, eds. Handbook of clinical neurology. Amsterdam: Elsevier, 1993;19:71–91.

37. Spence JD, Arnold JMO, Gilbert n. Consequences of hypertension and effects of antihypertensive therapy. In: Robertson JIS, ed. *Handbook of hypertension*. Amsterdam: Elsevier, 1992;15:621–654.

38. Gilbert N, Vinters HV. Cerebral amyloid angiopathy: Incidence and complications in the aging brain. i: Cerebral hemorrhage. Stroke 1983;14:915–923.

39. Vinters HV, Gilbert JJ. Cerebral amyloid angiopathy: Incidence and complications in the aging brain. ii. The distribution of amyloid vascular changes. Stroke 1983;14:924–928.

40. Tegeler CH, Fenglin S, Morgan T. Carotid stenosis in lacunar stroke. Stroke 1991;22:1124–1128 (See also Mazagri R, Hrapchak M, Denath F, et al. The type of TIA does not predict the degree of carotid stenosis. Can J Neurol Sci 1991;19:249.)

41. Barnett HJM. Symptomatic carotid artery stenosis: A solvable problem. Stroke 1992;23:1048–1053.

42. Toole JF, Hobson RW, Howard VJ, et al. Nearing the finish line?: The asymptomatic carotid atherosclerosis study. Stroke 1992; 4:1054–1055.

43. Hachinski VC, Potter P, Merskey PH. Leuko-araiosis: An ancient term for a new problem. Can J Neurol Sci 1987;13:533–534.

44. Floras JS. Antihypertensive treatment, myocardial infarction, and nocturnal myocardial ischemia. Lancet 1988;2:994–996.

45. Berglund G. Goals of antihypertensive therapy: Is there a point beyond which pressure reduction is dangerous? Am J Hypertens 1989;2:586–593.

46. Fletcher AE, Bulpitt CJ. How far should blood pressure be lowered? N Eng J Med 1992;326;251–254.

47. Stamler J. Research opportunities and directions on the blood pressure problem. Am J Hypertens 1991;4:646S–660S.

48. SHEP Cooperative Research Group. Prevention of stroke by antihypertensive drug treatment in older persons with isolated systolic hypertension. Final results of the Systolic Hypertension in the Elderly Program. (SHEP). JAMA 1991;265:3255–3264.

49. Kaplan NM. The case for low dose diuretic therapy. Am J Hypertens 1991;4:970–971.

50. Spence JD. Stepped care therapy for hypertension is dead, but what will replace it? Can Med Assoc J 1989;140:1133–1136.

51. Christensen KL. Reducing pulse pressure in hypertension may normalize small artery structure. Hypertension 1991;18:722–727.

52. Messerli FH, Ventura HO, Amodeo C. Osler's maneuver and pseudohypertension: N Engl J Med 1985;312:1548–1551.

53. Spence JD. Pseudohypertension. In: Laragh JH, Brenner BM, eds. *Hypertension: Pathophysiology, diagnosis and management*. New York: Raven 1990:1407–1414.

54. Spence JD. Ischemic cerebrovascular disease. In: Rakel RE, ed. *Conn's current therapy*. Philadelphia: Saunders, 1993;844–847.

55. Britton M, Carlsson A, de Faire U. Blood pressure course in patients with acute stroke and matched controls. Stroke 1986;17: 861–864.

CHAPTER 25

The Patient with Renal Failure

Eberhard Ritz
Danilo Fliser

Hypertension is a hallmark of renal failure. On the one hand, hypertension is the consequence of renal disease. On the other hand, hypertension accelerates progression of renal failure. In the management of renal patients with hypertension, some specific recommendations regarding diagnostic procedures, concurrent therapy, indications for antihypertensive therapy, target blood pressure, and selection of antihypertensive medication differ from those for hypertensive patients without renal problems. These points will be briefly discussed in this chapter.

MAGNITUDE OF THE PROBLEM

Before antihypertensive treatment was available, renal failure was seen in approximately 5% of patients with primary (essential) hypertension.[1] This was mainly due to the occurrence of accelerated hypertension (malignant phase), which has become infrequent in recent years, at least in non-black patients. Although full-blown renal failure has become rare in patients with primary hypertension, renal dysfunction is quite frequent even in the absence of renal disease; e.g., microalbuminuria or albuminuria, elevated serum uric acid concentration, and elevation of serum creatinine.[2] With aging of the general population, end-stage renal failure caused by nephrosclerosis (i.e., the renal lesions thought to reflect hypertension-induced damage) now accounts for up to 20% of patients over age 50 who are hospitalized for renal replacement therapy. Therefore, signs of renal involvement should be carefully looked for, especially in elderly patients with hypertension. Hypertension is also common among patients with primary renal disease. As shown in Table 1,[3] patients with glomerulonephritis have a several-fold higher prevalence of hypertension than the age-matched general population, even if serum creatinine is still within the normal range. In renal failure, virtually all patients are hypertensive, except in renal disease with severe renal sodium

TABLE 1. PREVALENCE OF HYPERTENSION IN FEMALE
PATIENTS (N = 102) WITH PRIMARY CHRONIC
GLOMERULONEPHRITIS.

	Serum Creatinine (mg/dL)		
	<1.1	1.1 to 1.4	>1.4
Patients with chronic glomerulonephritis; median age 35 years (15 to 62 years)	35.5%	64.3%	75.0%
General Population			
Age 30 to 39	7.4%		
Age 40 to 49 years	21.0%		

Modified from Rambausek M, Rhein C, Waldherr R, et al. Hypertension in chronic idiopathic glomerulonephritis: Analysis of 311 biopsied patients. Eur J Clin Invest 1989;19:176–180.

loss. Finally, progression of renal failure is accelerated by the presence of hypertension.[4] Figure 1 illustrates that the fall in glomerular filtration rate was more marked in patients who had diastolic blood pressure levels consistently above 90 mm Hg. However, it has been clearly demonstrated that lowering of blood pressure with medication effectively attenuates the gradual fall in glomerular filtration. There is consensus among nephrologists that normalization of blood pressure is the single most important measure to prevent failure in patients with renal disease.

DIAGNOSTIC MEASURES

If one is confronted with a hypertensive patient with evidence of renal dysfunction, the following points should be checked: (1) Does the patient have malignant hypertension; that is, the accelerated phase of hypertension with arteriolar

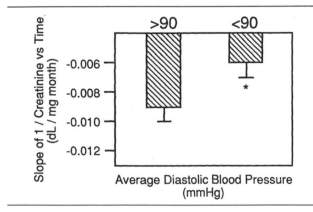

Figure 1. *Slope of 1: Serum creatinine versus time (as an index of loss of glomerular filtration rate) as a function of blood pressure. Note more rapid loss of renal function at diastolic pressures above 90 mm Hg From Brazy PC, Stead WW, Fitzwilliam JF. Progression of renal insufficiency: Role of blood pressure. Kidney Int 1989;35:670–674. Reprinted from Kidney International with permission.*

TABLE 2. POTENTIALLY CURABLE UNILATERAL RENAL DISEASES AS A CAUSE OF SECONDARY HYPERTENSION.

Occlusion of the renal artery

Reflux nephropathy

Segmental hypoplasia

Postobstructive kidney

Thrombosis of the renal artery
   or perirenal hematoma after renal trauma

Renin-producing tumor

Hydronephrosis (rare)

Tuberculosis (rare)

Giant single renal cyst (rare)

Malignant tumor (renal cell carcinoma, Wilms' tumor)

TABLE 3. RECOMMENDED DIAGNOSTIC PROCEDURES IN HYPERTENSIVE PATIENTS WITH SUSPECTED PRIMARY RENAL DISEASE.

---

1. Urine

    Albuminuria (dip stix, nephelometry, enzyme-linked immunosorbent assay, radioimmunoassay)

    Proteinuria (dip stix, biuret)

    Microhematuria (dip stix)

    Erythrocyte morphology and cellular casts (phase-contrast microscopy)

2. Serum chemistry: Creatinine

3. Renal sonography

---

necrosis and rapid deterioration of renal function? Malignant hypertension can be identified with fundoscopy, which shows swelling of the papilla, striated retinal hemorrhages, cotton wool exudates, and perimacular star figure (Sternspritzerfigur). (2) Does the patient have potentially curable unilateral renal disease causing hypertension? The most common causes are listed in Table 2. (3) Does the patient have primary renal disease? Pertinent diagnostic procedures are summarized in Table 3. The most common diseases to consider are: primary glomerulonephritis and systemic disease (systemic lupus erythematosus, vasculitis) with renal involvement, diabetic nephropathy, polycystic kidney disease, urinary tract malformation, obstruction, renal stone disease, and analgesic nephropathy.[5]

Serum creatinine provides a first approximation of glomerular filtration rate (GFR) because elevated serum creatinine indicates reduced glomerular filtration. However, one should be aware that creatinine, a product of muscle metabolism, depends on muscle mass. Serum creatinine is, therefore, higher in males than in females. Because of the broad normal range, values in the upper normal range are entirely consistent with quite marked reduction of GFR, as illustrated in Figure 2. If a more accurate assessment of renal function is required, endogenous creatinine clearance (from timed urine collections) or clearance measurements are necessary.

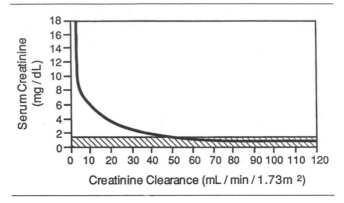

Figure 2. *Relation between glomerular filtration rate, estimated by creatinine clearance, and serum creatinine concentration. Note hyperbolic relationship. This implies that great changes in filtration rate initially cause only modest changes in serum creatinine concentration. Conversely, in advanced renal failure, modest changes in filtration rate cause marked changes in serum creatinine.*

Urine Analysis

Glomerular involvement (that is, primary glomerular disease or secondary glomerular involvement; e.g., glomerulosclerosis in advanced analgesic nephropathy) can be recognized from urinary analysis. The hallmarks of glomerular disease, pointing to a "leaky" glomerulus, are proteinuria, erythrocyturia (and/or leukocyturia), and cylindruria.

The normal range of *protein* excretion is 150 mg/day. Most of the proteins are of postglomerular origin, synthesized in the distal nephron (such as the Tamm Horsfall glycoprotein, which is the matrix of urinary casts) or in the urinary tract. Because of the admixture of nonglomerular proteins, urinary protein excretion is a relatively insensitive index of renal disease. Recently, sensitive and specific tests to measure urinary albumin have been developed (radioimmunoassay, enzyme-linked immunosorbent assay, specific dip stix) that make it possible to recognize even a slight increase in albumin excretion above baseline. This is particularly helpful in patients with diabetes mellitus. The upper normal range is 30 mg/24 hours or 20 µg/min in 24-hour collections or 20 µg/mL, respectively, in morning urine collections.

To monitor protein excretion, protein can be quantitated in spot urine or in 24-hour urine collections. Because of the wide variation of urine flow rates (0.51 to 31 per 24 hours), measurements of spot urine collection are not sensitive. Concentration values below the upper limit of normal (20 mg/dL) are consistent with elevated rates of protein excretion if urinary flow is high.[6]

Microhematuria is a frequent but nonspecific sign of glomerular disease. Of specific value are dysmorphic erythrocytes; i.e., akanthocytes, as illustrated in Figure 3. The upper normal range for urinary erythrocytes is approximately 5,000 mL in females and 3,000 mL in males.

The most important item in the evaluation of urine are casts upon microscopic evaluation of urinary sediment, preferably by phase contrast microscopy. Casts represent

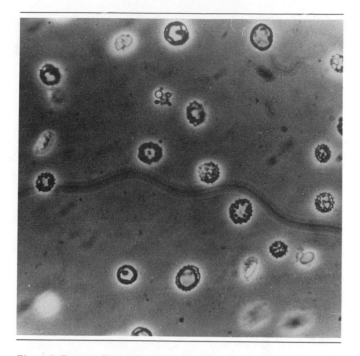

Figure 3. Dysmorphic erythrocytes in the urinary sediment of a patient with glomerulonephritis (phase-contrast microscopy × 400). Note rupture of erythrocyte membrane and misshapen contour (the small crenations are caused by osmotic shrinkage). Courtesy of Dr. Giovanni B. Fogazzi, Milan, Italy.

replicas of the collecting duct in which Tamm Horsfall glyco-protein, synthesized in the loop of Henle may precipitate at low pH and high osmolality. Cellular debris or cells passing through the nephron are trapped within the forming cylinders. Cellular casts in the afebrile patient who is not undergoing strenuous physical exercise are virtually diagnostic of glomerular disease. Examples are given in Figures 4 and 5.

In cases of proteinuria with or without nephritic sediment, serologic investigation is indicated (antinuclear antibodies [ANA], double-stranded deoxyribonucleic acid [dsDNA] antibodies, antineutrophil cytoplasmic antibodies [ANCA], complement, immunoelectrophoresis) and renal biopsy may be necessary to make the diagnosis.

Renal Imaging

Renal imaging is indispensable in the evaluation of hypertensive patients with suspected or known renal disease. Although ultrasonography does not permit diagnosis of renal vascular hypertension, it may provide useful diagnostic hints: asymmetry of renal size (>1 cm difference in length) and/or unilateral rarification of renal parenchymal width. Other unilateral diseases in which hypertension may be cured by intervention (see Table 2) are also readily demonstrable by ultrasonography. Of particular importance is prompt recognition of the rare patient with renal cell carcinoma that may present as hypertension of recent onset and unknown origin. Bilateral disease can often be identified

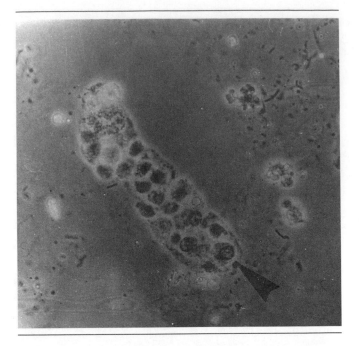

Figure 4. Cellular cast in the urinary sediment of a patient with chronic glomerulonephritis. Note numerous nucleated cells within the matrix of the cast, which is a replica of the collecting duct. Cells passing through the collecting duct at the time of gel formation are trapped in the cylinder. Most cells are degenerated, and their nature is not identifiable; one cell (arrow) is, however, clearly a tubular cell (phase-contrast microscopy × 400).

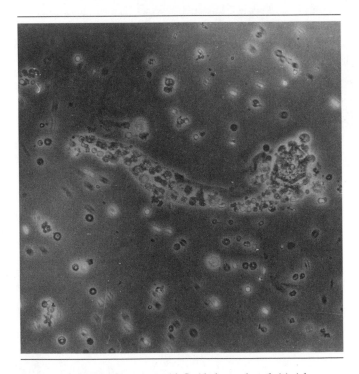

Figure 5. Sediment of a patient with florid glomerulonephritis (phase-contrast microscopy × 200). The sediment contains numerous dysmorphic erythrocytes, few leukocytes, and one cellular cast. In the cast matrix, tubular cells and erythrocytes have been trapped.

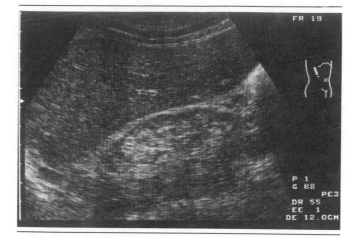

Figure 6. Right kidney of a hypertensive patient with proteinuria. Note shrunken size, reduced parenchymal width, and heightened echogenicity (approaching that of the adjacent liver).

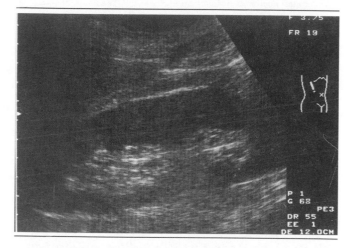

Figure 7. Hypertensive patient with diabetes mellitus. Note enlarged right kidney (length 135 mm, parenchymal width 10 mm) with unremarkable echogenicity of parenchyma. Nephromegaly is typical of diabetes mellitus.

with ultrasonography. Some useful hints are given in the legends to Figures 6 and 7. Further work-up may necessitate an excretory urogram, renal arteriography (digital subtraction angiography), computed tomography, or magnetic resonance imaging.

Measurement of Blood Pressure

Even minor increases in blood pressure are thought to be deleterious to the kidneys. It is, therefore, important to adequately evaluate blood pressure in renal patients. This is confounded by the problem that, in renal patients, circadian rhythm is frequently abnormal even in an early stage of disease, showing an attenuated nocturnal decrease in blood pressure (Figure 8).

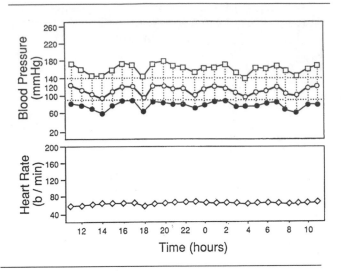

Figure 8. *Twenty-four-hour ambulatory blood pressure monitoring in a patient with renal hypertension. Note absence of the nocturnal decline in blood pressure.*

The circadian blood pressure profile must be taken into account to adequately assess the blood pressure burden to the kidney. Ambulatory blood pressure measurement should also be complemented by echocardiographic evaluation to assess left ventricular mass.

ANTIHYPERTENSIVE TREATMENT

In principle, the therapeutic strategies are similar in nonrenal and renal patients. In renal patients, however, numerous specific points must be considered.

When to Treat, and At Which Pressure to Aim

Both in diabetic nephropathy and in other primary renal diseases, renal function begins to deteriorate when blood pressure starts to rise. At first, blood pressure in such patients may still be within the range of normotension as defined by the World Health Organization; that is, 140/90 mm Hg. There is consensus that in the presence of renal disease such patients should be treated, preferably to attain values in the mid-normal range, or approximately 120/70 mm Hg.[7] It is important that currently there is no controlled evidence for the efficacy of this recommendation. Furthermore, such rigorous lowering of blood pressure necessitates careful patient instruction and monitoring to avoid excessive lowering of blood pressure, which may expose the patient to dangers related to traffic, construction work, etc. Important and necessary practical points are to (1) instruct the patient how to measure blood pressure, (2) recognize hypovolemia by measuring blood pressure with the patient in the standing position, and (3) adjust medication when blood pressure decreases excessively (for example, at high environmental temperatures or during periods of reduced food intake—for instance,

TABLE 4. ACCUMULATION OF ANTIHYPERTENSIVE DRUGS
IN RENAL FAILURE.

	Plasma Half-life (Hours)	
	Normal Function	Renal Failure
Amiloride	6	8 to 144*
Atenolol	6 to 9	15 to 35
Nadolol	12 to 24	45
Sotatol**	5 to 8	30 to 50
Clonidine	6 to 23	39 to 42
Hydralazine	2 to 5	7 to 16
Captopril	0.5 to 2	12 to 40
Enalapril	10 to 12	15 to 36

*Contraindicated in renal failure
**Sotalol is used for antiarrhythmic therapy in the renal patient; it may cause
Torasade de point arrhythmias even at normal plasma concentrations.

during intercurrent diseases—or sodium loss from vomiting,
diarrhea, etc.).

Renal Excretion of Antihypertensive Agents (or Their Active Metabolites)

Some antihypertensive agents (or their active metabolites)
are eliminated by the kidney. Adjustment of dose may,
therefore, be necessary in patients with impaired renal function. This is not a major problem in most cases because
dosage is titrated according to the antihypertensive effect,
but complications may arise from accumulation of
hydrophilic beta-blockers (bradycardia) and angiotensin-
converting enzyme (ACE) inhibitors (exanthema, blood cell
dyscrasia, hyperkalemia). Table 4 provides more detailed
information about accumulation of antihypertensive agents
in renal failure.

Antihypertensive Treatment and Progression of Renal Failure

In principle, blood pressure is lowered by antihypertensive
agents in the same way in patients with and without renal
disease. Some specific considerations, however, concern the
potential selective benefit provided by ACE inhibitors (and,
less well documented, calcium channel blockers) on the progression of renal failure.

In experimental models of renal damage, renal function
was better preserved with ACE inhibitors than with alternative antihypertensive agents despite similar lowering of systemic blood pressure. This led to the concept of renoprotective action of ACE inhibitors.

Recently, large prospective randomized and placebo-
controlled trials have provided evidence for renoprotective
action of ACE inhibitors in patients with diabetic[8] and nondiabetic[9,10] renal disease and proteinuria; fewer patients
reached the renal endpoint despite nearly identical values of
achieved blood pressure. Hence, ACE inhibitors should be
part of the antihypertensive treatment in any renal patient, at
least if he or she has proteinuria.

The antiproteinuric and renoprotective action of ACE inhibitors is only seen when a dietary excess of sodium is avoided. Furthermore, because of the role of sodium retention in the genesis of hypertension of patients with renal disease, reduction of dietary sodium intake, treatment with diuretics, or both, appears to be indicated.

The effects of calcium channel blockers in this respect are less consistent. Because calcium channel blockers dilate intrarenal vessels, it appears important to normalize systemic blood pressure when renal patients are treated with calcium channel blockers in order to avoid intrarenal hypertension. Because ACE inhibitors reduce the generation of angiotensin II, and calcium channel blockers reduce the intrarenal response to angiotensin II, it also seems reasonable to combine the two classes of antihypertensive agents.[11]

The renal effects (progression) of the angiotensin II-receptor subtype 1 have been extensively investigated in animal experiments. In humans, the acute effects of inhibitors of the angiotensin II-receptor subtype 1 (i.e., AT1-receptor-blockers) and of ACE inhibitors are identical. Whether AT1-receptor-blockers are superior with respect to progression is currently under investigation in several large trials. A definite indication for AT1-receptor-blockers are side effects of ACE inhibitors, e.g., cough and angioedema; such patients can be safely switched to AT1-receptor-blockers.

Practical Recommendations

Hypertension in the renal patient is usually salt sensitive, and salt retention plays a crucial role in the genesis of renal hypertension. Dietary sodium restriction to approximately 5 g/day (approximately 80 mmol sodium daily) is, therefore, indicated. This can be achieved by avoiding addition of salt to food and avoiding food items with high salt content (e.g., processed meats, canned foods, salted bread). Even in the nonedematous patient, dietary salt restriction is indicated (1) because salt restriction, at least in animal experiments, has beneficial effects on preservation of renal function that cannot be imitated by diuretics, and (2) because salt restriction permits the use of lower doses of diuretics and, therefore, causes fewer side effects from diuretic treatment.

In the nonedematous patient with serum creatinine below approximately 2.5 mg/dL, *thiazide* monotherapy (e.g., chlorthalidone 25 mg/day to 100 mg/day) is sufficient. At higher serum creatinine levels, *furosemide* or other loop diuretics in higher doses are required (40 mg/day to 500 mg/day in divided doses). Coadministration of thiazide diuretics and furosemide potentiates the effect of loop diuretics and reduces some of their side effects, such as calciuria.[12]

ACE Inhibitors

ACE inhibitors are indicated to reduce progression of renal disease. With few exceptions (e.g., fosinopril), all ACE inhibitors are eliminated via the kidney, so dose adjustment is necessary. ACE inhibitors may reversibly decrease glomerular filtration and increase *serum creatinine* in states in which GFR is dependent on angiotension II; furthermore, particularly in patients with hyporeninemic hypoaldosteronism, *hyperkalemia* may supervene. It is, therefore, indispensable to closely monitor urinary volume, serum creatinine, and serum potassium in the first week of administration. When ACE inhibition is begun in patients with decreased renal function, serum creatinine may increase by up to 70% without apparent reason. If the rise in serum creatinine is more marked, one should exclude the following conditions:

- Bilateral renal artery stenosis (or renal artery stenosis in single kidneys, for example in renal transplants)
- Severe hypovolemia (usually from overzealous diuretic treatment)
- Congestive heart failure
- Bilateral hyperreninemic renal state; for example, polycystic kidney disease, scleroderma, endarteritis of transplant rejection, treatment with cyclosporin A, etc.

In patients with preterminal renal failure, that is serum creatinine above approximately 6 mg/dL, ACE inhibitors are no longer the first choice for initial antihypertensive treatment. An ACE inhibitor-induced increase in serum creatinine by 70% may transform the patient acutely from a person who does not require dialysis to one who does.

Using ACE inhibitors and diuretics alone, one is only rarely successful in controlling blood pressure. When further antihypertensive agents are required, good candidates are calcium antagonists and alpha-adrenergic antagonists. Arguments for the former are a good safety record in renal patients and potential benefit as agents conferring renal protection by non-hemodynamic actions. Arguments for the latter are the common presence of additional metabolic risk factors in uremic patients and the recent demonstration of excess sympathetic activity in the patient with renal failure. However, the patient should be monitored for orthostatic hypotension during treatment with alpha-adrenoreceptor blockers, particularly when receiving high-dose diuretic treatment.

It has been recently recognized that uremia is a state of sympathetic overactivity.[13] This may explain why centrally sympathoplegic agents, e.g., clonidin or the imidazoline receptor blocker moxonidine, are very effective antihypertensive agents in patients with renal disease.

If hypertension and advanced renal failure are refractory to multidrug treatment, it is often useful to start hemodialysis even if this is not rigorously required on the basis of serum urea values. In most patients, hemodialysis brings hypertension rapidly under control.

Assessment of Progression during Antihypertensive Treatment

It is useful to monitor proteinuria after the start of antihypertensive treatment. Proteinuria is blood pressure dependent, and reduction of proteinuria points to successful treatment.[14] For any given amount of blood pressure reduction, ACE inhibitors reduce proteinuria more than alternative antihypertensive agents.

It is useful to serially assess serum creatinine or creatinine clearance. The reciprocal of serum creatinine concentra

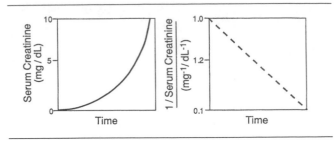

Figure 9. Schema of change in serum creatinine with time (A) and change of ratio 1/serum creatinine with time (B). The decrease in 1/serum creatinine with time usually yields a linear line in patients with progressive renal failure. Changes in the slope indicate changes in the evolution of renal failure.

tion (l/serum creatinine) when plotted versus time (Figure 9) usually yields a linear relationship and provides an imprecise but useful index to assess progression. It permits one to recognize departure from the predicted course, which usually implies acceleration of progression.

Recognition of Associated Risk Factors

In the renal patient, mortality from cardiac causes is several-fold higher than that in the general population. It has been shown that the number of patients with renal failure who die prematurely from cardiovascular causes is similar to the number of patients who reach end-stage renal failure.[15] It is therefore, desirable to look for associated cardiovascular risk factors such as smoking and dyslipidemia and treat them accordingly. Dyslipidemia is a feature of nephrotic-range proteinuria (predominately elevation of low-density lipoprotein) and of renal failure (impaired function of lipoproteinase with accumulation of beta-very-low-density lipoprotein and low high-density lipoprotein).

REFERENCES

1. Perera GA. Hypertensive vascular disease—description and natural history. J Chronic Dis 1995;1:33–42.

2. Klahr S, Schreiner G, Ichikawa I. The progression of renal disease. N Engl J Med 1988;318:1657–1666.

3. Rambausek M, Rhein C, Waldherr R, et al. Hypertension in chronic idiopathic glomerulonephritis: Analysis of 311 biopsied patients. Eur J Clin Invest 1989;19:176–180.

4. Brazy PC, Stead WW, Fitzwilliam JF. Progression of renal insufficiency: Role of blood pressure. Kidney Int 1989;35:670–674.

5. Lewin A, Blaufox MD, Castle H, et al. Apparent prevalence of curable hypertension in the Hypertension Detection and Follow-up Program. Arch Intern Med 1985;145:424–427.

6. Bigazzi R, Bianchi S, Campese VM, et al. Prevalence of microalbuminuria in a large population of patients with mild to moderate hypertension. Nephron 1992;61:94–97.

7. Parving HH, Anderson AR, Schmidt UM, et al. Early aggressive antihypertensive treatment reduces rate of decline in kidney function in diabetic nephropathy. Lancet 1982;1:1175–1179.

8. Lewis EJ, Hunsicker LG, Bain RP, Rohde RD. The effect of angiotensin converting enzyme inhibition on diabetic nephropathy. the Collaborative Study Group. New Engl J Med 1993;329: 1456–1462.

9. Maschio G, Albert D, Janin G, Locatelli F, Mann JFE, Motolese M, Ponticelli C, Ritz E, Zucchelli P. Angiotensin conveting enzyme inhibition in progressive renal insufficiency study group. Effect of the angiotensin converting enzyme inhibitor benazepril on the progression of chronic renal insufficiency. New Engl J Med 1996;334: 939–945.

10. The GISEN study. Randomised placebo-controlled trial of effects of ramipril on decline in glomerular filtration rate and risk of terminal renal failure in proteinuric, non-diabetic nephropathy. Lancet 197;349:1857–1863.

11. Bakris GL, Williams B, Angiotensin converting enzyme inhibitors and calcium antagonists alone or combined: does the progression of diabetic renal disease differ? J Hypertens 1995;13:S95–S101.

12. Fliser D, Schröter M, Neubeck M, Ritz E. Coadministration of thiazides increases the efficacy of loop diuretics even in patients with advanced renal failure. Kidney Int 1994;46.482–488.

13. Converse RL, Jacobsen TN, Toto RD, Jost CMT, Cosentino F, Tarazi FF, Victor GG. Sympathetic overactivity in patients with chronic renal failure. N Engl J Med 1992;327:1912–1918.

14. Peterson JC, Adler S, Burkart JM, Green T, Hebert LA, Hunsicker LG, King AJ, Klahr S, Massry SG, Seifter JL: MDRD Study Group: Blood pressure control, proteinuria and the progression of renal disease. Ann Intern Med 1995;123:754–762.

15. Fliser D, Schweizer C, Ritz E. How many patients with renal insufficiency survive until end-stage renal failure. Nephrol Dial Transplant 1991;6:600–604.